NEUROPSYCHIATRY AND MENTAL HEALTH SERVICES

NEUROPSYCHIATRY AND MENTAL HEALTH SERVICES

Edited by

Fred Ovsiew, M.D.

*Associate Professor of Clinical Psychiatry,
University of Chicago;
Chief, Clinical Neuropsychiatry Service, and
Medical Director, Adult Inpatient Psychiatry Service,
University of Chicago Hospitals, Chicago, Illinois*

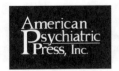

American Psychiatric Press, Inc.

Washington, DC
London, England

Copyright © 1999 American Psychiatric Press, Inc.
ALL RIGHTS RESERVED
Manufactured in the United States of America on acid-free paper
02 01 00 99   4   3   2   1
First Edition

American Psychiatric Press, Inc.
1400 K Street, N.W., Washington, DC   20005
www.appi.org

Library of Congress Cataloging-in-Publication Data
Neuropsychiatry and mental health services   /   edited by Fred Ovsiew.
    p.   cm.
   Includes bibliographical references and index.
   ISBN 0-88048-730-5 (alk. paper)
   1. Neuropsychiatry. 2. Mental health services. I. Ovsiew, Fred, 1949–   .
   [DNLM: 1. Brain Diseases. 2. Mental Disorders. WL 348N4942 1999]
RC341.N43545 1999
616.8—dc21
DNLM/DLC
for Library of Congress   98-39584
                                                  CIP

British Library Cataloguing in Publication Data
A CIP record is available from the British Library.

CONTENTS

Contributors ix

Introduction. xiii

CHAPTER 1

Neuropsychiatry in the History of Mental Health Services . . . 1

Fred Ovsiew, M.D., and Thomas H. Jobe, M.D.

CHAPTER 2

**Epidemiology and Recognition of
Neuropsychiatric Disorders in Mental Health Settings 23**

Barbara L. Yates, M.D., and Lorrin M. Koran, M.D.

CHAPTER 3

Neuropsychiatry in Public Mental Health Settings 47

Barry S. Fogel, M.D., M.S.

CHAPTER 4

Dementia in Public Mental Health Settings 69

*Patricia Hanrahan, Ph.D., Daniel J. Luchins, M.D., and
Fred Ovsiew, M.D.*

CHAPTER 5

Neuropsychiatry of Substance Abuse. 105

E. Jane Marshall, M.R.C.P.(I), M.R.C.Psych.

CHAPTER 6

A Neuropsychiatric Approach to Aggressive Behavior. . . . 149

Sheldon Benjamin, M.D.

CHAPTER 7

Neuropsychiatry in the Prison 197

Fred Ovsiew, M.D., and Peter B. C. Fenwick, M.B.,
B.Chir.(Cantab.), D.P.M., F.R.C.Psych.

CHAPTER 8

Neuropsychiatry of Human Immunodeficiency Virus
Infection 221

Joel K. Levy, Ph.D., Francisco Fernandez, M.D.,
Barbara L. Lachar, Ph.D., Ann L. Friedman, Ph.D., J.D., and
Zishan Samiuddin, M.D.

CHAPTER 9

Neuropsychiatry and Persons With
Developmental Disabilities 259

Ruth M. Ryan, M.D.

CHAPTER 10

Neuropsychiatry of Late-Onset Psychosis and
Depression 291

Ira M. Lesser, M.D., and J. Randolph Swartz, M.D.

CHAPTER 11

Neuropsychiatry and the Homeless 319

Jonathan M. Silver, M.D., and Alan Felix, M.D.

CHAPTER 12

**Neuropsychiatric and Mental Health Services
Aspects of Tardive Dyskinesia** 335

*Dilip V. Jeste, M.D., David Naimark, M.D.,
Maureen C. Halpain, M.S., and Brian Cuffel, Ph.D.*

CHAPTER 13

Neuropsychiatry of Sexual Deviations 363

Jeffrey L. Cummings, M.D.

Index 385

CONTRIBUTORS

Sheldon Benjamin, M.D.
Associate Professor of Psychiatry and Neurology, University of Massachusetts Medical School; Director of Neuropsychiatry and Director of Psychiatric Education and Training, University of Massachusetts Medical Center, Worcester, Massachusetts

Brian Cuffel, Ph.D.
Assistant Vice President for Research and Evaluation, United Behavioral Health, San Francisco, California

Jeffrey L. Cummings, M.D.
Professor of Neurology and Psychiatry and Biobehavioral Sciences, UCLA School of Medicine; Neurobehavioral Consultant, Neurobehavior and Neuropsychiatry Section, Psychiatry Service, West Los Angeles Veterans Affairs Medical Center, Los Angeles, California

Alan Felix, M.D.
Associate Clinical Professor of Psychiatry, Columbia University College of Physicians and Surgeons; Director, Critical Time Intervention Mental Health Program, New York–Presbyterian Hospital, New York, New York

Peter B. C. Fenwick, M.B., B.Chir.(Cantab.), D.P.M., F.R.C.Psych.
Senior Lecturer, Institute of Psychiatry; Consultant Neuropsychiatrist, Bethlem and Maudsley NHS Trust, London; Honorary Research Consultant Neurophysiologist, Broadmoor Hospital, England

Francisco Fernandez, M.D.
Professor and Chairman, Department of Psychiatry, Loyola University Stritch School of Medicine, Maywood, Illinois

Barry S. Fogel, M.D., M.S.
Attending Neuropsychiatrist, Brigham Behavioral Neurology Group, Brigham and Women's Hospital, Boston, Massachusetts; Visiting Professor of Psychiatry, Harvard Medical School, Boston, Massachusetts; Adjunct Professor of Community Health, Brown University, Providence, Rhode Island; Executive Vice President, LTCQ, Inc., Providence, Rhode Island; Managing Director, Synchroneuron, L.L.C.

Ann L. Friedman, Ph.D., J.D.
Psychologist in independent practice, Houston, Texas

Maureen C. Halpain, M.S.
Program Manager, Geriatric Psychiatry Clinical Research Center,
University of California, San Diego, San Diego Veterans Affairs Medical
Center, San Diego, California

Patricia Hanrahan, Ph.D.
Research Associate and Assistant Professor of Psychiatry, University of
Chicago; Director of Clinical Program Evaluation, Illinois Department of
Mental Health and Developmental Disabilities, Chicago, Illinois

Dilip V. Jeste, M.D.
Professor of Psychiatry and Neurosciences, and Director, Geriatric
Psychiatry Clinical Research Center, University of California, San Diego,
San Diego Veterans Affairs Medical Center, San Diego, California

Thomas H. Jobe, M.D.
Associate Professor of Psychiatry, College of Medicine, University of
Illinois at Chicago; Associate Director, Division of Neuropsychiatry,
University of Illinois at Chicago Hospital and Clinics, Chicago, Illinois

Lorrin M. Koran, M.D.
Professor of Psychiatry, Stanford University; Director,
Obsessive-Compulsive Disorders Clinic, Stanford University Medical
Center, Stanford, California

Barbara L. Lachar, Ph.D.
Psychologist in independent practice, Houston, Texas

Ira M. Lesser, M.D.
Professor of Psychiatry, UCLA School of Medicine; Director of
Residency Training in Psychiatry and Vice Chair for Academic Affairs,
Harbor-UCLA Medical Center, Torrance, California

Joel K. Levy, Ph.D.
Assistant Professor of Neurology, Psychiatry and Behavioral Sciences,
and Physical Medicine/Rehabilitation, Baylor College of Medicine;
Consulting Neuropsychologist, St. Luke's Episcopal Hospital; Consulting
Neuropsychologist, Harris County Hospital District, Houston, Texas

Daniel J. Luchins, M.D.

Associate Professor of Psychiatry, Director of the Geriatric Psychiatry Clinic, and Chief of Extramural Adult Psychiatry, University of Chicago; Associate Director for Clinical Services, Illinois Department of Mental Health and Developmental Disabilities, Chicago, Illinois

E. Jane Marshall, M.R.C.P.(I), M.R.C.Psych.

Senior Lecturer and Consultant Psychiatrist in the Addictions, National Addiction Center, Institute of Psychiatry and the Maudsley Hospital, London, England

David Naimark, M.D.

Staff Psychiatrist, Scripps Clinic, and County of San Diego Forensic Evaluation Unit, San Diego, California

Fred Ovsiew, M.D.

Associate Professor of Clinical Psychiatry, University of Chicago; Chief, Clinical Neuropsychiatry Service, and Medical Director, Adult Inpatient Psychiatry Service, University of Chicago Hospitals, Chicago, Illinois

Ruth M. Ryan, M.D.

The Community Circle, Denver, Colorado

Zishan Samiuddin, M.D.

Assistant Professor of Psychiatry and Behavioral Sciences, Baylor College of Medicine; Director, Psychiatry Outpatient Clinic, Thomas Street Clinic, Harris County Hospital District, Houston, Texas

Jonathan M. Silver, M.D.

Clinical Professor of Psychiatry, New York University School of Medicine; Chief, Ambulatory Services, Lenox Hill Hospital, New York, New York

J. Randolph Swartz, M.D.

Assistant Professor of Psychiatry, UCLA School of Medicine; Co-Ward Chief, Inpatient Psychiatry, Harbor-UCLA Medical Center, Torrance, California

Barbara L. Yates, M.D.

Clinical Faculty, Department of Psychiatry, University of California Medical Center, San Francisco, California

INTRODUCTION

Neuropsychiatry encompasses both the care of the patient with overt brain disease (such as Alzheimer's disease or the sequelae of traumatic brain injury) and an approach to the care of patients with the major psychiatric disorders traditionally considered nonorganic or "functional" (such as schizophrenia and the mood disorders). This volume grew out of the experience of the Clinical Neuropsychiatry Service at the University of Chicago in developing a neuropsychiatric consultation service at an affiliated state hospital. The physicians directly involved in that project, Drs. Jeffrey I. Bennett and Carol Black, and I were impressed by the high prevalence of organic psychopathology in that setting. Preliminary research efforts demonstrated that abnormal clinical findings suggestive of organic states were equally frequent in the acute patients referred for neuropsychiatric consultation and in chronic patients randomly selected from the population resident at the hospital for more than 5 years (C. Black, J. I. Bennett, and F. Ovsiew, unpublished data, 1992–1993). We thought that this tentative finding might indicate the importance of organic contributions to psychopathology, leading to treatment refractoriness and long hospitalizations. Further, we guessed that such organic contributors to psychopathology not only were seen in the state hospital but might be clinically important in many public settings.

We were then fortunate to be able to invite several speakers to discuss aspects of neuropsychiatry in the public health setting. (The clinical work and the invitations were supported by a State of Illinois Department of Mental Health and Developmental Disabilities grant for a "Public Psychiatry Experience for Psychiatric Residents.") Drs. Sheldon Benjamin, Barry S. Fogel, Dilip V. Jeste, Ira M. Lesser, Ruth M. Ryan, and Jonathan M. Silver were our invited speakers, and their talks, suitably reworked and referenced, are included here.

Each of the contributors to this book was asked to maintain a triple focus of attention. Each chapter was to address the subject within a public health framework, with due attention to the epidemiology and costs of the disorder under discussion; to provide clinical guidance for those working in public settings; and to draw implications from the neuropsychiatric data for policy-making in public facilities. The contributors, most of whom spend much of their working lives in public institutions, responded well to this challenge.

I hope that this volume can be of use to clinicians and policymakers alike in improving the understanding and care of our patients.

Fred Ovsiew, M.D.

CHAPTER 1

Neuropsychiatry in the History of Mental Health Services

Fred Ovsiew, M.D.
Thomas H. Jobe, M.D.

> One of the by-products of the founding of mental hospitals was the creation of the specialty of psychiatry. This fact is of crucial significance, for it means that psychiatric thought and practice were not dominant in shaping the structure and function of these institutions. Instead the reverse was true. Psychiatry, for the most part, was shaped by the institutional setting within which it was born and grew to maturity. Many of the dominant characteristics of psychiatric thought were but rationalizations of existing conditions within mental hospitals.
>
> Gerald Grob (1985, p. 2)

This historical perspective on the place of neuropsychiatry in public mental health psychiatry is meant to be disconcerting. We all tend to accept our customary concepts and practices as natural or inevitable. To see how concepts evolved and what practice was or might have been may occasion a sense of accomplishment, even triumph. Our accomplishments are real, but if we forego the Whiggish perspective of inexorable progress, a view of the past can help us understand the frailty of our concepts and the mutability of our institutions. Our review focuses on the 19th century, with its crucial developments of the public asylum and the professional structures of neurology and psychiatry.

An unreflective view of the place of neuropsychiatry in relation to general psychiatry and neurology might assume that at one time neurology and psychiatry were one (as indicated by the joint American Board of Psychiatry and Neurology). But, so the story would go, with neurology's organic emphasis, a split developed, as psychiatry cared for "functional" mental disorder and focused on psychological conceptions of mental illness, whereas neurology made its contribution to the understanding and treatment of organic brain diseases that produced mental illness. Neuropsychiatry, then, is the revivification of an old unity, with the contemporary neuroscientific backing that our forebears could not have had.

This story is wrong or misleading in almost every respect. Neurology and psychiatry arose on entirely separate foundations. When neurology developed within general medicine and the general hospital some decades after the profession of psychiatry took shape, there was criticism of the asylum doctors for their care of patients with mental illness in public asylums; however, neurologists never had an important role in the care of these patients, even when organic brain disease was known by all to be present.

To be sure, psychiatrists and neurologists fully concurred that "lunacy" or "insanity" was a result of brain disease. More important, however, than the largely speculative 19th-century assumption of the cerebral origin of insanity is an underappreciated fact: a sizable proportion of the population cared for by asylum physicians had organic brain disease ascertainable even by the limited tools of the last century. Neurology, nonetheless, set its sights on a different population, generally drawn from the educated classes, who were suffering from "neurasthenia": the range of emotional and somatic complaints for which an organic basis was not to be found and that were therefore thought "nervous" (Oppenheim 1991; Shorter 1992).

> The neurologists of the late nineteenth century had little in common with their present-day namesakes. . . . They were much nearer to being forerunners of twentieth-century psychiatrists than of modern neurologists because of their emphasis on the emotions and the social origins of stress. (Gosling 1987, p. 17)

Despite what may seem by today's standards an odd division of labor, by which neurotic illness belonged to neurology and severe organic disorders belonged to psychiatry, neurology made enormous progress in the understanding of brain disease, whereas psychiatry failed to do so. Neurology's speculations about the effects of "mental strain and emotional disturbance" on "nerve force" (Hammond 1878) in neurasthenic patients are now fortunately forgotten, and psychiatry's gains in the psychological understanding of neurotic illness have produced little benefit for the patients entrusted to psychiatric care in public settings.

Origins of the Asylum

The care of people with mental illness has been a problem each society has had to address from time immemorial. Why large public institutions for their care arose in the 19th century has been a matter of historical controversy. Hare's (1983, p. 451) provocative explanation was that schizophrenia was a new disease: "The real increase in insanity made urgently necessary the establishment and increasing provision of a specialized system of care." Others (Jeste et al. 1985; Scull 1984) took issue with Hare's data and conclusions. Any simplistic theory of a societal wish for control of people who were poor and mentally ill is refuted by the important and early role of institutional solutions for people who were rich and mentally ill. Exclusive and expensive private institutions played a prominent role in the development of theories and practices in the care of people with mental illness. Such institutions included the York Retreat (Digby 1985), where moral therapy arose under the Tukes, and the Ticehurst House Asylum (McKenzie 1992) in England and the Pennsylvania Hospital for the Insane (Tomes 1984) and the McLean Hospital (Sutton 1986) in the United States. Moreover, the same theories and practices that were applied to the poor were brought into play by the mental illness of King George III, a foundational episode for the nascent psychiatric profession at the end of the 18th century (Macalpine and Hunter 1969).

Undoubtedly, a number of social changes in the 19th century made care of people with mental illness in the community more problematic. The rapid growth of the population and its urbanization encouraged the development of specialized public institutions of many kinds, asylums included (Rothman 1990). The development of a market economy meant less room for nonproductive family members and less time available for their care by relatives who now worked outside the home (Scull 1993). At the same time, a service economy was developing in which

> entrepreneurs sprouted in many fields. . . . Madhouses and mad-doctors arose from the same soil which generated demand for general practitioners, dancing masters, man midwives, face painters, drawing tutors, estate managers, landscape gardeners, architects, journalists and that host of other white-collar, service, and quasi-professional occupations which a society with increased economic surplus and pretensions to civilization first found it could afford, and soon found it could not do without. (Porter 1987, p. 164)

Foucault's (1965) thesis of a "great confinement" beginning in the 17th century, the asylum and the prison being similar manifestations of the triumph of rationality over unreason (*déraison*), has been celebrated (Rousseau 1970), disputed (Arieno 1989; Doerner 1981; Midelfort 1980; Porter 1990; Scull 1992), and defended (Gordon 1990; Gutting 1994). To its detractors, Foucault's thesis seems to owe more to poetry or philosophy (or, in Scull's (1989c, p. 17) phrase, Foucault's "overactive imagination") than to validated historical evidence. Foucault's focus, to the extent that it is chronological, is on a period earlier than the 19th century and, to the extent that it is geographical, is on France more than on the Anglo-American tradition we are considering. Furthermore, Foucault is seemingly truly interested in something other than mental illness, as he implied in an essay attached to the 1972 French edition of *Histoire de la folie à l'âge classique* (Foucault 1972). Now that modern literature has made available new forms of discourse, he argued, "madness [*folie*] is undoing its kinship . . . with mental illness [*maladie mentale*]. The latter . . . is going to move into a better and better regulated technical area: in hospitals, pharmacology has already transformed violent wards into large lukewarm aquariums." Madness, he said, is the "lyrical halo of illness . . . far from the pathological" (pp. 581–582, our translation). In any event, the goal of this chapter is far less ambitious than Foucault's reconstruction of the *episteme* of post-Enlightenment culture. Possibly the evidence we adduce is relevant in a limited way to a judgment on the empirical adequacy of Foucault's thesis.

For whatever reason, in the early 19th century in both the United States and the United Kingdom, specialized institutions for poor people with mental illness arose, were legally mandated, and spread widely. Beyond doubt, the institutions satisfied the need for respite felt by the families and the communities of the mentally ill (Fox 1978, p. 97). However, these facilities at their outset did not aim just at care or custody, but at cure. Moral—we might today say, psychological—therapy was the method by which the new institutions were to bring about their humanitarian aims. Moral therapy entailed a kindly attitude toward people with mental illness, the careful elicitation of their life experiences, the provision of activities aimed at social reintegration, and reeducation of the mind by contact with the forceful personality of the medical superintendent (Dain and Carlson 1960). Abjuring not just overt violence but to the greatest possible extent any measures of mechanical restraint was seen as inherent in this form of treatment.

The grand hopes for the early asylums to cure patients gave way to custodial realities (Grob 1994; Rothman 1990; Scull 1993). The growing number of chronically ill patients made impossible the practices that asylum superintendents extolled. Carefully planned small, even intimate, institutions were overwhelmed by crowding. Milieus designed for those recently fallen ill, whose chances of cure and discharge were high, found themselves addressing chronically ill patients who would never leave. In this setting, the psychiatric profession came into being (McGovern 1985).

In large part, the confinement of people with mental illness in specialized facilities represented a "transinstitutionalization" of people who were mentally ill and poor, who until then had been cared for—or had languished—in prisons, workhouses, poorhouses, and other public facilities (Rothman 1990). In England, a thriving private "trade in lunacy" (Parry-Jones 1972) by the 19th century comprised profit-making facilities perhaps not too different from today's nursing homes or "intermediate care facilities" for the mentally ill. In the United States, such a private industry had not yet arisen (Tomes 1988).

The Nature of Insanity

The prescientific roots of concepts of the relations between brain structure and function and normal and abnormal behavior are ancient. These concepts began to assume a recognizably modern form at the beginning of the 19th century. Gall and his system of phrenology were crucial in the development of our ideas about the relation of brain function to abnormal behavior, and many of the founders of the British and American psychiatric professions were phrenologists (Carlson 1958; Cooter 1981). Phrenology is now known mostly for its practice of cranioscopy, the inference of personality traits from the shape of the cranium. This method seems ludicrous today, but the true intellectual contribution of phrenology to the advance of the neuroscientific understanding of behavior is otherwise. Gall asserted that the brain was the organ of the mind. Though this claim now seems self-evident, its "materialism" led to Gall's exile from Vienna by Emperor Francis I and the proscription of his writings by the pope (Marshall 1980). In other words, Gall claimed psychology for the biological sciences, rather than for speculative philosophy. More specifically, he offered for anatomical analysis a set of psychological functions (such as musical ability or a sense of spatial relations) that were biologically relevant or adaptive (Young 1970/1990), in lieu of the traditional general categories such as perception or reasoning. Today this tradition continues as theories of the "modularity of mind" (Fodor 1983; Marshall 1980). The interest of many 19th-century psychiatrists in phrenology must therefore be seen as indicating their commitment to a neurobiological understanding of mental function and abnormal behavior.

In fact, the asylum doctors of the 19th century believed "with complete confidence and virtual unanimity" (Scull 1989b, p. 155) that insanity was a result of brain disease (Bynum 1981). In the fourth edition of their authoritative *A Manual of Psychological Medicine*, Bucknill and Tuke (1879, p. vii) announced with satisfaction that since their first edition, "[t]he great principle that Mental Disease depends solely upon cerebral conditions . . . has now become so thoroughly established that it is no longer questioned." The English alienist Henry Maudsley (1898, pp. 41–42) wrote,

> Mental disorders are neither more nor less than nervous diseases in which mental symptoms predominate. . . . When a blow on the head has paralyzed sensibility and movement, in consequence of the disease in the brain which it has initiated, the patient is sent to the hospital; but when a blow to the head has caused mental derangement, in consequence of the disease of brain which it has initiated, the patient is sent to an asylum. In like manner, one man who has unluckily swallowed the eggs of a taenia, and has got a cysticercus in the brain, may go to the hospital; another who has been similarly unlucky goes to an asylum. Syphilitic disease of the brain or its arteries lands one person in an asylum with mental symptoms predominant, another in a hospital with sensory and motor disorder predominant. The same cause produces different symptoms, according to the part of the brain which it particularly affects. No doubt it is right that mental derangements should have, as they often require, the special appliances of an asylum, but it is certainly not right that the separation which is necessary for treatment should reach to their pathology and to the methods of its study.

Dain (1964, p. 64) wrote of the early American psychiatric community, "They all agreed that insanity was a physical disorder, usually a morbid irritation of the brain," and cited as "typical" the opinion that the superintendent of the Friends' Asylum expressed in 1837:

> Insanity, in its various forms and degrees, has its origin in some disturbance of the brain, either structural or functional—which disturbance may spring from either a moral or physical source. Let it arise, however, from which it may, the proximate cause producing the deranged manifestation of mind, is always located in the brain. (Dain 1964, p. 66)

As this quotation suggests, asylum doctors held that, although brain disease was the proximate cause of insanity, social factors often operated to produce mental illness. Especially in the United States, alienists were sure that the tumultuous social life of the modern world was the source of much mental illness (Rothman 1990). The endorsement of moral therapy should not, however, be mistaken for a belief on the part of asylum doctors in a doctrine of psychogenesis of severe mental illness. The asylum doctors favored moral treatment for humane as well as pragmatic reasons and applied it to patients with known brain disease as well as to those whose brain disease was speculatively though confidently assumed (Bynum 1981). Dr. Morrill Wyman, the first superintendent of the McLean Hospital, made this explicit in a lecture given in 1830: "[M]oral treatment is indispensable even in cases arising from organic disease" (quoted in Scull 1989a, p. 103).

As a matter of day-to-day clinical practice, asylum doctors knew that both somatic and psychological factors operated to bring patients into their care. In the York and North Riding Asylums, for example, religious excitement, business and financial anxieties, and family stresses such as bereavement were recognized as causes of admission in the 1880s (Renvoize and Beveridge 1989). Similarly, at the Utica Asylum in New York State, annual reports charted the numbers of patients admitted because of emotional and economic stress (Dwyer 1987). Interestingly, differences between private and public settings in how often such factors were identified are striking. Renvoize and Beveridge (1989) were able to compare data from the first half of the 1880s from the private and influential York Retreat, the York Asylum with its mixed public and private patients, and the North Riding Asylum for people who were poor and mentally ill. With regard to what the asylum doctors took to be the cause of illness, business anxieties and overwork were ascribed importance in 53% of the private patients at the York Retreat but in only 12% of patients in the public asylum; in the mixed setting, an intermediate figure of 34% was noted.

Masturbation was confidently believed to be an etiologic factor by Anglo-American psychiatrists of the Victorian era. The rise and fall of the hypothesis that masturbation causes insanity was chronicled by Hare (1962). Turner (1992) described the place of so-called masturbatory insanity in the diagnostic thinking of the doctors of the private Ticehurst House Asylum in the 19th century. Masturbatory insanity still held a prominent place in diagnosis in California at the beginning of the 20th century, after which it faded (Fox 1978, pp. 154–155).

Heredity also was considered an important factor in the origin of insanity and was commonly implicated in the Utica cases in the mid-19th century, though it was less favored as a diagnosis before and after this time (Dwyer 1987). In the comparative English material already referred to (Renvoize and Beveridge 1989), a hereditary cause was alleged in a full quarter of the public patients—but in none of those in the exclusive York Retreat.

Organic Psychiatry in the Asylum

By the mid-19th century, cases of insanity resulting from organic conditions such as epilepsy, neurosyphilis, senile dementia, and substance abuse were recognized, tabulated, and managed.

Epilepsy was a disorder of particular concern to asylum doctors in the United States and the United Kingdom. Bucknill and Tuke (1879, p. 97) estimated that epilepsy was the cause of some 6% of cases of insanity. In a few elite private institutions (Tomes 1984, p. 133), and at the ancient Bethlem Hospital (Hare 1959), epilepsy was grounds for exclusion (because it presaged incurability), but for the most part it was regarded as a common phenomenon among the mentally ill, and indeed status epilepticus was a common cause of death in the asylum.

Hunter and Macalpine (1974) calculated that at the Colney Hatch Asylum in London during 1855, 140 of the men confined (21% of the total) and 184 women (23%) had among them a total of 82,962 seizures. This amounts to some 227 generalized convulsions observed daily at the asylum—during the daytime, because during the night shift, 8 P.M. to 6 A.M., the patients were unmonitored. (We have recalculated some of the numbers in Hunter and Macalpine's text.) In the much smaller Buckinghamshire Asylum, in 1861, 43 patients (16% of the asylum population) experienced on average 10 seizures a month each, though 1 patient had 10 times this number, a total of 1,183 in the year (Crammer 1990, p. 58). Epilepsy was the cause of death in 4 of the 32 patients who died in 1868 (p. 126). At the Hanwell Asylum in England, a quarter of epileptic patients died in status epilepticus (Hunter and Macalpine 1974, p. 203). At the County of Lancaster Asylum, Rainhill, epilepsy was diagnosed in 8% of admissions during 1890; review of the case notes resulted in a modern diagnosis of epilepsy in 6% (Parker et al. 1993). In the Utica Asylum in New York State, the proportion of patients whose illness was taken to be caused by epilepsy averaged approximately 3% in the middle of the 19th century (our rough calculation from the tables provided by Dwyer 1987, p. 100). The incidence of epilepsy in new admissions to Kraepelin's German asylum in 1908 was 10.5% (Jablensky et al. 1993).

Moreover, epilepsy was a public hospital disorder. With regard to the category including epilepsy (as well as "congenital defect, over-exertion, and sunstroke"), the contrast among the settings reviewed by Renvoize and Beveridge (1989) is striking. At the York Retreat, 2.8% of male cases were thought to result from this physical origin; at the public asylum, 12.5%, more than four times as many; and in the intermediate setting, 6.5%. The eminent

London neurologist William Gowers, working chiefly at the National Hospital for the Paralysed and Epileptic (now the National Hospital for Neurology and Neurosurgery, Queen Square), noted that he had never seen death from status epilepticus and believed that such a phenomenon is "very rare, at any rate out of asylums for the insane" (Gowers 1881, p. 194). His work was roughly contemporaneous with the data cited above, but he gave no explanation for the known and regular occurrence of death from status epilepticus in the asylums.

The term *general paresis of the insane* (GPI) implies a close connection between neurosyphilis and the mental hospital. Indeed, both English and American asylums admitted and managed patients with GPI and witnessed their inevitable deaths. Hare (1959), in his magisterial overview of this illness, noted that

> in some asylums in England and Wales there were whole decades when a quarter or more of all the male admissions were paretic. These cases pursued a slow but relentless course to complete dementia and death, and it is not hard to imagine that the unrewarding and dispiriting task of nursing them was one reason why the high standards of humane care set up by the pioneers of non-restraint and moral management seem gradually to have deteriorated during the latter half of the nineteenth century. (p. 608)

Hare (1981, 1983) reckoned the rate of GPI in the mid-19th century to be 10%–20% of asylum admissions, and through the latter decades of the 19th century, 7%–8%. In the County of Lancaster Asylum, Rainhill, 14% of patients in 1890 had general paresis recognized at admission (Parker et al. 1993). In a Scottish asylum for the poor in the last quarter of the 19th century, 1.5% of female patients and 7.6% of male patients had GPI (Doody et al. 1996). Even at the exclusive Ticehurst House Asylum, where efforts were made to exclude incurable cases, at least 7% of patients in the mid-19th century had GPI (Turner 1992). With GPI, as with epilepsy, we see a disparity in rates between the public and the private sectors: as a cause of death, GPI was recognized in 14% of those in the York Retreat, in 15.2% of those in the York Asylum with its mixed public and private population, and in 21.4% of those in the public North Riding Asylum (Renvoize and Beveridge 1989).

Similar magnitudes are seen in the American material. At the Utica Asylum, between 7% and 16% of male patients during the 1870s and 1880s were assessed to have mental illness caused by paresis; much lower rates, 1%–4%, were seen in the female patients (Dwyer 1987). At the private McLean Hospital at the beginning of the 20th century, some 10% of patients had paresis

(Sutton 1986, p. 167). Among patients committed to mental hospitals in early 20th century California, 16% of those with a cause of mental illness assigned were diagnosed as having syphilis as that cause (though only a quarter of all commitment documents listed a cause) (Fox 1978, p. 159). Grob (1994, p. 125) assessed the rate of GPI among first admissions to New York State mental hospitals in the second decade of the 20th century as approximately 20% of male patients, and one-third that number of female patients (about 7%). (His comment on these data has a contemporary ring: "[F]ew households were prepared to cope with paretic members. Nor could general hospitals pick up the slack; their concern with acute illnesses and short patient stays rendered them unsuitable for the care of paretic patients.")

The story of general paresis has important conceptual implications. The syndrome of GPI was identified well before its link with syphilis could be made (Quétel 1986/1990). Most of the varied causal attributions made in the 19th century can be seen in retrospect to reflect the moral judgments of the doctor rather than any scientific data. Confusion and prejudice reigned until developments in histological and serological methods put paid to fanciful explanations such as dram-drinking and venery. In Hare's (1959, p. 615) words, "There was no sure path through the speculative labyrinth until the autumn of 1912, when, in the paretic brain sections sent to Noguchi by Moore, the pale visage of a few spirochaetes sufficed to disinherit chaos."

Similarly today, we are more able to identify behavioral syndromes than to elucidate their causes, and not a few of our ideas may prove better to reflect our cultural milieu than to evince our scientific acumen. Psychiatry chose to focus on behavioral syndromes for nosological purposes. By contrast, general medicine and neurology identified diseases by pathoanatomical-clinical correlation, as prescribed by the Paris school of the early 19th century (Ackerknecht 1967; Ovsiew and McClelland 1995). This choice was adumbrated in the debate over the work of Bayle, who first linked GPI to an anatomical substrate of chronic meningitis (Brown 1994). Presumption can perhaps be seen in Bayle's further assertion that "the majority of mental illnesses are the symptom of a primary chronic inflammation of the membranes of the brain" (quoted in Brown 1994, p. 248). Yet the attitude of Bayle's opponents was that of subsequent psychiatric nosologists and possibly was a brake on progress over the decades. Pinel and Georget insisted that most mental illness is idiopathic, not symptomatic of identifiable pathological changes in the brain, and believed that detailed behavioral description and Linnaean classification on the basis of behavior were the paths of progress (Brown 1994; Duffy 1995).

One reason for the explosive growth of asylums in the later 19th and early

20th centuries was their increasing populations of older people. The poorhouse gave way to the mental hospital as the setting for the chronic care of the older population. The increase in the number and proportion of older people in the general population was then and remains today another factor in the increasing requirement for institutional care. In state hospitals, the proportion of the population over age 60 rose by 300%–400% in the first decades of the 20th century (Grob 1994, p. 120). For these patients, the early enthusiasm for the ability of the asylums to cure was clearly inappropriate.

The management of inebriety was a problem faced by asylums from early in their existence. The development of small private and large public institutions specifically for inebriety formed a counterpoint to the general-purpose mental hospitals, which also saw no lack of alcoholism and other substance-related disorders (Baumohl 1990; Brown 1985). Some physician superintendents believed that alcohol and other substance abuse was a vice, not an illness, and simply refused, as best they could, to admit inebriate patients; such was the case at the Utica Asylum under the leadership of the prominent alienist John Gray (Dwyer 1987, p. 103). Intemperance was the diagnosed cause of insanity in as many as a quarter of patients in English asylums (Renvoize and Beveridge 1989). Even when alcohol abuse was not specifically diagnosed or tabulated, case notes make clear that it was a common problem and that typical cases of delirium tremens and other alcohol-related mental disorders were frequently seen (Crammer 1990). Hare (1981) estimated that 5% of admissions to English asylums in the late 19th century were for alcoholic insanity. Present-day rediagnosis from case notes of patients at the County of Lancaster Asylum suggested that 8% of patients in 1890 had alcohol-related illness (Parker et al. 1993).

Similarly, mental retardation both contributed a substantial number of patients to the asylums and gave rise to a separate institutional development (Trent 1994). The Buckinghamshire County Pauper Lunatic Asylum recorded the admission of 4 patients (5%) with severe mental retardation of 79 admitted in 1861; in 1911, mental handicap accounted for 11% of admissions (Crammer 1990, pp. 62–63). Similarly, in the County of Lancaster Asylum, mental retardation can be retrospectively recognized in 9% and was contemporaneously diagnosed in 6% of admitted patients (Parker et al. 1993). Epilepsy was commonly present in the mentally retarded, and one can easily imagine both the difficulty these patients posed to the institutions and the inadequacy of the care they received.

The diagnosis of illnesses among these early psychiatric patients was undertaken with limited tools. Turner (1992) noted that the doctors at Ticehurst House Asylum probably underestimated the prevalence of GPI because the presentation could be mistaken for an idiopathic manic state and early discharge might prevent the deteriorating course from being evident. Not until the Wassermann reaction became available at the beginning of this century could early diagnoses of syphilitic disease be confidently made. The estimates of prevalence of epilepsy in the asylum as reviewed above do not take account of Hughlings Jackson's later description of the "uncinate group of fits," which we would today call complex partial seizures. Often still difficult today, the recognition of organic illness was rudimentary in the 19th century. Yet it is likely that by the early years of this century, in one-third to one-half of all first admissions to state mental hospitals, the mental disorder was attributable to organic disease (Grob 1994, p. 126). For example, Evenson and his colleagues (Evenson et al. 1994a, 1994b) reviewed records from 1886 through 1904 from the St. Louis City Insane Asylum. With contemporary rediagnosis, 25.5% of patients had "organic brain syndrome," in addition to 6.3% who suffered from mental retardation. Similarly, organic rediagnoses were made in 26% of patients admitted to the Fife and Kinross District Asylum in Scotland during the last quarter of the 19th century (Doody et al. 1996). Because these organic disorders often had an unremitting or declining course, the number of such patients in the early asylums may have been even greater.

Conclusion

Many writers have considered psychiatry an agency of social control, and in particular the "discovery" of the asylum a product of the social needs of its time (Rothman 1990; Scull 1993). In contrast, few writers have examined the consequences of the prominent social role of psychiatry for its development as a profession, for its theories as well as its practices—a matter perhaps of more concern to psychiatrists than to sociologists or historians. Yet our review of the 19th-century data supports Grob's statement quoted as the epigraph to this chapter. Psychiatry does bear the stamp of its origins. Without, we hope, committing the genetic fallacy of believing that only the origins of the asylum and of the profession of psychiatry contain relevant lessons, we have focused on the 19th century and have not taken into account the important changes in professional practice between then and now. We realize that psychiatry later took root in the general hospital, that outpatient treatment became preeminent, that deinstitutionalization took hold, that psychoanalysis had profound effects on psychiatry's self-conception, and so on. Still, the stamp placed on psychiatry by its public origins is a story that has perhaps not been fully told, and one relevant to this volume in particular.

Although all of medical practice may be a social phenomenon and all diagnoses socially constructed (Wright and Treacher 1982), it is psychiatric diagnoses that have drawn the most sociological attention. The argument that mental illness is a myth or a form of social deviance depends in large measure on the claim that mental illness is not truly medical; few consider that epilepsy or syphilis is mythical or deviant. Some commentators saw "no immediately compelling argument for putting physicians in charge of moral treatment" (Tomes 1988, p. 8) and in charge of the asylums in which that treatment took place; Jacyna (1982) and Scull (1989b) argued that it was "entrepreneurship" on the part of medical men to arrogate the asylum to themselves and that the belief that brain disease underlay mental illness was so much ideology toward that goal.

The data presented here certainly give no support to such arguments. Doctors took care of patients with epilepsy or syphilis in the asylum, just as they did patients with epilepsy or syphilis outside the asylum. "Hospital and asylum served different patient populations for basically the same conditions" (Hunter and Macalpine 1974, p. 203). As Maudsley said, the accident of a mental presentation sent some to the asylum and its alienist, rather than to the hospital and its physician. What Maudsley did not say is that the accident of poverty and social need played an equal role. "The difficult and dirty, the unmanageable and the incurable" (Hunter and Macalpine 1974, p. 203) were the province of the asylum doctor. If the explosive growth of mental institutions resulted disproportionately in the incarceration of the poor (Scull 1984), this does not gainsay the significance of somatic disease: poor families and communities are less able to compensate for aberrant behavior and lost abilities, whatever the causes.

What were the consequences for psychiatry of this social assignment? One was sheer overwork. Hunter and Macalpine (1974) compared the workload of the Colney Hatch Asylum doctor with that of a contemporary at the National Hospital, Queen Square. At the former, 5 medical officers had charge of 2,250 patients, 1 medical officer for every 450 patients; at Queen Square, 12 physicians and their junior doctors worked in a 75-bed hospital, 1 senior physician for every 6 patients. It is no surprise that publications chronicling remarkable insights into epilepsy originated at the latter, not the former. Overwork is not a thing of the past, as many doctors in public mental health settings today can testify. The way that the psychiatric profession has complied with this social understanding of the medical needs of people who are mentally ill and poor should be scrutinized.

Asylum superintendents grew expert in ventilation and architecture and the management of farmland and large staffs, the better to pursue the institutional basis of moral therapy. Even if one discounts venal motives of power in this professional specialization, it is hard not to see such concerns as distracting asylum doctors from scientific advances. As late as the 1930s, psychiatrists in at least some English settings led a peculiarly insular life, as recounted by the late eminent British psychiatrist Eliot Slater (1975, p. 71):

> The hospitals were planned as little villages, nearly self-supporting, isolated from the countryside by their high stone walls and great locked gates with lodge and weigh-bridge. Inside were a fair-sized farm and vegetable gardens, power house, bakeries, kitchens, laundries, as well as the hospital buildings proper and the houses for the staff. Within this island fortress the medical superintendent was the highest authority. . . . He would commonly take great pride in the management of the farm and the quality of the pigs and poultry and garden produce. . . . Life could be quite leisured, and at that time it was still possible for the "super" to live the life of a gentleman farmer, invited to tennis parties at the Rectory, fishing and even riding to hounds.

Psychiatry adapted itself to its social role, perhaps seduced by the power and prestige offered by the position of guardian of the social order. Especially in the elite private institutions, often the home of opinion makers and theoreticians in psychiatry, practitioners had to meet the needs of their patients' families (D'Antonio 1990; Tomes 1984). Dowbiggin (1992) described how the prominent psychiatrist G. Alder Blumer ceased to support eugenic measures when he left the chronic and deteriorated patients of the Utica State Hospital in 1899 to become medical superintendent of the private Butler Hospital in Rhode Island. Instead of eugenics, he favored emphasizing the "'nerve' element in the case" (Dowbiggin 1992, p. 392), which was more agreeable to the wealthy clientele, who also received thorough physical and mental examinations and frequently lumbar punctures. Turner (1992, p. 33) remarked that diagnosis "had a strong social pressure behind it," because recognizing and avoiding chronicity was essential in the private asylum. Social misdemeanor and dangerousness have long been important psychiatric diagnostic issues (Fox 1978). Chronicity, dangerousness, and other socially important psychiatric concepts may not be heuristically valuable from a neurobiological perspective.

Further, the socially imposed separation between severe mental illness and milder forms of mental disorder—the latter, in the 19th century, often falling into the care of neurologists—may have been an obstacle to an adequate psychiatric nosology. Mapother, then superintendent of the Maudsley Hospital in London, made this point more than 70 years ago:

The distinction between what are termed neuroses and psychoses has really grown out of practical differences, particularly as regards certification and asylum treatment. It has become customary to call those types and degrees of mental disorder which rarely call for such measures by the name of neuroses. (Mapother 1926, p. 872)

Eventually neuroses were seen as psychogenic, and the possible biological continuity between mild and severe disturbances of mood or thinking was ignored. Although psychiatry laudably developed a commitment to the chronic care of the severely ill (Wing 1990), its social role may have led it conceptually astray.

As asylums grew custodial, asylum doctors grew to be custodians. In its origins, psychiatry was the medical specialty caring for those whose minds were severely affected by brain diseases. Yet as the medical understanding of these illnesses was growing, the psychiatric profession of the 19th century grew away from a concern with medical understanding. S. Weir Mitchell, the most eminent American neurologist of his day, spoke to the 50th annual meeting of the American Medico-Psychological Association in 1894 (Mitchell 1894). He apologized profusely for his impoliteness in coming as a guest and criticizing his hosts, and then he said:

You were the first of the specialists and you have never come back into line. It is easy to see how this came about. You soon began to live apart, and you still do so [p. 414]. . . . When we ask for your asylum notes of cases, or by some accident have occasion to look over your case books, we are too often surprised at the amazing lack of complete physical study of the insane, at the failure to see obvious lesions, at the want of thorough day by day study of the secretions in the newer cases, of blood-counts, temperatures, reflexes, the eye-ground, color-fields, all the minute examination with which we are so unrestingly busy. (Mitchell 1894, p. 424)

Other American neurologists who criticized asylum doctors were less gentlemanly. Spitzka (1878, p. 209) was

inclined to believe that certain superintendents are experts in gardening and farming (although the farm account frequently comes out on the wrong side of the ledger), tin roofing (although the roof and cupola is usually leaky), drain-pipe laying (although the grounds are often moist and unhealthy), engineering (though the wards are either too hot or too cold), history (though their facts are incorrect, and their inferences beyond all measure so); in short, experts at everything except the diagnosis, pathology and treatment of insanity.

The neurologists' motives were humanitarian, scientific, political, and financial—Spitzka considered asylum doctors to hold an "unjust monopoly" (1878, p. 204) on patients with mental illness (Blustein 1981). Whatever the motives, the critique must be judged in retrospect largely accurate. Yet American neurologists themselves had little to offer asylum patients. Their textbooks lacked chapters on mental illness; their practices lacked contact with patients with mental illness who were hospitalized. Their interests were primarily in the grand themes of the stresses of modern life and the consequent depletion of nerve force. At the end of the 19th century, the St. Louis neurologist Hughes said that

> America breeds and develops neurologists as the water breeds and develops fishes. . . . It cannot yet be said that we are a neuropathic people, though we are tending that way; but neurology is advancing with equal pace with neuropathic breakdown, and will, it is hoped, ultimately enlighten and save the people from their neuropathic sins. (Blustein 1979, p. 177)

It was not inevitable that one professional group should provide custodial and psychological care for those with severe organic lesions of the brain and another professional group should learn to understand, diagnose, and treat those lesions. That it might have been otherwise is shown by the example of the West Riding Lunatic Asylum in Yorkshire, England (Oppenheim 1991; Todd and Ashworth 1991; Viets 1938). Under the leadership of Dr. (later Sir) James Crichton Browne, a remarkable program of research into the cerebral diseases of asylum patients was initiated and, in the *West Riding Lunatic Asylum Medical Reports* of the 1870s, was brought to the attention of the medical community. Much of the pioneering work of Dr. (later Sir) David Ferrier on cerebral localization was done in the laboratories of the West Riding Lunatic Asylum. Ferrier reported on the clinical application of this work in West Riding patients with epilepsy, brain tumor, and stroke (Ferrier 1874)—as we have seen, not unusual findings in the asylum population. The *West Riding Lunatic Asylum Medical Reports* contained several papers by Hughlings Jackson as well as a number of other contributions on epilepsy (George and Trimble 1992). Publication ceased in 1876 after only 6 years, when Crichton Browne took on new public responsibilities, but in 1879 *Brain*—which continues today as a leading neurological journal—was founded by Crichton Browne, Hughlings Jackson, Ferrier, and the alienist Bucknill (Henson 1978).

In the preface to the first issue of the *West Riding Lunatic Asylum Medical Reports*, Crichton Browne (1871) repeated, with the aim of parrying but the impression of acknowledging, the charges of medical critics that too little scientific work was done in asylums. In a later volume, he wrote,

> It is upon Asylum medical officers that the obligation to watch and interrogate nervous diseases most heavily falls, for their opportunities of doing so are peculiarly great and excellent. Our lunatic hospitals are stored with only too vast an accumulation of pathological material. (Crichton Browne 1875, p. vi)

Although patients with mental illness in public mental health settings now find themselves in many locations other than the "lunatic hospital"—as the chapters of this book document—Crichton Browne's words ring true today.

References

Ackerknecht EH: Medicine at the Paris Hospital, 1794–1848. Baltimore, MD, Johns Hopkins University Press, 1967

Arieno MA: Victorian Lunatics: A Social Epidemiology of Mental Illness in Mid-Nineteenth-Century England. Selinsgrove, Susquehanna University Press, 1989

Baumohl J: Inebriate institutions in North America, 1840–1920. British Journal of Addiction 85:1187–1204, 1990

Blustein BE: New York neurologists and the specialization of American medicine. Bull Hist Med 53:170–183, 1979

Blustein BE: "A hollow square of psychological science": American neurologists and psychiatrists in conflict, in Madhouses, Mad-doctors, and Madmen: The Social History of Psychiatry in the Victorian Era. Edited by Scull A. Philadelphia, PA, University of Pennsylvania Press, 1981, pp 241–270

Brown EM: "What shall we do with the inebriate?" Asylum treatment and the disease concept of alcoholism in the late nineteenth century. J Hist Behav Sci 21:48–59, 1985

Brown EM: French psychiatry's initial reception of Bayle's discovery of general paresis of the insane. Bull Hist Med 68:235–253, 1994

Bucknill JC, Tuke DH: A Manual of Psychological Medicine: Containing the Lunacy Laws, the Nosology, Ætiology, Statistics, Description, Diagnosis, Pathology, and Treatment of Insanity With an Appendix of Cases, 4th Edition. Philadelphia, PA, Lindsay & Blakiston, 1879

Bynum WF: Rationales for therapy in British psychiatry, 1780–1835, in Madhouses, Mad-doctors, and Madmen: The Social History of Psychiatry in the Victorian Era. Edited by Scull A. Philadelphia, PA, University of Pennsylvania Press, 1981, pp 35–57

Carlson ET: The influence of phrenology on early American psychiatric thought. Am J Psychiatry 115:535–538, 1958

Cooter R: Phrenology and British alienists, ca. 1825–1845, in Madhouses, Mad-doctors, and Madmen: A Social History of Psychiatry in the Victorian Era. Edited by Scull A. Philadelphia, PA, University of Pennsylvania Press, 1981, pp 58–104

Crammer J: Asylum History: Buckinghamshire County Pauper Lunatic Asylum—St John's. London, Gaskell, 1990

Crichton Browne J: Preface. West Riding Lunatic Asylum Medical Reports 1:iii–v, 1871

Crichton Browne J: Preface. West Riding Lunatic Asylum Medical Reports 5:v–vi, 1875

Dain N: Concepts of Insanity in the United States, 1789–1865. New Brunswick, NJ, Rutgers University Press, 1964

Dain N, Carlson ET: Milieu therapy in the nineteenth century: patient care at the Friend's Asylum, Frankford, Pennsylvania, 1817–1861. J Nerv Ment Dis 131: 277–290, 1960

D'Antonio P: The need for care: families, patients, and staff at a nineteenth-century insane asylum. Trans Stud Coll Physicians Phila 12:147–366, 1990

Digby A: Madness, Morality and Medicine: A Study of the York Retreat, 1796–1914. Cambridge, UK, Cambridge University Press, 1985

Doerner K: Madmen and the Bourgeoisie: A Social History of Insanity and Psychiatry. Oxford, England, Basil Blackwell, 1981

Doody GA, Beveridge A, Johnstone EC: Poor and mad: a study of patients admitted to the Fife and Kinross District Asylum between 1874 and 1899. Psychol Med 26:887–897, 1996

Dowbiggin I: "An exodus of enthusiasm": G. Alder Blumer, eugenics, and US psychiatry, 1890–1920. Med Hist 36:379–402, 1992

Duffy JD: General paralysis of the insane: neuropsychiatry's first challenge. J Neuropsychiatry Clin Neurosci 7:243–249, 1995

Dwyer E: Homes for the Mad: Life Inside Two Nineteenth-Century Asylums. New Brunswick, NJ, Rutgers University Press, 1987

Evenson RC, Holland RA, Cho DW: A psychiatric hospital 100 years ago, I: a comparative study of treatment outcomes then and now. Hospital and Community Psychiatry 45:1021–1025, 1994a

Evenson RC, Holland RA, Johnson ME: A psychiatric hospital 100 years ago, II: patients, treatment, and daily life. Hospital and Community Psychiatry 45: 1025–1029, 1994b

Ferrier D: Pathological illustrations of brain function. West Riding Lunatic Asylum Medical Reports 4:30–62, 1874

Fodor JA: The Modularity of Mind. Cambridge, MA, MIT Press, 1983

Foucault M: Madness and Civilization: A History of Insanity in the Age of Reason. New York, Random House, 1965

Foucault M: Histoire de la folie à l'âge classique: suivi de mon corps, ce papier, ce feu et la folie, l'absence d'œuvre. Paris, Gallimard, 1972

Fox RW: So Far Disordered in Mind: Insanity in California, 1870–1930. Berkeley, CA, University of California Press, 1978

George MS, Trimble MR: The changing 19th-century view of epilepsy as reflected in the *West Riding Lunatic Asylum Medical Reports*, 1871–1876, vols 1–6. Neurology 42:246–249, 1992

Gordon C: *Histoire de la folie*: an unknown book by Michel Foucault. History of the Human Sciences 3:3–26, 1990

Gosling FG: Before Freud: Neurasthenia and the American Medical Community, 1870–1910. Urbana, IL, University of Illinois Press, 1987

Gowers WR: Epilepsy and Other Chronic Convulsive Diseases: Their Causes, Symptoms, and Treatment. London, J & A Churchill, 1881

Grob GN: The Inner World of American Psychiatry, 1890–1940. New Brunswick, NJ, Rutgers University Press, 1985

Grob GN: The Mad Among Us. New York, Free Press, 1994

Gutting G: Michel Foucault's *Phänomenologie des Krankengeistes*, in Discovering the History of Psychiatry. Edited by Micale MS, Porter R. New York, Oxford University Press, 1994, pp 331–347

Hammond WA: Cerebral Hyperæmia: The Result of Mental Strain or Emotional Disturbance. New York, G. P. Putnam's Sons, 1878

Hare EH: The origin and spread of dementia paralytica. Journal of Mental Science 105:594–626, 1959

Hare EH: Masturbatory insanity: the history of an idea. Journal of Mental Science 108:1–25, 1962

Hare E: The two manias: a study of the evolution of the modern concept of mania. Br J Psychiatry 138:89–99, 1981

Hare E: Was insanity on the increase? Br J Psychiatry 142:439–455, 1983

Henson RA: The editors of *Brain*. The Practitioner 221:639–644, 1978

Hunter R, Macalpine I: Psychiatry for the Poor: 1851 Colney Hatch Asylum—Friern Hospital 1973. London, Dawsons, 1974

Jablensky A, Hugler H, Von Cranach M, et al: Kraepelin revisited: a reassessment and statistical analysis of dementia praecox and manic-depressive insanity in 1908. Psychol Med 23:843–858, 1993

Jacyna LS: Somatic theories of mind and the interests of medicine in Britain, 1850–1879. Med Hist 26:233–258, 1982

Jeste DV, del Carmen R, Lohr JB, et al: Did schizophrenia exist before the eighteenth century? Compr Psychiatry 26:493–503, 1985

Macalpine I, Hunter R: George III and the Mad-Business. New York, Random House, 1969

Mapother E: Discussion on manic-depressive psychosis. Br Med J ii:872–879, 1926

Marshall JC: The new organology. Behav Brain Sci 3:23–25, 1980

Maudsley H: Body and Mind: An Inquiry Into Their Connection and Mutual Influence, Specially in Reference to Mental Disorder. New York, D Appleton, 1898

McGovern CM: Masters of Madness: Social Origins of the American Psychiatric Profession. Hanover, VT, University Press of New England, 1985

McKenzie C: Psychiatry for the Rich: A History of Ticehurst Private Asylum, 1792–1917. London, Routledge, 1992

Midelfort HCE: Madness and civilization in early modern Europe: a reappraisal of Michel Foucault, in After the Reformation: Essays in Honor of J. H. Hexter. Edited by Malament BC. Philadelphia, PA, University of Pennsylvania Press, 1980, pp 247–265

Mitchell SW: Address before the 50th annual meeting of the American Medico-Psychological Association, held in Philadelphia, May 16th, 1894. J Nerv Ment Dis 21:413–437, 1894

Oppenheim J: "Shattered Nerves": Doctors, Patients, and Depression in Victorian England. New York, Oxford University Press, 1991

Ovsiew F, McClelland R: Anglo-American neuropsychiatry in historical perspective. Current Opinion in Psychiatry 8:45–47, 1995

Parker RR, Dutta A, Barnes R, et al: County of Lancaster Asylum, Rainhill: 100 years ago and now. History of Psychiatry 4:95–105, 1993

Parry-Jones WL: The Trade in Lunacy: A Study of Private Madhouses in England in the Eighteenth and Nineteenth Centuries. London, Routledge & Kegan Paul, 1972

Porter R: Mind-Forg'd Manacles: A History of Madness in England From the Restoration to the Regency. Cambridge, MA, Harvard University Press, 1987

Porter R: Foucault's great confinement. History of the Human Sciences 3:47–54, 1990

Quétel C: History of Syphilis [1986]. Baltimore, MD, Johns Hopkins University Press, 1990

Renvoize EB, Beveridge AW: Mental illness and the late Victorians: a study of patients admitted to three asylums in York, 1880–1884. Psychol Med 19:19–28, 1989

Rothman DJ: The Discovery of the Asylum: Social Order and Disorder in the New Republic, Revised Edition. Boston, MA, Little, Brown, 1990

Rousseau GS: Michel Foucault. Madness and civilization: a history of insanity in the age of reason (book review). Eighteenth Century Studies 4:90–95, 1970

Scull A: Was insanity increasing? a response to Edward Hare. Br J Psychiatry 144:432–436, 1984

Scull A: The discovery of the asylum revisited: lunacy reform in the new American republic, in Social Order/Mental Disorder: Anglo-American Psychiatry in Historical Perspective. Edited by Scull A. Berkeley, CA, University of California Press, 1989a, pp 95–117

Scull A: From madness to mental illness: medical men as moral entrepreneurs, in Social Order/Mental Disorder: Anglo-American Psychiatry in Historical Perspective. Edited by Scull A. Berkeley, CA, University of California Press, 1989b, pp 118–161

Scull A: Reflections on the historical sociology of psychiatry, in Social Order/Mental Disorder: Anglo-American Psychiatry in Historical Perspective. Edited by Scull A. Berkeley, CA, University of California Press, 1989c, pp 1–30

Scull A: A failure to communicate? on the reception of Foucault's *Histoire de la folie* by Anglo-American historians, in Rewriting the History of Madness: Studies in Foucault's *Histoire de la folie*. Edited by Still A, Velody I. London, Routledge, 1992, pp 150–163

Scull A: The Most Solitary of Afflictions: Madness and Society in Britain 1700–1900. New Haven, CT, Yale University Press, 1993

Shorter E: From Paralysis to Fatigue: A History of Psychosomatic Illness in the Modern Era. New York, Free Press, 1992

Slater E: Psychiatry in the 'thirties. Contemporary Review 226:70–75, 1975

Spitzka EC: Reform in the scientific study of psychiatry. J Nerv Ment Dis 5:201–229, 1878

Sutton SB: Crossroads in Psychiatry: A History of the McLean Hospital. Washington, DC, American Psychiatric Press, 1986

Todd J, Ashworth L: James Crichton-Browne and the West Riding Asylum, in 150 Years of British Psychiatry, 1841–1991. Edited by Berrios GE, Freeman H. London, Gaskell, 1991, pp 389–418

Tomes N: A Generous Confidence: Thomas Story Kirkbride and the Art of Asylum-Keeping, 1840–1883. Cambridge, England, Cambridge University Press, 1984

Tomes N: The Anglo-American asylum in historical perspective, in Location and Stigma: Contemporary Perspectives on Mental Health and Mental Health Care. Edited by Smith CJ, Giggs JA. Boston, MA, Unwin Hyman, 1988, pp 3–20

Trent JW: Inventing the Feeble Mind: A History of Mental Retardation in the United States. Berkeley, CA, University of California Press, 1994

Turner TH: A diagnostic analysis of the Casebooks of Ticehurst House Asylum, 1845–1890. Psychological Medicine Monograph (suppl) 21:1–70, 1992

Viets HB: West Riding, 1871–1876. Bulletin of the Institute of the History of Medicine 6:477–487, 1938

Wing JK: The functions of asylum. Br J Psychiatry 157:822–827, 1990

Wright P, Treacher A (eds): The Problem of Medical Knowledge: Examining the Social Construction of Medicine. Edinburgh, Edinburgh University Press, 1982

Young RM: Mind, Brain, and Adaptation in the Nineteenth Century: Cerebral Localization and Its Biological Context From Gall to Ferrier (1970). New York, Oxford University Press, 1990

CHAPTER 2

Epidemiology and Recognition of Neuropsychiatric Disorders in Mental Health Settings

Barbara L. Yates, M.D.
Lorrin M. Koran, M.D.

Mental and physical health are often linked (Lipowski 1987). Mental health professionals, therefore, must consider whether an organic condition is causing or exacerbating each patient's psychiatric symptoms. For many patients in a public mental health setting, moreover, the mental health system provides their only contact with medical personnel. This contact creates a high-payoff opportunity to detect important physical disorders in a symptomatic population.

In this chapter, we examine the importance of an integrated approach to neuropsychiatric conditions and the difficulties in assessing medical disorders in psychiatric populations. We also review studies of the prevalence of medical disorders in patients in psychiatric settings, discuss screening strategies, and alert clinicians to situations in which an organic cause for a psychiatric syndrome should be strongly considered. Finally, we make recommendations for implementing medical screening in public mental health settings.

Psychiatric Symptoms and Medical Diseases

The links between psychiatric symptoms and medical diseases have long been noted. For example, in 1840 Basedow described psychotic reactions associated with exophthalmic goiter, and in 1855 Addison described changes in the behavior and mood of patients with Addison's disease (Koranyi 1982). Psychiatric symptoms can be directly related to neurological, vascular, degenerative, toxic, infectious, and neoplastic processes as well as to endocrine or nutritional disorders affecting brain function.

Physical disease can cause mental disorders in less direct ways as well. The illness may disrupt normal mental functioning by disrupting sleep, body image, or physical functioning. It may exacerbate environmental stressors by limiting the patient's ability to provide economically for himself or herself or others. The illness's meanings—for example, impending mortality—may also contribute to the onset of mental disorder, such as severe anxiety or depression, or its signs, such as denial or substance abuse (Lipowski 1975).

Psychiatric treatments can also cause medical disorder. For example, psychiatric medications can induce or exacerbate diabetes, hypothyroidism, systemic lupus erythematosus, liver dysfunction, and sexual difficulties (Ananth 1984). Disentangling the symptoms of an iatrogenic medical condition from those of the patient's psychiatric condition can be difficult. For example, the patient with bipolar disorder who complains of weight gain, weakness, and low energy could be having these symptoms as a result of a worsening depression, lithium use, or lithium-induced hypothyroidism (Ananth 1984).

Substantial rates of mortality and medical morbidity in psychiatric patients also support the need to be alert for medical conditions. Most studies have found in psychiatric patients modestly increased mortality rates, which vary with psychiatric diagnosis (Martin et al. 1985; Tsuang and Simpson 1985). In general, patients with organic brain syndromes have elevated mortality rates from natural causes (Black et al. 1985; Innes and Millar 1970; Martin et al. 1985). Mortality from suicide and homicide is higher among patients with alcoholism, antisocial personality, or drug addiction and among gay patients, but whether mortality from natural causes is elevated remains uncertain (Martin et al. 1985). In other psychiatric patient populations, confounding variables have prevented clear conclusions; patients frequently had other risk factors for increased mortality and morbidity, such as poverty and poor access to health care, or the sample selection was biased. Kendler (1986) attempted to sort out some of these factors using the National Academy of Sciences–National Research Council Twin Registry. Kendler found excess mortality from both trauma and medical disease in patients with schizophrenia or broadly defined "neurosis" compared with their twins.

In summary, the professional and legal obligation to investigate the presence of physical disease in mental health patients stems from several sources. First, physical diseases may cause the patient's mental disorder. Second, physical disease may worsen a mental disorder, either by affecting brain function or by giving rise to a psychopathological reaction. Third, patients with mental illness are often unable or unwilling to seek medical care and frequently harbor undiscovered physical disease. Finally, a patient's visit to a mental health program creates an opportunity to screen for physical disease in a symptomatic population. The yield of disease from such screening is usually higher than the yield in an asymptomatic population.

Difficulties in Assessing Physical Illness

Psychiatrists should always examine the evidentiary basis for the appellations *medically clear* or *no significant disease* applied to patients who are referred by other physicians. For example, patients presenting with psychiatric complaints have a low but significant rate of unrecognized organic brain syndrome even when they have recently been medically evaluated (Dubin et al. 1983; Hoffman and Koran 1984; Waxman et al. 1984). Bunce and his colleagues (1982) found that 92% of chronically ill psychiatric patients transferred to a medical/psychiatric unit had at least one previously undiagnosed disease in addition to the problem that had prompted the transfer. An average of three unexpected disorders per patient was found. Hoffman (1982) examined 215 patients on a medical/psychiatric unit and found that a thorough neuropsychiatric evaluation changed the diagnosis in 41% of patients. Although these percentages may be unrepresentative of inpatient settings in general, they highlight the need for careful medical evaluation of psychiatric inpatients.

In outpatient settings, undetected physical disease is also common, even when the patient has been followed by a primary care physician (Davies 1965; Hall et al. 1978; Karasu 1980; Koranyi 1972). For example, of patients referred by medical services, Koranyi (1972) found that only 70% of their physical diseases were known to the referring service. Hall and his colleagues (1978) reported that 77% of their sample had illnesses that were previously unrecognized, although approximately two-thirds of the patients had seen a family physician regularly. The careful psychiatrist will often detect important physical disease missed by his or her colleagues (Eilenberg and Whatmore 1961; Weissberg 1979). Reviewing the specifics of the prior medical evaluation and supplementing when necessary are crucial for correct diagnosis and treatment.

Why is it difficult to assess medical disorders in psychiatric patients? Problems can be divided into four categories: those related to the physical disease, to the psychiatric disorder, to the physician, and to organizational factors. One of the most important reasons that physical diseases are missed is that they can masquerade as psychiatric disorders. Moreover, symptoms such as weakness, fatigue, and anorexia can be the result of either or both of these kinds of pathology. In addition, organically induced symptoms may precede signs of the physical disease. And physical disease itself, especially if it affects the brain, may interfere with the patient's ability to provide an adequate history (Hoffman and Koran 1984).

Psychiatric illness may also impair history giving. Psychotic patients may have problems communicating discomfort or pain. Symptoms of physical disease may be masked by psychotropic medications (Ananth 1984). Psychodynamic defense mechanisms such as denial may interfere with the patient's ability to cooperate with the physician. Psychiatric illness may produce poor hygiene, and this may lead the examiner to examine the patient with less than usual thoroughness.

Psychiatrists may miss medical diagnoses if they rely too heavily on a medical consultant's opinion or lack faith in their own ability to perform a physical examination (Ananth 1984; Koranyi 1982). A physician's negative emotional reaction to a patient may also interfere with medical decision making (Saravay and Koran 1977). In addition, psychiatrists (and other mental health professionals) may uncover medical conditions by obtaining collateral information and by repeating examinations over time in patients with puzzling symptoms (Hoffman and Koran 1984). Hoffman and Koran (1984) advised that physicians avoid plausible but dangerous assumptions such as that 1) the current episode is simply a recurrence of a past psychiatric disorder, 2) the episode is explained by psychosocial stressors, and 3) the symptoms are directly reflective of their cause (e.g., depressive symptoms are necessarily the result of major depression).

Finally, from an organizational perspective, psychiatric patients may have more difficulty gaining access to health care, because of, for example, inability to navigate a complex system or financial limitations (Browning et al. 1974).

Prevalence

Table 2–1 displays the prevalence of medical illness in psychiatric patients, as uncovered in modern studies, organized by type of setting. Although the range of prevalence figures is wide, physical disease is common, and many of the diseases found were previously unrecognized. In studies of outpatient clinics, it was commonly found that half of the patients presented with physical diseases (results ranged from 26% to 79%). Inpatient studies showed greater variation in prevalence, but again physical disease was often found in one of every two patients. The prevalence of medical disorders in state hospital patients and in older populations was especially high, with some studies showing prevalences of 80% or greater. The need for medical care for state hospital patients was further documented by Tardiff and Deane (1980), who found that at least one-third of these patients required skilled nursing care daily or more often.

The variance in results probably reflects differences both in the populations studied and in study design. For example, Barnes and colleagues (1983) believed that the low prevalence they observed reflected exclusion of patients who had a physical examination in the prior year and also the long-term care the patients in their sample received. Study designs involved widely varying medical evaluation methods. For example, some studies undoubtedly underestimated physical disease prevalence because the evaluation method consisted mainly of chart review (Karasu 1980; Muecke and Krueger 1981; Weingarten et al. 1982).

Prevalence figures also vary because of differing criteria for the inclusion of physical diseases. Koran and his colleagues (1989) suggested that attention be focused on active, important organic diseases—that is, those that require treatment or surveillance; are life-threatening or communicable; could cause, mimic, or interact with psychiatric conditions; interact with psychotropic medication; have significant long-term health consequences; or affect self-esteem through disfigurement, social stigma, or loss of role function.

Establishing whether an uncovered medical condition has caused the patient's psychiatric disorder can be difficult. Related time of onset, known pathophysiological mechanisms, absence of life stress, and parallel courses imply such a relationship, but treating the medical condition may not alleviate the psychiatric symptoms, and this makes judgment difficult. For example, myxedema psychosis may persist for some time even after the thyroid disease is treated (Ananth 1984).

Psychiatric patients have the same medical conditions—cardiovascular, endocrine, infectious, genitourinary, nutritional, metabolic, and neurological diseases—that affect psychiatrically well populations. Interestingly enough, diabetes is frequently missed, and the unrecognized brain tumor dreaded by every psychiatrist is not common (Hoffman and Koran 1984).

TABLE 2–1. Prevalence of physical disease in psychiatric patients

Setting and study	No. of patients	Physical disease (%)	New diagnosis (%)	Causal or related (%)	Causal (%)
Outpatient					
Forsythe et al. 1977	677 out 433 in	56	29	—	—
Hall et al. 1978	658	—	4	9	
Koranyi 1979	2,090	43	20	32	8.3
Karasu 1980	200	52	42		
Muecke and Krueger 1981	910	—	20	—	0
Barnes et al. 1983	147	26	13	—	<1
Farmer 1987	59	—	53	—	—
Maricle et al. 1987	43	79	51	22.1	3.5
Koran et al. 1989	136	42	13	—	—
Bartsch et al. 1990	175	46	20	16	—
Honig et al. 1989	156	53	32	—	—
Honig et al. 1992	73	36	0	—	—
Inpatient					
Burke 1972	202	43	—	—	—
Allodi and Cohen 1978	—	50	—	—	—
Karasu 1980	612	15	—	—	—
Summers et al. 1981	75	65	—	—	—
Ferguson and Dudleston 1986	650	17			
Koran et al. 1989	63	44	17	—	—
Chandler and Gerndt 1988	224	77	—	—	—
Chatham-Showalter 1992	524	50	27	—	—
State hospital					
Hall et al. 1981	100	80	46	46	—

(continued)

TABLE 2–1.   Prevalence of physical disease in psychiatric patients
(*continued*)

Setting and study	No. of patients	Physical disease (%)	New diagnosis (%)	Causal or related (%)	Causal (%)
State hospital *(continued)*					
Kurucz 1983	100	92	—	41	—
Koran et al. 1989	53	57	8	—	—
Emergency room					
Eastwood et al. 1970	100	40	16	—	1
Carlson et al. 1981	2,000	—	—	4.6	—
24-hour nonhospital					
Koran et al. 1989	55	36	15	—	—
Community care (board and care)					
Koran et al. 1989	40	33	20	—	—
Day treatment					
Burke 1978	133	50	30	—	—
Roca et al. 1987	42	93	46	—	—
Koran et al. 1989	58	28	12	—	—
Brugha et al. 1989	121	41	5.8	—	—
Skilled nursing facilities					
Koran et al. 1989	51	25	6	—	—
Elderly					
Weingarten et al. 1982	49	—	20	51	24
Kolman 1985	68	60	—	—	—
Sheline 1990	95	92	—	—	—

Screening

The content of medical evaluations in different settings is influenced by legal mandates, organizational policy, local custom, and professional standards regarding quality of care and individual training and motivation. *We recommend that a medical history be taken of every patient admitted to any mental health setting.* Half or more of physical disease can be detected by history taking (Kolman 1985), which can be accomplished, in part, by nonphysician staff and subsequently reviewed and expanded by the psychiatrist. Physician and nonphysician staff must, however, be educated about the utility of searching for physical disease. Otherwise, screening will be seriously compromised. For example, physicians' physical examinations will often be incomplete and may omit an adequate neurological examination (Koran et al. 1989). In some settings, approximately half of all abnormal laboratory results may be ignored (Berber and McFeely 1991) or not followed up appropriately (Anfinson and Kathol 1992; Dolan and Mushlin 1985).

A physical examination is particularly important in inpatient settings, in older patients, and in those with signs of organic brain syndrome (e.g., delirium, dementia, amnestic disorders, or other cognitive impairments). A physical examination can also be helpful in outpatient settings. For example, Koranyi (1980) found that 12% of psychiatric outpatients with negative medical histories had physical examination findings that changed their psychiatric diagnosis or treatment. In an inpatient setting, physical examination led to a change in psychiatric diagnosis or treatment in 8.8% of patients (Chandler and Gerndt 1988). In this study, the physical examination was the most important predictor of need for treatment of concurrent medical problems in that it identified 44% of the patients who required medical treatment. In a state hospital study, the physical examination also uncovered the greatest number of significant findings (Kurucz 1983).

Which laboratory tests to use in screening depends on the population being screened. In choosing a screening laboratory battery, certain considerations should be kept in mind: cost per case detected, test sensitivity and specificity, and the expected prevalence of test-related disease in the population to be screened (because prevalence strongly affects sensitivity and specificity). In some cases, laboratory screening has led to a referral rate of 27.8% (Beresford et al. 1985). The use of individual laboratory tests is thoroughly reviewed by Anfinson and Kathol (1992). We do not recommend using laboratory tests alone because this produces a high false-positive rate. For example, when 651 patients in a nursing home were screened for thyroid abnormalities (Drinka et al. 1991), all instances of elevated free thyroxine index were normal on reevaluation and were judged to be the result of other chronic illness or malnourishment. In addition, many abnormal laboratory findings do not affect treatment. Berber and McFeely (1991) found that although 7.8% of 515 patients admitted to a psychiatric hospital had laboratory abnormalities, only 4 patients (0.8%) had laboratory abnormalities that affected treatment. In a study of older inpatients, 23% had laboratory abnormalities, and 60% of the patients needed treatment for medical disorders; however, the diagnosis was made solely from laboratory values in only 1.4% (Kolman 1985). Although these results suggest that laboratory tests by themselves are of limited usefulness, many of the findings were unexpected. In Kolman's study, only 28% of the abnormal results were correctly predicted by psychiatric residents caring for the patients.

If a routine set of laboratory tests is implemented, research suggests that a reasonable battery would be a complete blood cell count (CBC); a chemistry panel that includes electrolytes, glucose, calcium, and thyroid-stimulating hormone (TSH); hepatic and renal function tests; erythrocyte sedimentation rate (ESR); a urinalysis; the fluorescent treponemal antibody absorption test (FTA-ABS) for syphilis (Hart 1986); and measures of levels of B_{12} and folate (Hoffman and Koran 1984). Hoffman and Koran (1984) further recommend a toxicology screen and plasma levels of medications if there are indications of organic brain dysfunction. A purified protein derivative (PPD) skin test is probably indicated in many public mental health settings. Dolan and Mushlin (1985) found that a more limited set of tests would have found all abnormalities in their private inpatients and suggested checking CBC, serum thyroxine, calcium, aspartate aminotransferase, alkaline phosphatase, and syphilis serology, and, in men, a urinalysis. Screening for human immunodeficiency virus infection would be reasonable in psychiatric patients who are intravenous drug users, engage in high-risk sexual behaviors such as unprotected sex with multiple partners, or are health care workers. Recommendations of expert panels for screening tests to apply to patients presenting with a new-onset dementia syndrome are discussed in Chapter 4.

Some investigators recommended routine electrocardiograms (ECGs), but evidence of their utility in asymptomatic patients is limited. ECGs may be of more use in certain patient populations, such as older populations or acutely hospitalized patients (Hall 1982; Hoffman 1982; Kolman 1985). Although a chest X ray is sometimes used in screening algorithms (Ananth 1984; Kolman 1985), findings from such X rays are usually associated with symptoms (Anfinson and Kathol 1992); therefore, routine chest X rays for asymptomatic patients are not indicated.

More extensive procedures such as an electroencephalogram (EEG), computed tomography (CT) scan, or lumbar puncture are useful only in patients with suggestive findings on history or physical examination. A CT scan is unlikely to reveal treatable lesions unless patients show abnormalities on careful neurological examination (Hoffman 1982) and, therefore, cannot be recommended as a cost-effective screening method to be used for all patients with new-onset psychosis, for example. A CT scan may be indicated, however, if the patient has focal neurological findings, cranial ecchymosis, or palpable cranial lumps. Lumbar puncture should be considered when a patient presents with an altered level of consciousness, especially if this is accompanied by headache, fever, or leukocytosis. The use of these tests in patients presenting with dementia is discussed in Chapter 4. In the presence of infection with human immunodeficiency virus, the likelihood of infection is markedly increased; the appropriate workup in this circumstance is discussed in Chapter 8.

Although widespread use of extensive laboratory batteries may not be indicated for screening, normal results have value in ruling out medical conditions, in establishing baseline values for individual patients, and in monitoring known medical conditions (Sheline and Kehr 1990). They can also be useful when mental illness impairs the patient's ability to provide reliable information or to comply with physical examination.

The cost-effectiveness of a facility's medical evaluation methods should be studied, both to seek improvement and to increase staff motivation. Determination of which evaluation methods to employ should take into account the characteristics of the facility and its patient population. For example, a facility in which patients are seen regularly by their internists, the patients' complaints are chronic, and the psychiatric unit and the facility's internists work closely together may conclude that screening can be initiated by the primary care physician (Honig et al. 1992).

Other facilities may wish to compare an algorithmic approach with their current procedures. The work of Sox and his colleagues (1989) provides an excellent starting point. They evaluated with a complete medical history, physical examination, and laboratory screening tests 509 patients in California's mental health system. Patients who were believed to have previously unrecognized disease were referred to community internists or neurologists, and a final diagnosis was made on the basis of the evaluation and referral findings. Sox and his colleagues then used the data from the evaluation and referrals to create a series of screening algorithms by using data from the first 343 patients. Recursive partitioning placed screening items into decision nodes on the basis of their likelihood of indicating the presence of physical disease. These algorithms were then tested on the remaining 166 patients. The algorithms are presented in Table 2–2. The mental health system had identified only 59% of the sick patients found by the study's complete screening. When data from all six branch points of the algorithmic model were used to identify medically ill patients (algorithm node F), up to 90% of patients with an active, important physical disease had their condition correctly diagnosed. The algorithm's cost per patient screened was similar to the cost incurred by the

TABLE 2–2. Algorithm for detecting active physical disease in psychiatric patients

Node A

Serum T_4 <4.5 µg/dL or free T_4 <1 ng/dL
Hematocrit <39% (m) or <35% (f)
Hematocrit >56% (m) or 52% (f)
White blood cell count <4,100/mm^3
Serum aspartate aminotransferase   Yes (to any)   Disease likely
   (SGOT) >150 IU/L   LR = 6.4
Serum albumin <2.0 g/dL
Serum calcium >12.0 mg/dL
Glycosuria (by dipstick)

                                          No (to all)

                                              Disease less likely
                                              LR = 0.82

Node B

History of epilepsy
History of emphysema   Yes (to any)   Disease likely
History of blood or pus in the urine   LR = 5.7
Hematuria (by dipstick) in male,
   age over 50 years

                                          No (to all)

                                              Disease less likely
                                              LR = 0.58

Node C

History of diabetes
Serum T_4 >12.5 µg/dL or
   free T_4 >4.4 ng/dL   Yes (to any)   Disease likely
Proteinuria (by dipstick)   LR = 2.75
Serum aspartate aminotransferase
   (SGOT) >60 IU/L or serum alanine
   aminotransferase (SGPT) >75 IU/L

                                          No (to all)
                                              Disease less likely
                                              LR = 0.58

(continued)

Table 2–2.   Algorithm for detecting active physical disease in psychiatric patients *(continued)*

Node D

History of asthma		
History of high blood pressure	Yes (to any)	Disease likely
Diastolic blood pressure >94 mm Hg		LR = 2.2
Serum vitamin B_{12} <200 pg/L		
	No (to all)	
	Disease less likely	
	LR = 0.39	

Node E

Pain in the chest while at rest		
Headaches associated with vomiting	Yes (to any)	Disease likely
History of thyroid disease		LR = 1.9
Serum albumin <3.9 g/L		
	No (to all)	
	Disease less likely	
	LR = 0.34	

Node F

Loss of control of urine or stool		
White blood cell count >11,000/mm³		
Serum cholesterol >320 mg/dL or	Yes (to any)	Disease likely
serum triglyceride >400 mg/dL		LR = 1.7
Serum potassium >5.5 mEq/L		
Serum sodium <134 mEq/L		
	No (to all)	
	Disease less likely	
	LR = 0.21	

Note.   The algorithm depicted places a patient in one and only one subgroup. To obtain the odds that a patient has active physical disease, multiply the odds of physical disease in the patient's mental health program by the likelihood ratio (LR) enclosed in the box corresponding to the patient's subgroup. For example, suppose that a day treatment patient has none of the findings in branch node A but has a history of seizures (branch node B). The prevalence of disease for patients in day treatment is 0.28 (the corresponding odds are 0.39 to 1). The likelihood ratio for a positive finding at branch node B is 5.7. The odds of disease are therefore 2.22 to 1, which corresponds to a 0.69 probability of active disease. If the same patient has none of the findings at any of the branch nodes A through F, the odds of disease would be the product of the prior odds (0.39 to 1) and the likelihood ratio if no findings are present (0.21), or 0.08 to 1. The corresponding probability of active disease is 0.07, as given by the formula probability = odds/(1v + odds).
m = male; f = female.
Source.   Adapted from Sox HC, Koran LM, Sox CH, et al.: "A Medical Algorithm for Detecting Physical Disease in Psychiatric Patients." *Hospital and Community Psychiatry* 40:1270–1276, 1989. Used with permission.

mental health system's evaluation methods ($59.16 vs. $57.00), and the algorithm's cost per case detected was considerably less ($155.68 vs. $230.78).

Analyzing screening data to discover which information best predicts the presence of physical disease in a given patient population allows cost-effective algorithms to be developed. The data (10 medical history items, a blood pressure reading, and 16 laboratory tests) recommended by Sox and his colleagues can be obtained by mental health staff and do not require a physician's presence for the decision whether to refer a patient for complete medical evaluation. Although this study shows that a systematic approach to screening for physical disease could improve patients' health care, any algorithm should be tested for utility and validity before being widely implemented. Note that Sox et al. (1989) used serum thyroxine (T_4) and free T_4 as their screening measure of thyroid function. We recommend using a TSH test because it is a more sensitive and specific measure of hypothyroidism, which is a more common cause of psychiatric morbidity than is hyperthyroidism.

Organic Masqueraders

Although patients with physical diseases can present with a wide range of psychiatric symptoms, clinicians should be alert to certain aspects of the history, mental status examination, physical examination, and laboratory evaluation that suggest that patients are at high risk of having an organic cause for their psychiatric symptoms. A number of clues to organic causation of psychiatric symptoms are shown in Table 2–3.

Estimates of the percentage of patients in mental health settings with a physical disorder directly causing their psychiatric symptoms vary greatly (as shown in Table 2–1) but may be as high as 10% in some outpatient settings, in state hospitals, or in the older population. The prevalence may also be higher among patients whose conditions were diagnosed as hysteria, now termed *somatization disorder* or *conversion disorder*. For example, in 10 of 40 patients presenting with what were originally diagnosed as "conversion" symptoms, the symptoms proved to have organic etiologies on long-term follow-up (Watson and Buranen 1979).

When taking a history, the clinician should be quicker to initiate a medical workup in patients who are 40 or older or who present with psychiatric symptoms for the first time. Asking about chronic medical conditions; about all medications, including nonprescription medications; and about alcohol or

TABLE 2–3.   Selected clues to organic causes of mental disorders

First episode of major psychiatric illness

Onset of psychiatric symptoms after age 40

Psychiatric symptoms

  During a major medical illness

  While taking drugs that can cause mental symptoms

  In the absence of apparent life stress or psychiatric history

History of

  Alcohol or drug abuse

  Physical illness impairing organ function (neurological, endocrine, renal, hepatic, cardiac, pulmonary)

  Use of multiple prescribed or over-the-counter drugs

Family history of

  Degenerative or inheritable brain disease

  Inherited metabolic disease (e.g., diabetes, pernicious anemia, porphyria)

Mental signs that include

  Altered level of consciousness

  Fluctuating mental status

  Cognitive impairment

  Episodic, recurrent, or cyclic (menstrual) course

  Visual, tactile, or olfactory hallucinations

Physical signs that include

  Signs of organ malfunction that can affect the brain

  Focal neurological deficits

  Diffuse subcortical dysfunction (e.g., slowed speech/mentation/movement, ataxia, incoordination, tremor, chorea, asterixis, dysarthria)

  Cortical dysfunction (e.g., dysphasia, apraxias, agnosias, visuospatial deficits, or defective cortical sensation)

Poor response to seemingly appropriate psychiatric treatment, whether psychotherapeutic or pharmacological. (In this case, rethink the diagnosis, reexamine the patient, and obtain appropriate consultative advice.)

Source.   Adapted from Hoffman RS, Koran LM: "Detecting Physical Illness in Patients With Mental Disorders." *Psychosomatics* 25:654–660, 1984. Used with permission.

drug abuse is important (Dietch 1981). Perinatal or developmental events may prove significant. Neurological symptoms, unusual diet, recent falls, and head trauma should be explored. Family history and broader psychosocial issues such as self-neglect and life stresses also require exploration. Information from collateral sources should be actively sought, because it may yield additional or connected diagnoses (Hoffman and Koran 1984; Taylor 1990).

All psychiatric patients should be asked whether they have had a head injury. If they have, severity is assessed by asking about loss of consciousness or hospitalization. Inquiry regarding headache, vertigo, irritability, and ability to concentrate is also indicated. Collateral information can prove informative, not only when the patient is cognitively impaired but also when subtle emotional or personality changes are noted by the family (Silver 1992).

There are many ways to evaluate for signs of organicity in the mental status examination, and several excellent sources of information are available (La Bruzza 1981; Lishman 1987; Rickler 1983; Strub and Black 1985; Taylor 1990). Fluctuating or altered levels of consciousness are particularly significant (Karasu 1980). Cognitive functions must be examined; recent memory, remote personal memory, and fund of information can help distinguish organic from functional diseases, as can speech and language skills or the ability to construct simple figures (Hoffman and Koran 1984). Visual and olfactory hallucinations and illusions suggest underlying physical disorder (Forsythe et al. 1977; Karasu 1980).

On performing a physical examination, the clinician should be alert to signs of major organ impairment. Abnormal neurological findings may be subtle, such as a downward drift of an extremity, mild pronator drift, or problems with stereognosis or two-point discrimination. Anderson (1980) discussed the specific findings to look for in examining patients who present with psychosis, possible substance abuse, or toxic effects of psychotropic medication. Ovsiew (1992) provided a thorough review of the aspects of history taking and examination that can point to cerebral dysfunction. Psychiatric symptoms occurring in a variety of medical illnesses together with physical findings suggesting the correct diagnoses are reviewed elsewhere (Hall 1982; Lishman 1987; Martin 1983; Skuster et al. 1992).

Once information is obtained, several general guidelines should be kept in mind. First, one must avoid the bias invited by unattractive or difficult patients (Johnson and Ananth 1986; La Bruzza 1981; Saravay and Koran 1977). Koranyi (1972), for example, found that a typical patient in whom physical illness was missed was a middle-aged, poorly educated or not very bright woman with a depressive disorder and inadequate or passive-aggressive personality. Second, information must not only be obtained but also be utilized. Several studies have found that more than half of abnormal laboratory values were ignored (Berber and McFeely 1991). Similarly, the meaning of all physical examination abnormalities must be explored (Johnson and Ananth 1986; Saravay and Koran 1977). Information regarding the patient's prescription and over-the-counter medications should not be ignored.

Third, the temporal sequence of the patient's symptoms must be considered. Patients who do not describe prior stressors or prior episodes of similar psychiatric symptoms must be examined exceptionally closely. Approximately 80% of psychiatric symptoms caused by primary mental disorder have a gradual onset and develop slowly over a fairly long time, whereas 70%–80% of psychiatric symptoms caused by a medical disorder have a clearly defined onset and a shorter time course (Hall et al. 1979). Another temporal pattern that suggests an underlying medical disorder is episodic exacerbation with intervening asymptomatic periods (Koran 1991). Diseases such as porphyria, systemic lupus erythematosus, or multiple sclerosis may present in this way. Finally, the usual time course of recovery must be considered; an underlying medical disorder should be reconsidered if the response to psychiatric treatment is poor (Ananth 1984; Koran 1991).

Thinking in an organized manner about possible etiologies for psychiatric symptoms can increase the likelihood that organic masqueraders will be recognized. One helpful mnemonic is DIVE AT TEN MD SIN. Each letter stands for a major disease category (*MD* can also be thought of as standing for *missed diagnosis*) as follows:

D:	Degenerative
I:	Infectious
V:	Vascular
E:	Endocrine
A:	AIDS
T:	Toxic
T:	Traumatic
E:	Epileptic
N:	Neoplastic
M:	Metabolic
D:	Drug
S:	Structural
I:	Inflammatory
N:	Nutritional

Remembering this mnemonic or dividing medical diseases into other broad categories will help the clinician to review a broad range of potentially causal medical disorders.

Recommendations for Implementing a Medical Screening Program

The first step in providing psychiatric patients with medical evaluations is to decide where screening will take place. Possible sites in public mental health systems include outpatient clinics, local hospitals, psychiatric health facilities, state hospitals, skilled nursing facilities, and crisis facilities (Sheline and Kehr 1990). This decision should be influenced not only by the resources available in a given setting but also by the frequency and nature of medical conditions in the facility's patients. The *Medical Evaluation Field Manual* describes in detail how to create and operate a screening program (Koran 1991). In some settings, an outside medical system of which the members are closely integrated with the mental health team, have experience working with psychiatric patients, and are aware of the links between psychiatric and medical conditions may provide cost-effective medical evaluation (Honig et al. 1992).

In other settings, a mobile medical evaluation van staffed by physician's assistants or nurse practitioners can mitigate problems that discourage screening. Such problems include lack of space, physicians' lack of interest in medical screening, and too few new patients to justify hiring screening personnel for each program. The mobile screening team can use as its examination space a motor home converted into a medical screening facility (Koran 1991; Koran et al. 1984).

If a facility has decided to screen its psychiatric patients, the next decision is when to screen. Sheline and Kehr (1990) recommended delaying routine screening until the second or third visit, especially in outpatient clinics where many patients do not return for a second visit. Although some patients' physical disorders would then be missed, this strategy avoids the logistical problems of trying to refer patients who do not have an ongoing relationship with the facility. Decisions must also be made about screening patients who are readmitted to a program. These patients may have had interim exposure to new disease-causing agents (Sheline and Kehr 1990). Finally, patients may recently have been medically evaluated in another setting, especially if they are transferred from an inpatient to an outpatient setting. Copies of the evaluation records for these patients must be obtained for review.

When a mental health program institutes a medical screening program, a standardized form for recording data is helpful. This form can help ensure that evaluations are adequate and that records are not too brief and do not omit important information (Sheline and Kehr 1990). An Essential Medical Information Form should include information about *any* past medical problems. These include problems that might cause or exacerbate the patient's mental disorder, require ongoing treatment, or interact with psychotropic drug treatments. Placing the form directly behind the clinical record's *face sheet* (containing identifying data and insurance information) would bring the information to staff attention (Koran 1991). Auditing the number of forms completed as well as their degree of completion (Sheline and Kehr 1990) is necessary to ensure compliance. Further suggestions regarding documentation can be found in the *Medical Evaluation Field Manual* (Koran 1991).

A screening program must recruit staff who can care for patients with both mental and physical disorders. Bartsch and colleagues (1990) suggested that a physician who is knowledgeable regarding the connections between mental and physical disorders be involved in patient-care planning sessions to ensure proper integration between medical screening results and psychiatric care. Medical consultants who are willing to carry out evaluations for patients with mental disorder must also be found. The mental health program will need mechanisms to ensure that indicated medical consultations are completed and that the consultation results are received by the program.

Patients with mental disorders often fail to seek recommended medical care. Several steps can increase the likelihood that the patient will see the referral physician (Koran 1991):

1. Explain to the patient the reason for the referral.
2. Ask the patient about any concerns about the referral.
3. Help the patient to complete any forms necessary and make the appointment.
4. Give the patient written confirmation of the referral.
5. Provide information about the costs involved.
6. Help the patient arrange transportation.

Ensuring acceptance of medical screening by mental health facility staff is essential to the screening program's success. People resist change because it demands attention and energy and because the advantages of new procedures are not always apparent. Mental health facility staff may resist the introduction of a medical screening program because it creates additional work, interferes with mental health program activities, or represents the threat of uncovering errors in diagnosis (the failure to detect physical diseases masquerading as mental disorders). Program leaders can take several steps to minimize staff resistance:

1. Motivate the staff by teaching them about the prevalence of physical disease in patients with mental disorders.

2. State explicitly the mental health program's obligation: helping patients with their basic medical needs is as much a part of community-based mental health care as helping them with social supports, protection, housing, and transportation.
3. Involve the staff in planning.
4. Allay fears by assuring the staff that the discovery of unsuspected physical disease by the screening program will not result in negative staff evaluations.
5. Create incentives for rewarding staff members who recognize physical disease.
6. Provide feedback about successes; for example, a monthly review of successful medical interventions could help maintain staff support for the screening program.
7. Set goals and audit their attainment.
8. Announce and provide leadership support of the program (Koran 1991).

Does a mental health program, in mounting a screening program, become legally liable when a patient is unable to obtain recommended follow-up care? The answer is unclear but is probably *no* (Busch and Cavanaugh 1985). Mounting a physical disease screening program in settings other than emergency rooms and inpatient psychiatric facilities is beyond the standard of community mental health care, so failure of such a screening program to ensure perfect results would not be evidence of negligence. The program's responsibility probably ends with informing legally competent patients and the conservators of incompetent patients who are not receiving emergency or inpatient care that they should seek further evaluation. The advice of legal counsel, however, should be sought on this point. In emergency room and inpatient settings, inadequate medical evaluation can result in findings of liability (Busch and Cavanaugh 1985; Koran 1991).

Conclusion

Overwhelming evidence shows that undiagnosed physical illness is prevalent in patients with psychiatric disorders. Medical conditions in this population are overlooked for many reasons, but in some cases these conditions directly cause the patients' psychiatric symptoms. Public mental health programs, especially programs for the seriously mentally ill, may be the patient's primary source of health care. Even with patients who have a primary care physician, the possibility of undetected, important physical disease remains substantial.

Therefore, administrators in all mental health settings should review the potential benefits of screening for physical disorders in their program's patients or of integrating medical and psychiatric care in other ways. The frequency of misdiagnosis can be decreased by 1) always considering the possibility that physical disease is causing a patient's psychiatric symptoms; 2) performing complete assessments, including physical examination and laboratory screening as indicated; and 3) performing serial examinations when the clinical picture is confusing (Hoffman and Koran 1984).

The artificial labeling of patients as *psychiatric* or *medical* can lead to poor care, both psychiatric and medical. Psychiatrists in public mental health settings who wish to provide comprehensive care for their patients must maintain their medical skills, including the art of physical examination. They must also lobby for adequate space and appropriate resources for conducting complete physical examinations. Finally, continuing to educate all public health care professionals regarding the value of considering physical disease in patients with mental disorders is critical to serving these patients well.

References

Allodi F, Cohen M: Physical illness and length of psychiatric hospitalization. Canadian Psychiatric Association Journal 23:101–106, 1978

Ananth J: Physical illness and psychiatric disorders. Compr Psychiatry 25:586–593, 1984

Anderson WH: The physical examination in office practice. Am J Psychiatry 137:1188–1192, 1980

Anfinson TJ, Kathol RG: Screening laboratory evaluation in psychiatric patients: a review. Gen Hosp Psychiatry 14:248–257, 1992

Barnes RF, Mason JC, Greer C, et al: Medical illness in chronic psychiatric outpatients. Gen Hosp Psychiatry 5:191–195, 1983

Bartsch DA, Shern DL, Feinberg LE, et al: Screening CMHC outpatients for physical illness. Hospital and Community Psychiatry 41:786–790, 1990

Berber MJ, McFeely N: Efficacy of routine admission urinalyses in psychiatric hospitals. Can J Psychiatry 36:190–193, 1991

Beresford TP, Hall RCW, Wilson FC, et al: Clinical laboratory data in psychiatric outpatients. Psychosomatics 26:731–744, 1985

Black DW, Warrack G, Winokur G: The Iowa record-linkage study, III: excess mortality among patients with "functional" disorders. Arch Gen Psychiatry 42:82–88, 1985

Browning CH, Miller SI, Tyson RL: The psychiatric emergency: a high-risk medical patient. Compr Psychiatry 15:153–156, 1974

Brugha TS, Wing JK, Smith BL: Physical health of the long-term mentally ill in the community: is there unmet need? Br J Psychiatry 133:22–27, 1989

Bunce DFM, Jones LR, Badger LW, et al: Medical illness in psychiatric patients: barriers to diagnosis and treatment. South Med J 75:941–944, 1982

Burke AW: Physical illness in psychiatric hospital patients in Jamaica. Br J Psychiatry 121:321–322, 1972

Burke AW: Physical disorder among day hospital patients. Br J Psychiatry 133:22–27, 1978

Busch KA, Cavanaugh JL: Physical examination of psychiatric outpatients: medical and legal issues. Hospital and Community Psychiatry 36:958–961, 1985

Carlson RJ, Nayar N, Suh M: Physical disorders among emergency psychiatric patients. Can J Psychiatry 26:65–67, 1981

Chandler JD, Gerndt JE: The role of medical evaluation in psychiatric inpatients. Psychosomatics 29:410–416, 1988

Chatham-Showalter PE: Medical disorders among young acutely ill psychiatric patients in a military hospital. Hospital and Community Psychiatry 43:511–514, 1992

Davies DW: Physical illness in psychiatric out-patients. Br J Psychiatry 111:27–33, 1965

Dietch JT: Diagnosis of organic anxiety disorders. Psychosomatics 22:661–669, 1981

Dolan JG, Mushlin AI: Routine laboratory testing for medical disorders in psychiatric inpatients. Arch Intern Med 145:2085–2088, 1985

Drinka PJ, Nolten WE, Voeks S, et al: Misleading elevation of the free thyroxine index in nursing home residents. Arch Pathol Lab Med 115:1208–1211, 1991

Dubin WR, Weiss KJ, Zeccardi JA: Organic brain syndrome: the psychiatric imposter. JAMA 249:60–62, 1983

Eastwood MR, Mindham RHS, Tennent TG: The physical status of psychiatric emergencies. Br J Psychiatry 116:545–550, 1970

Eilenberg MD, Whatmore PB: Physical disease and psychiatric emergencies. Compr Psychiatry 2:358–363, 1961

Farmer S: Medical problems of chronic patients in a community support program. Hospital and Community Psychiatry 38:745–749, 1987

Ferguson B, Dudleston K: Detection of physical disorder in newly admitted psychiatric patients. Acta Psychiatr Scand 74:485–489, 1986

Forsythe RJ, Ilk CR, Bard J, et al: Primary medical care in psychiatry, in Current Psychiatric Therapies. Edited by Masserman JH. New York, Grune & Stratton, 1977, pp 91–97

Hall RC: The medical care of psychiatric patients. Hospital and Community Psychiatry 33:25–34, 1982

Hall RCW, Popkin MK, Devaul RA, et al: Physical illness presenting as psychiatric disease. Arch Gen Psychiatry 35:1315–1320, 1978

Hall RCW, Gruzenski WP, Popkin MK: Differential diagnosis of somatopsychic disorders. Psychosomatics 20:381–389, 1979

Hall RCW, Gardner ER, Popkin MK, et al: Unrecognized physical illness prompting psychiatric admission: a prospective study. Am J Psychiatry 138:629–635, 1981

Hart G: Syphilis tests in diagnostic and therapeutic decision making. Ann Intern Med 104:368–376, 1986

Hoffman RS: Diagnostic errors in the evaluation of behavioral disorders. JAMA 248:964–967, 1982

Hoffman RS, Koran LM: Detecting physical illness in patients with mental disorders. Psychosomatics 25:654–660, 1984

Honig A, Pop P, Tan ES, et al: Physical illness in chronic psychiatric patients from a community psychiatric unit: the implications for daily practice. Br J Psychiatry 155:58–64, 1989

Honig A, Pop P, de Kemp E, et al: Physical illness in chronic psychiatric patients from a community psychiatric unit revisited: a three-year follow-up study. Br J Psychiatry 161:80–83, 1992

Innes G, Millar WM: Mortality among psychiatric patients. Scott Med J 15:143–148, 1970

Johnson R, Ananth J: Physically ill and mentally ill. Can J Psychiatry 31:197–201, 1986

Karasu TB: The medical care of patients with psychiatric illness. Hospital and Community Psychiatry 31:463–472, 1980

Kendler KS: A twin study of mortality in schizophrenia and neurosis. Arch Gen Psychiatry 43:643–649, 1986

Kolman PBR: Predicting the results of routine laboratory tests in elderly psychiatric patients admitted to hospital. J Clin Psychiatry 46:532–534, 1985

Koran LM: Medical Evaluation Field Manual, prepared for the California Department of Mental Health and Local Mental Health Programs, Pursuant to Chapter 376, Statutes of 1988, Assembly Bill 1877, Stanford, CA, 1991 (Available from California Department of Mental Health, Office of the Director, 1600 9th Street, Sacramento, CA 95814.)

Koran LM, Sox HC, Marton KI, et al: Mobile medical screening teams for public programs. Hospital and Community Psychiatry 35:1151–1152, 1984

Koran LM, Sox HC, Marton KI, et al: Medical evaluation of psychiatric patients, I: results in a state mental health system. Arch Gen Psychiatry 46:733–740, 1989

Koranyi EK: Physical health and illness in a psychiatric outpatient department population. Canadian Psychiatric Association Journal 17:S109–S116, 1972

Koranyi EK: Morbidity and rate of undiagnosed physical illnesses in a psychiatric clinic population. Arch Gen Psychiatry 1979:414–419, 1979

Koranyi EK: Somatic illness in psychiatric patients. Psychosomatics 21:887–891, 1980

Koranyi EK: Undiagnosed physical illness in psychiatric patients. Annu Rev Med 33:309–316, 1982

Kurucz J: The incidence and significance of physical illness in chronic psychiatric patients. Columbia/Creedmoor Quality Assurance Grand Rounds, Queens Village, NY, 1983

La Bruzza AL: Physical illness presenting as psychiatric disorder: guidelines for differential diagnosis. Journal of Operational Psychiatry 1:23–31, 1981

Lipowski ZJ: Psychiatry of somatic diseases: epidemiology, pathogenesis, classification. Compr Psychiatry 16:105–124, 1975

Lipowski ZJ: The interface of psychiatry and medicine: towards integrated health care. Can J Psychiatry 32:743–748, 1987

Lishman WA: Organic Psychiatry: The Psychological Consequences of Cerebral Disorder. Oxford, UK, Blackwell Scientific, 1987

Maricle RA, Hoffman WF, Bloom JD, et al: The prevalence and significance of medical illness among chronically mentally ill outpatients. Community Ment Health J 23:81–89, 1987

Martin MJ: A brief review of organic diseases masquerading as functional illness. Hospital and Community Psychiatry 34:328–332, 1983

Martin RL, Cloninger R, Guze SB, et al: Mortality in a follow-up of 500 psychiatric outpatients. Arch Gen Psychiatry 43:643–649, 1985

Muecke LN, Krueger DW: Physical findings in a psychiatric outpatient clinic. Am J Psychiatry 138:1241–1242, 1981

Ovsiew F: Bedside neuropyschiatry: eliciting the clinical phenomena of neuropsychiatric illness, in Textbook of Neuropsychiatry, 2nd Edition. Edited by Yudofsky SC, Hales RE. Washington, DC, American Psychiatric Press, 1992, pp 89–126

Rickler KC: Neurological diagnosis in psychiatric disease. Psychiatric Annals 13:408–411, 1983

Roca R, Breakey WR, Fischer PJ: Medical care of chronic psychiatric outpatients. Hospital and Community Psychiatry 38:741–745, 1987

Saravay SM, Koran LM: Organic disease mistakenly diagnosed as psychiatric. Psychosomatics 18:6–11, 1977

Sheline YI: High prevalence of physical illness in a geriatric psychiatric inpatient population. Gen Hosp Psychiatry 12:396–400, 1990

Sheline Y, Kehr C: Cost and utility of routine admission laboratory testing for psychiatric inpatients. Gen Hosp Psychiatry 12:329–334, 1990

Silver JM: Neuropsychiatric aspects of traumatic brain injury, in Textbook of Neuropsychiatry, 2nd Edition. Edited by Yudofsky SC, Hales RC. Washington, DC, American Psychiatric Press, 1992, pp 363–396

Skuster DZ, Digre KB, Corbett JJ: Neurological conditions presenting as psychiatric disorder. Psychiatr Clin North Am 15:311–333, 1992

Sox HC, Koran LM, Sox CH, et al: A medical algorithm for detecting physical disease in psychiatric patients. Hospital and Community Psychiatry 40:1270–1276, 1989

Strub RL, Black FW: The Mental Status Exam in Neurology. Philadelphia, PA, FA Davis, 1985

Summers WK, Munoz RA, Read MR: The psychiatric physical examination, II: findings in 75 unselected psychiatric patients. J Clin Psychiatry 42:99–102, 1981

Tardiff K, Deane K: The psychological and physical status of chronic psychiatric inpatients. Compr Psychiatry 21:91–97, 1980

Taylor RL: Distinguishing Psychological From Organic Disorders: Screening for Psychological Masquerade. New York, Springer, 1990

Tsuang MT, Simpson JC: Mortality studies in psychiatry. Should they stop or proceed? Arch Gen Psychiatry 42:47–54, 1985

Watson CG, Buranen C: The frequency and identification of false positive conversion reactions. J Nerv Ment Dis 167:243–247, 1979

Waxman HM, Dubin W, Klein M, et al: Geriatric psychiatry in the emergency department, II: evaluation and treatment of geriatric and nongeriatric admissions. J Am Geriatr Soc 32:343–349, 1984

Weingarten CH, Rosoff LG, Eisen SV, et al: Medical care in a geriatric psychiatry unit: impact on psychiatric outcome. J Am Geriatr Soc 30:738–743, 1982

Weissberg MP: Emergency room medical clearance: an educational problem. Am J Psychiatry 136:787–790, 1979

CHAPTER 3

Neuropsychiatry in Public Mental Health Settings

Barry S. Fogel, M.D., M.S.

State and county mental hospitals in the United States are the locus of care for numerous patients with neuropsychiatric disorders. According to the Center for Mental Health Services' annual statistical abstract (Atay et al. 1994), 254,932 patients were admitted to state and county mental hospitals in 1992. Of these, 11,210 (4.4%) received diagnoses of organic mental disorders, and an additional 1,211 (0.5%) received a diagnosis of mental retardation. A tabulation of individuals resident on December 31, 1992, indicated that of 83,320 total patients, 7,418 (8.9%) had diagnoses of organic mental disorders, and 2,575 (3.1%) had a diagnosis of mental retardation. Thus, patients with organic mental disorders or mental retardation have substantially longer stays than those with primary mental disorders and contribute disproportionately to the overall cost of public sector mental health care.

However, these numbers substantially underestimate the prevalence and relevance of brain diseases and brain dysfunction in the state mental hospital population. Among patients with primary diagnoses related to substance abuse (14% of admissions and 4.3% of residents), there are many with memory impairment, dementia, seizures, or past traumatic brain injury. Among patients with primary diagnoses of schizophrenia and other psychoses (39.1% of admissions and 52.8% of residents), common neuropsychiatric problems include involuntary movements such as tremors and dyskinesias, cognitive impairment, and epilepsy. Patients age 65 and over account for 4.4% of all admissions but 14.8% of residents. Older persons have the highest prevalence of brain diseases and systemic diseases that affect brain function, so assessment for causal or contributory medical conditions is essential to their psychiatric diagnosis. Yet resident patients age 65 and over have a higher rate of missing or deferred diagnoses than any other age group—13.1% in the 1992 data.

State hospitals are variably equipped to address their patients' neuropsychiatric problems (American Psychiatric Association Task Force on Geriatric Psychiatry in the Public Mental Health Sector 1993). Some have neuropsychiatrists or behavioral neurologists available on staff or as consultants. Commonly, however, neurologists available for consultation do not have special expertise in behavioral neurology or neuropsychiatry, and there is a relative separation of psychiatric and general medical and neurological care. Patients without gross brain disease may escape neurological evaluation (by any qualified specialty), and such functionally relevant concerns as frontal lobe dysfunction and parkinsonism may go undiagnosed.

Over the past 10 years, I have visited numerous state mental hospitals and have examined hundreds of state mental hospital patients. In this chapter, I offer suggestions for improving the quality of neuropsychiatric care in state mental hospitals. The ideas arise from my work as consultant, but in many cases they can be supported by published studies of specific issues. Studies specifically evaluating the benefit of a neuropsychiatric approach in improving the health and function of a state hospital patient population have not been done.

The Nature of the State Hospital Patient Population

Fifty years ago, state hospitals were the primary locus of care for persons with severe mental illness of any kind. As general hospital psychiatry units and private psychiatric hospitals proliferated, acute mental disorders increasingly were treated in these settings, leaving the state hospitals with more chronically ill patients (Dorwart and Epstein 1993). The dissemination of drug therapies and the development and refinement of intensive community-based care options led to community placement for large numbers of people with continued symptoms of mental illness but with sufficient behavioral control and functional capacity for safety and self-maintenance outside a hospital setting. The Medicaid nursing home benefit and the development of neuroleptics tolerable to older persons led to nursing home placement for many patients with behaviorally complicated dementia or late-life psychotic conditions (APA Task Force 1993).

The role of state mental hospitals in treating patients with acute mental illness varies greatly among states. In some states, *all* acute hospital care for persons with mental illness—including involuntary and indigent patients—is provided by general hospitals and private psychiatric hospitals. In others, voluntary patients with health insurance coverage are treated in general hospitals and private psychiatric hospitals, whereas involuntary and indigent patients are treated in state or county facilities. In all states, however, public hospitals have a special role in the treatment of severe and chronic mental illness.

States vary also in which patients with severe and chronic mental illness receive treatment in state hospitals rather than in nursing homes or community-based settings. Several patient characteristics increase the likelihood that a patient with chronic mental illness will be hospitalized (Barber et al. 1988; Holohean et al. 1993):

1. Recurrent or continual aggressive or self-injurious behavior
2. Severe impairment in function, especially of instrumental activities of daily living necessary for self-maintenance and safety
3. Involuntary status, legal incompetence, or a history of criminal behavior associated with mental illness
4. Active general medical problems
5. Recurrent or continual nonadherence to prescribed treatment
6. Lack of financial resources
7. Lack of social supports
8. A strong preference for continued hospitalization by the patient (Drake and Wallach 1988)

Apart from these considerations, a lack of community-based alternatives will keep patients in the hospital who might be successfully treated elsewhere if the continuum of care were more fully developed (Okin et al. 1990). For example, consider the state of Alabama, which in 1994 had fewer nursing home beds per capita and many fewer assisted living beds per capita than the average state. In Alabama, nursing homes routinely have 97.5% occupancy (Hardwick et al. 1994) and are free to reject prospective residents with behaviorally complicated dementia. Many of the state's general hospitals either do not have psychiatric units or do not accept older persons on them. Some large community mental health centers have minimal services for older persons. Alabama's mental health law permits the commitment of older persons with dementia and agitated behavior if someone gets hurt. In this context, Alabama's rate of state hospital admissions for older people with dementia is almost twice the national average (Atay et al. 1994).

The character of the population treated by a state hospital directly determines the neuropsychiatric issues of greatest relevance. The themes of this chapter are therefore organized by the patient characteristics just enumerated. Before management can be considered, however, a correct diagnosis must be made.

Diagnostic Considerations in State Hospital Patients

Because many patients in state hospitals have been hospitalized for months or years, and because most of the patients who are acute admissions to state hospitals have had previous psychiatric treatment of some kind, most patients carry a psychiatric diagnosis when they are first encountered by the neuropsychiatrist. These diagnoses should be regarded with skepticism by the neuropsychiatrist in terms of both their validity and their completeness. For example, Wilson (1989) reported on a systematic reassessment and rediagnosis of 72 chronically ill state hospital patients who had received the diagnosis of schizophrenia. When all available data were evaluated and DSM-III-R (American Psychiatric Association 1987) criteria were applied, 27 patients (one-third) had the diagnosis reclassified. Of these, 7 received diagnoses of organic mental disorders, 1 had mental retardation, and 1 had pervasive developmental disorder. The issue of completeness comprises both psychiatric and general medical comorbidity. Regarding psychiatric comorbidity, the issue of greatest concern is *diagnostic overshadowing* (Reiss et al. 1982). Applied originally to clinicians' failure to diagnose mental illness in persons with mental retardation, this phrase is an apt description of clinicians' failing to diagnose any other mental condition once a diagnosis of schizophrenia is made. Thus, major depression, panic disorder, or dementia might be undiagnosed in a person with schizophrenia, or obsessive-compulsive disorder might be undiagnosed in a person with pervasive developmental disorder. The diagnosis of comorbid medical conditions poses at least two problems. First, the necessarily limited *medical clearance* that patients receive before referral to a state mental hospital often is accepted as more definitive than it is. Numerous studies of general medical illness in psychiatric patients in public mental health settings have established that active and relevant new medical diagnoses will be made if such patients are systematically examined (Anfinson and Kathol 1993). (This issue is discussed extensively in Chapter 2.) Second, long-stay patients can develop new medical conditions that will not be detected unless new symptoms are carefully evaluated and periodic screening examinations are performed as they would be in a community population of the same age and health risks.

The implication for neuropsychiatric practice is that a newly encountered state hospital patient should be approached as an undiagnosed patient. Recorded diagnoses should be regarded as important data but not necessarily a sufficient basis for treatment planning.

Setting Priorities

State hospital patients often have multiple problems, and resource constraints are the rule. Setting priorities for diagnosis and treatment is necessary. Ensuring the safety of the patient and caregivers and addressing acute or unstable general medical problems must be the top priorities. Next, the management of the patient's chronic medical conditions must be optimized, with attention to potential effects of medical treatments on the patient's mental and behavioral symptoms. Once these tasks have been accomplished, the most salient issues are those related to the need for continued hospitalization. To recommend a focus on identifying and addressing the issues that keep the patient in the hospital is not to give trivial advice, because inpatient services can and often do concern themselves with diagnoses and prominent symptoms, even when these are not what keeps the patient in the hospital. For example, persistent hallucinations in themselves do not imply that hospitalization is necessary, but recurrent assaultiveness triggered by those hallucinations is likely to make hospitalization necessary for safety. Neuropsychiatric intervention that stopped the patient's violent behavior might permit community-based treatment, even if the hallucinations continued. Although community-based treatment is not always better than hospital treatment (Munetz and Geller 1993) and may, if inadequate, lead to homelessness (Belcher and Toomey 1988), most patients prefer living in the community, and the cost of such treatment is lower (Thornicroft 1993).

Neuropsychiatric Approaches to Problems Responsible for Continued Hospitalization

Aggressiveness and Self-Injurious Behavior

More than any other symptom, continual or recurrent aggressive or self-injurious behavior is responsible for patients' being placed in psychiatric institutions. Yet even when a patient is admitted to an institution or kept there because of violent or self-injurious behavior, the patient's *primary* diagnosis is a mental disorder, rather than the behavioral problem leading to hospitalization. At times, this leads to treatment being directed to the diagnosis, with the hope that the problem behavior will diminish, rather than direct neuropsychiatric and behavioral assessment and treatment of the problem behavior itself. An unfortunate example is when self-injurious behavior in a patient with schizophrenia is related to akathisia; in this situation, increasing the neuroleptic dosage to treat positive symptoms of schizophrenia may actually aggravate the most problematic behavior.

Behavioral assessment of aggressive and self-injurious behaviors focuses on determining the usual antecedents and consequences of the problem behavior; therapy aims to reduce both triggers and reinforcers of the behavior. Neuropsychiatric assessment, which is complementary to traditional behavioral analysis, focuses on the following questions (Fogel and Stone 1992):

- Is the problem behavior goal-directed?
- What is the target of the aggressive behavior?
- Is there an external provocation?
- Is the reaction commensurate?
- Are there internal stimuli driving the behavior?
- Is the behavior associated with general dysphoria and/or irritability?
- Are there physiological, chronobiological, or pharmacological correlates of the behavior?

The systematic investigation of such considerations is described in Chapter 6. This assessment leads to inferences about possible problems with the function of the hypothalamus, limbic system, or frontal executive control systems and often suggests specific treatment strategy. For example, aggressive behavior not directed at a specific target and always associated with extreme autonomic arousal suggests a hypothalamic problem and might be treated with an agent, such as a β-blocker or clonidine, that would attenuate the autonomic arousal. Or it might be observed that self-injurious behavior in a patient with pervasive developmental disorder occurred when someone attempted to interfere with the patient's ritual behavior of arranging objects. The hypothesis would be one of serotonergic deficit, and the attempted treatment would be administration of a serotonin reuptake inhibitor. Further discussion of these matters is found in Chapter 6. The critical observation here is that nonspecific psychiatric hospital interventions, such as seclusion and restraint or increased dosages of neuroleptics, may be less useful than precisely targeted interventions that consider underlying brain functions as well as their behavioral manifestations.

Functional Impairment

In many state hospitals, a wide range of instrumental functions are carried out for the patient by the institution, which provides food; administers medication; arranges transportation for appointments, activities, and passes; and even assists patients with telephone calls if necessary. As a consequence, not only may patients get little practice in carrying out the instrumental activities of daily living (e.g., shopping, cooking, household maintenance, money management, self-medication, use of telephones and mail), but there may be little occasion for clinicians to observe whether patients are capable in these areas. Mental illnesses that affect executive cognitive functions (i.e., frontal system functions) can cause major deficits in these activities, independently of the magnitude of other disorder-specific symptoms (Fogel 1994; Fogel et al. 1994; Royall et al. 1993). Executive functions include the ability to maintain a mental set in the face of distraction, to resist an immediate impulse to action when the context is inappropriate, to organize activities in a rational time sequence, and to generalize from specific experiences. Deficits in specific executive functions can be documented and quantitated by neuropsychological testing. For example, the Wisconsin Card Sorting Test (Heaton et al. 1993) assesses a combination of abstract reasoning and the ability to shift mental set when new information provided by the examiner suggests that the patient's current method of sorting the cards is no longer correct (Berg 1948; Lezak 1995).

Dementing disorders, mental retardation, pervasive developmental disorder, and chronic schizophrenia are widely known to cause such impairments, but they also can be encountered in more severe and treatment-refractory cases of other conditions, including bipolar disorder and obsessive-compulsive disorder. Instrumental functions are crucial to self-maintenance and safety, and a patient's level of instrumental function is a major determinant of how much support will be required for the patient to live in the community. Therefore, assessment of instrumental functions by an occupational therapist is needed for optimal treatment planning in the state hospital population.

Executive cognitive function is one factor that influences patients' independence in instrumental functions; other important factors are physical impairments and disabilities, sensory loss, mood, and personality. Once a loss of instrumental function is identified, the relative contributions of these factors should be assessed. Remediation of vision and hearing impairment and treatment of depression are two of the most productive interventions to restore function. If impaired executive cognitive function is the result of central nervous system (CNS) side effects of medications, a change in the medications should be considered. If underarousal or apathy is prominent, pharmacological treatment with a stimulant or dopamine agonist might be entertained, particularly if the patient does not have severe deficits in cortical function (Marin et al. 1995). When an instrumental function is intermittent, slow, or fluctuating but not totally lost, practice and environmental cuing strategies implemented by an occupational therapist can help the patient recover function. The role of adaptive devices should also be explored; telephones that dial a short list of numbers automatically are a typical example.

Legal Status

The legal status of a state hospital patient can be problematic when a patient with severely impaired insight and/or judgment is not so acutely dangerous to require commitment or so overtly cognitively impaired that he or she clearly needs a guardian. If such patients are judged competent by a court, they can refuse medically necessary treatments in the hospital and doom a community-based treatment plan by nonadherence. From the point of view of the physician or family caregiver, such patients *ought* to be judged incompetent, but obtaining a guardianship may be difficult if traditional formal mental status testing (e.g., the Mini-Mental State Examination [Folstein et al. 1975]) does not show abnormality.

When one approaches this issue with attorneys, family members, administrators, and the courts, the neuropsychiatric concept of executive cognitive dysfunction can be extraordinarily useful, especially if combined with the observation (first pointed out to me by Dr. Brandon Krupp) that patients with specific neuropsychiatric disorders become incompetent in different, disease-specific ways. For some conditions, such as frontal lobe dementias and negative symptom schizophrenia, impairments in judgment and self-maintenance routinely exceed gross cognitive deficits or positive symptoms of psychosis. Faced with a patient with predominant impairment of frontal lobe functions who cannot take care of himself or herself but who rejects appropriate care, the psychiatrist can explain to those concerned that the patient's particular illness is associated with dysfunction of the frontal systems necessary for self-awareness, judgment, and persistence. If evidence of frontal lobe damage or dysfunction is available from imaging studies or neuropsychological tests, this is presented in support of the argument. If neuropsychological test data are not available and such testing is not feasible or clinically indicated, a structured measure of executive function, such as the Executive Interview Test (Royall et al. 1992), is performed to establish that the patient is not "normal on cognitive tests." (The instrument itself will be published by the Psychological Corporation in 1999 [Royall, in press].) A prospective guardian and the court are offered a sound rationale on which to conclude that the patient requires assistance with decision making. With a legal determination of incompetence and a responsible guardian, both hospital care and discharge planning can focus primarily on the patient's needs and not on the slim chance that a patient with severe executive impairment will both agree with an optimal treatment plan and carry it out on his or her own initiative.

General Medical Problems

Patients with chronic mental illness and active general medical problems raise several specifically neuropsychiatric concerns: 1) drug-drug interactions affecting the CNS, 2) drug-disease interactions affecting the CNS, and 3) the impact of cognitive impairment and denial of illness on the reporting of symptoms and on active participation in general medical follow-up. The first two concerns are of particular relevance in state hospitals, where patients may not be receiving the most up-to-date medical treatment, because older drugs for several common medical conditions have substantially greater CNS side effects than their contemporary replacements.

Screening a patient's drug list for potential drug-drug interactions can be carried out using a computer database or contemporary text. Special attention should be paid to potential *pharmacodynamic* interactions because these must be diagnosed clinically rather than by drug-level determinations. The most common example is aggravation of cognitive impairment by multiple anticholinergic agents, each of which is present at a therapeutic dosage and/or blood level (Tune et al. 1981). Other common examples are sedation with multiple antiepileptic drugs (Plaa 1989), an issue discussed below; insomnia or agitation when theophylline is combined with a stimulating antidepressant drug such as fluoxetine, bupropion, or desipramine; and the potentiation of extrapyramidal side effects of neuroleptics by carbamazepine or valproate (Fogel 1988).

Drug-disease interactions most familiar to psychiatrists are the relative medical contraindications to psychotropic drugs, for example, avoiding tricyclic antidepressants in patients with heart block or benzodiazepines in people with chronic lung disease who retain carbon dioxide. Drug-disease interactions in which a drug for a general medical condition aggravates a psychiatric disorder are equally important and may be neglected when the prescription of drugs for general medical conditions is completely delegated to an internist or family practitioner unfamiliar with psychiatry. Some important examples include the aggravation of anxiety or irritable or aggressive behavior by theophylline, the aggravation of depression or negative symptoms of schizophrenia by methyldopa, and the worsening of mood disorders by systemic corticosteroids. The increasing availability of alternative therapies for common chronic medical conditions makes the identification of these situations of more than theoretical interest. For example, most cases of chronic lung disease with bronchospasm can be managed with inhalers, an approach that avoids the regular use of theophylline and systemic corticosteroids (Barnes 1995). Hypertension, the most common chronic disease of all, can virtually always be controlled by agents that do not exacerbate mental illness or its symptoms (Levenson 1993).

The impairments in executive cognitive function that are frequently found in state hospital patients, whether they have dementia or a primary mental disorder, often include diminished self-awareness and impairment in consistent goal-directed behavior. At times, partial or complete denial of illness is present. Patients with these problems have diminished capacity to seek medical attention for physical symptoms (Fogel 1994), and some may express physical distress through an escalation of behavioral problems. Other patients have persistent somatic complaints or hypochondriasis that can mask new and relevant medical problems. Successful management of patients with diminished capacity to seek medical attention requires a proactive approach to recognizing medical problems. A useful strategy includes 1) identifying the patient's characteristic behavioral response to physical discomfort; 2) establishing and documenting the baseline symptoms of somatizing or hypochondriacal patients so that new symptoms can be recognized; 3) determining whether denial of illness, when present, reflects a fixed neurological deficit, such as a frontal lobe or right hemisphere lesion, or a psychological defense mechanism possibly modifiable by a psychological therapy; and 4) determining the patient's health risk factors and establishing a schedule for health maintenance examinations that is independent of the patient's complaints or lack of such.

Special advice can be offered regarding the problem of epilepsy, which is common in several state hospital populations. Epilepsy affects more than one-third of institutionalized people with mental retardation or developmental disabilities (Richardson et al. 1979, 1981), but is also found in nonretarded state hospital patients at rates well above community prevalence. Conversely, patients with epilepsy are more likely than the general population to develop an acute psychiatric disorder such as psychosis or major depression (Cockerell et al. 1996). In one Brazilian state hospital, 6% of patients with a primary psychiatric diagnosis had epilepsy (Trevisol-Bittencourt et al. 1990). Electroencephalograms showing focal temporal abnormalities were encountered in 20% of a group of violent male state hospital patients studied by Wong et al. (1994); in such patients, thorough clinical assessment for symptoms and signs of epilepsy is necessary.

The general principles of modern epilepsy management (e.g., Laidlaw et al. 1993), including avoidance of sedating antiepileptic drugs and use of monotherapy or rational polytherapy (Wilder 1995), apply with even greater force in patients who suffer from both epilepsy and mental illness. The vulnerability of such patients to functional deterioration with seizures and postictal states is greater than that of patients without mental disorders, and so control must be pursued vigorously. Patients with poorly controlled seizures who have never been tried on newer antiepileptic agents (such as lamotrigine and gabapentin) should receive trials of them because these agents sometimes can render a patient seizure-free. (See, for example, Schapel and Chadwick (1996) for evidence that lamotrigine can have this effect.). Moreover, such patients are sensitive to mental and behavioral side effects of sedating antiepileptic drugs and to drug interaction problems that grow exponentially with the total number of drugs prescribed. Some of the antiepileptic drugs, specifically carbamazepine, valproate, lamotrigine, and gabapentin, can have positive effects on mental and behavioral symptoms and thus are preferable to barbiturates or phenytoin in this population. Both barbiturates and phenytoin can cause or aggravate cognitive impairment, and barbiturates may disinhibit inappropriate behavior (Baker 1995; Fogel 1996; Stoudemire et al. 1991). These considerations sometimes necessitate changing antiepileptic drugs even when seizures are controlled, because the psychiatric syndrome is not controlled and is disabling. In this situation, leaving antiepileptic drug therapy to a general neurologist may not be satisfactory; either the epilepsy should be treated by a neuropsychiatrist or behavioral neurologist, or a dialogue between neurologist and psychiatrist should take place in which potential risks and benefits are balanced and an appropriate scheme for conducting, monitoring, and evaluating a drug trial is agreed on.

Nonadherence to Treatment

Treatment nonadherence in the state hospital population most often refers to noncompliance with neuroleptic therapy for schizophrenia or another psychosis or to noncompliance with lithium or other thymoleptic therapy for bipolar disorder. Adherence to prescribed medical treatment is a complex issue with multiple determinants; however, two neuropsychiatric perspectives deserve consideration. First, adherence to a prescription is an instrumental activity of daily living and, as such, requires both motivation and executive cognitive function. Patients who do not adhere to therapy may be apathetic, may lack the executive cognitive function to persist with adherent behavior despite distraction, or may have difficulty shifting their mental set from one therapeutic program to another. These deficits may be amenable to treatment or may be partly remedied by environmental cues or human assistance (Zgola 1987). Second, neurological side effects of major psychotropic agents, especially akathisia and parkinsonism, as well as neuroendocrine problems such as obesity and sexual dysfunction, may be so unpleasant to patients that they opt for a risk of relapse to avoid them. Parkinsonism can be experienced by the patient when it is not obvious to the clinician, as when akinesia, gait instability, bradykinesia, or cognitive slowing predominates over tremor and rigidity.

Side effects of neuroleptics often are unrecognized or misattributed, as when drug-induced obesity is ascribed to poor eating habits, akinesia is attributed to lack of motivation, or akathisia is seen as agitation based on anxiety. When recognized, they may be undertreated, most often because of concerns about polypharmacy or of aggravating the psychotic condition. In particular, dopamine agonists, despite their increasing role in the treatment of Parkinson's disease (Poewe and Caraceni 1995), are used infrequently by general psychiatrists to treat neuroleptic-induced extrapyramidal disorders because of concerns about precipitation of a relapse or aggravation of psychosis. However, several studies suggest that amantadine is at least as effective as anticholinergics in treating drug-induced parkinsonism, that it rarely aggravates the patient's psychosis, and that it may have fewer side effects (Friedman 1992). Bromocriptine and neuroleptics may have therapeutic synergy in some cases of schizophrenia (Lombertie et al. 1995). In the author's experience, agents such as amantadine or bromocriptine are less likely than anticholinergic agents to cause cognitive impairment and more likely to relieve apathy, anhedonia, and impaired libido. Stip (1996) emphasized that memory impairment is usually present in schizophrenia and that such impairment is aggravated by anticholinergic antiparkinson drugs.

Stip (1996) emphasizes that memory impairment usually is present in schizophrenia and that such impairment is aggravated by anticholinergic antiparkinson drugs. Dopamine agonists not only lack anticholinergic effects but may alleviate some negative symptoms and may counteract akinesia, apathy, and anhedonia induced by neuroleptics. Pramipexole, a recently approved nonergot dopamine agonist with relatively strong effects on limbic D_3

receptors, has been, in the author's experience, particularly helpful for neuroleptic-induced apathy and anhedonia. When used by the author in conjunction with atypical antipsychotics for the treatment of severe mood disorders, the drug has not provoked relapses of psychosis when given to patients in remission.

Akathisia, an extremely unpleasant motor side effect of neuroleptics, usually can be controlled by the use of β-blockers such as propranolol. A prompt and correct diagnosis of akathisia, with immediate prescription of a drug that relieves the condition, can both improve treatment adherence and increase the patient's confidence in the prescribing psychiatrist.

Other prescriptions that may improve patients' quality of life and, therefore, their treatment adherence include the following:

1. Lower-potency neuroleptics (e.g., thioridazine or mesoridazine) or atypical neuroleptics (e.g., olanzapine, risperidone, sertindole, quetiapine, and clozapine) instead of high-potency neuroleptics
2. Antianxiety agents to augment neuroleptics so that lower doses can be used
3. Alternatives to lithium, such as valproate or carbamazepine, when the side effects of lithium are unacceptable to the patient
4. Alternative thymoleptics or thymoleptic combinations rather than lithium-neuroleptic combinations when a nondelusional bipolar patient does not respond to lithium alone
5. Dopamine agonists such as bromocriptine, pergolide, or pramipexole to lower prolactin levels to the normal range in patients with gynecomastia, galactorrhea, menstrual irregularity, or sexual dysfunction
6. Molindone or adjunctive psychostimulants, fenfluramine, or amantadine for patients troubled by weight gain on neuroleptics
7. Thyroid hormone supplementation for patients on lithium and/or carbamazepine who are sluggish or cold intolerant with low or borderline low thyroid indices

The preceding list touches on a number of issues, two of which are somewhat controversial—adjunctive benzodiazepine use and thyroid supplementation in lithium-treated patients with borderline laboratory values. The suggested actions have support in the literature and have proved useful in my clinical practice, but readers are encouraged to examine alternative viewpoints for themselves. Marder (1996), in a review of the management of patients with treatment-resistant schizophrenia, stated that patients with persistent positive symptoms despite adequate neuroleptic dosage sometimes improve when benzodiazepines are added to their regimen. Carpenter (1996), another veteran schizophrenia researcher, includes benzodiazepine augmentation among relapse prevention strategies.

The question of thyroid augmentation in patients taking carbamazepine or lithium is not controversial when the thyroid-stimulating hormone (TSH) level is significantly elevated. Controversy arises when the TSH level is borderline. My recommendation that such cases be treated if symptomatic is based on the following considerations:

1. Patients taking these drugs for psychiatric indications usually have an affective or schizoaffective disorder, which makes them more sensitive to developing depression if they have mild hypothyroidism.
2. Patients with subclinical hypothyroidism who take lithium frequently progress to overt hypothyroidism.
3. Lithium can reduce the pharmacodynamic effect of a given level of thyroid hormone at the cellular level (Bolaris et al. 1995).
4. Carbamazepine lowers free triiodothyronine (T_3) and thyroxine (T_4) levels by displacing thyroid hormone from protein, and thus these levels are unreliable in the interpretation of borderline elevated TSH.
5. Like lithium, carbamazepine can antagonize some of the effects of thyroid hormone on central neurons, for example, in the hippocampus (Baumgartner et al. 1994).
6. The risk of a time-limited trial of thyroid supplementation is small. In my view, the risk of untreated motivational or cognitive impairment resulting from hypothyroidism is greater. Patients with preexisting brain dysfunction, regardless of whether the dysfunction results from demonstrable structural lesions, probably are more likely to show CNS symptoms of hypothyroidism than those with normal brain function.

Three additional points should be made regarding "controversial" treatment suggestions. First, recommended therapies should have meaningful support in the scientific literature and be related to a plausible pathophysiological hypothesis. Second, opponents of all such treatments might be reminded that carbamazepine was once a controversial treatment, not only for patients with bipolar disorder but for those epileptic patients whose seizures were controlled by phenobarbital, but at the expense of depressed mood, disinhibited behavior, or cognitive impairment. Third, state hospital patients seen in consultation by neuropsychiatrists usually have not responded to more conventional treatments or have exhibited troublesome or subjectively intolerable side effects from those treatments.

Lack of Financial Resources

Although at first the lack of financial resources would not appear to be a neuropsychiatric problem, the reassessment of a patient's problem from a neuropsychiatric standpoint may identify a potential new source of financial support, either Social Security Disability Insurance (SSDI) or a categorical program such as those for persons with developmental disabilities. As an example of the latter, consider the case of a person with the diagnosis of schizophrenia whose condition is rediagnosed as a pervasive developmental disorder. As a developmentally disabled person, he or she may be eligible for an array of community-based services, such as a group home with behavior therapy, that may be unavailable in his or her state to a person with a chronic mental illness. As an example of the former, consider a person with bipolar disorder who is found also to have multiple sclerosis. If the person's disability can be shown to derive from executive cognitive deficits attributable to cerebral lesions of multiple sclerosis, a successful claim for SSDI benefits might be made even if a prior claim based on bipolar disorder was unsuccessful.

Lack of Social Supports

Some patients who lack social supports have family or friends who could potentially assist in the support of a community placement but are reluctant to become involved. When this reluctance is directly related to the patient's behavior rather than to the circumstances or personalities of the individuals involved, the behavior responsible for the alienation of support should be analyzed. Apathy, frontal lobe syndromes, and behavioral manifestations of right hemisphere dysfunction, such as denial of deficits and impaired emotional communication, all can lead to alienation of support, especially if these problems are viewed as intentional on the patient's part (Campbell et al. 1994). Direct pharmacological or behavioral treatment for these problems is possible in some cases. When it is not, explanation to potential caregivers and supports, along with suggestions for management and formal family therapy if necessary, may enable caregivers to participate willingly in the patient's care. Moreover, the reduction of blame and resentment brought about by identifying a neurological basis for the patient's behavior is therapeutic for both the patient and the caregiver (Fogel and Ratey 1995).

Patient Preference for Hospitalization

Patients' preferences for continued hospitalization may reflect human attachments to professional and nonprofessional staff at the institution, general discomfort with change, fear of becoming ill under the stress of transfer, or a well-founded belief that community-based care will be inadequate to meet their needs. One reason why patients may appropriately fear a community placement that professionals think is appropriate is that patients may know that they lack the executive cognitive function to cope with some aspect of life outside the institution, whereas professionals, who have not assessed executive function, focus on the remission of conspicuous positive symptoms of mental illness. When patients express the fear that they will be unable to cope with such problems as maintaining a household or keeping appointments, testing of executive cognitive function and an assessment by an occupational therapist should be carried out. When patients appear able to carry out instrumental activities of daily living but fear *stress*, they should be assessed for anxiety disorders or prominent symptoms of anxiety. Drug treatment targeting the anxiety may facilitate a successful community placement. Because of diagnostic overshadowing, the importance of persistent anxiety in people with schizophrenia is sometimes neglected. Studies showing improved function in people with schizophrenia when benzodiazepines (Wolkowitz and Pickar 1991) or buspirone (Goff et al. 1991) is added to neuroleptics support this view. The development of new classes of antianxiety agents that may offer greater effectiveness and safety could increase the relevance of this point even further. More generally, a patient's objection to community placement should raise the suspicion that there is an inadequately treated comorbid condition, such as depression or an uncomfortable general medical problem, that is still troubling the patient.

Access to Neurodiagnostic Technology and Specialist Consultation

Neurodiagnostic testing, including electroencephalographic monitoring, computed tomography (CT), magnetic resonance imaging (MRI), single photon emission computed tomography (SPECT), and neuropsychological assessment, has increasingly become a standard component of neuropsychiatric evaluation. (Functional MRI may be added in the near future to this list.) Furthermore, general psychiatrists practicing neuropsychiatry may need neurological consultation to assist them in the management of epilepsy, movement disorders, and other primary neurological problems. Access to these services at state hospitals is variable, and problems with quality or cost of services may arise, even when those services are available.

Nonetheless, neuropsychiatric services can be developed at state hospitals even when there are limitations on the availability of diagnostic technology and specialist consultation. Such services can begin with approaching history taking, examination, and diagnostic formulation from a neuropsychiatric perspective. The hypotheses that emerge often narrow the list of tests and consultations deemed necessary and provide more convincing justification for the ones that are carried out.

Access to high-quality neurodiagnostic and consultative services may be facilitated by the following strategies:

1. Have neurodiagnostic tests done at a single general hospital, where those performing the tests can become familiar with neuropsychiatric questions and concerns and with the management of behavioral problems that might arise in the testing situation.
2. Arrange for costs of tests to be paid for by Medicaid or Medicare, programs that usually cover state hospital patients for nonpsychiatric services. In states with rigorous preauthorization or utilization review requirements, be prepared to state the diagnostic hypothesis to be tested by the diagnostic procedure ordered and how information from the test might alter treatment strategy.
3. Ensure that when tests are done at general hospitals, primary data (e.g., brain images, electroencephalogram [EEG] tracings, and detailed description with examples of abnormalities) are sent.
4. Seek quality when obtaining specialist consultation. If the patient is sent to a general hospital for the consultation, send detailed background information and a very specific question to be answered. If possible, recruit consultants to come to the state hospital for several hours at a time to see several patients and to teach the staff. Compensate the consultants at a reasonable flat hourly rate and do not burden them with billing or difficult documentation requirements. Use hospital education and quality assurance budgets to help finance consultants' activities.

Collaborative arrangements between general hospital psychiatry services and state hospitals are another reasonable option. Under such arrangements, the general hospital carries out the complete neurodiagnostic assessment, usually funded by Medicare or Medicaid, and the state hospital follows through on the therapeutic plan that arises from the evaluation. To be effective and efficient, such an arrangement should include both procedures for sharing medical records and laboratory data and periodic conferences that include psychiatric staff from both facilities (Goldberg and Fogel 1989).

Conclusion

The increase in the numbers of long-stay patients who cannot be safely or stably discharged into the community is a central problem for the administration of all state hospitals. A neuropsychiatric approach to the problems that prevent successful community placements holds the promise of enabling those placements. If this promise is realized, the place of neuropsychiatry at the institution is ensured.

References

American Psychiatric Association: Diagnostic and Statistical Manual of Mental Disorders, 3rd Edition, Revised. Washington, DC, American Psychiatric Association, 1987

American Psychiatric Association Task Force on Geriatric Psychiatry in the Public Mental Health Sector: State Mental Hospitals and the Elderly. Washington, DC, American Psychiatric Association, 1993

Anfinson TJ, Kathol RG: Laboratory and neuroendocrine assessment in medical-psychiatric patients, in Psychiatric Care of the Medical Patient. Edited by Stoudemire A, Fogel BS. New York, Oxford University Press, 1993, pp 105–138

Atay JE, Witkin MJ, Manderscheid RW: Additions and Resident Patients at End of Year, State and County Mental Hospitals, by Age and Diagnosis, by State, United States, 1992. Rockville, MD, U.S. Department of Health and Human Services, Public Health Service, Substance Abuse and Mental Health Services Administration, Center for Mental Health Services, 1994

Baker GA: Health-related quality-of-life issues. Neurology 45 (suppl 2):S29–S34, 1995

Barber JW, Kerler R, Kellogg EJ, et al: Clinical and demographic characteristics of chronic inpatients: implication for treatment and research. Psychiatr Q 59:257–270, 1988

Barnes PJ: Drug therapy: inhaled glucocorticoids for asthma. N Engl J Med 332: 868–875, 1995

Baumgartner A, Campos-Barrow A, Gaio U, et al: Carbamazepine affects triiodothyronine production and metabolization in rat hippocampus. Life Sci 54 (23):PL401–PL407, 1994

Belcher J, Toomey BG: Relationship between the deinstitutionalization model, psychiatric disability, and homelessness. Health Soc Work 13:145–153, 1988

Berg GE: A simple objective test for measuring flexibility in thinking. J Gen Psychol 39:15–22, 1948

Bolaris S, Margarity M, Valcana T: Effects of LiCl on triiodothyronine (T3) binding to nuclei from rat cerebral hemispheres. Biol Psychiatry 37:106–111, 1995

Campbell JJ, Duffy JD, Salloway SP: Treatment strategies for patients with dysexecutive syndromes. J Neuropsychiatry Clin Neurosci 6:411–418, 1994

Carpenter WT Jr: Maintenance therapy of persons with schizophrenia. J Clin Psychiatry 57 (suppl 9):10–18, 1996

Cockerell OC, Moriarty J, Trimble M, et al: Acute psychological disorders in patients with epilepsy: a nation-wide study. Epilepsy Res 25:119–131, 1996

Dorwart RA, Epstein SS: Privatization and Mental Health Care. Westport, CT, Auburn House, 1993

Drake RE, Wallach MA: Mental patients' attitudes toward hospitalization: a neglected aspect of hospital tenure. Am J Psychiatry 145:29–34, 1988

Fogel BS: Combining anticonvulsants with conventional psychopharmacologic agents, in Use of Anticonvulsants in Psychiatry: Recent Advances. Edited by McElroy SL, Pope HG. Clifton, NJ, Oxford Health Care, 1988, pp 77–94

Fogel BS: The significance of frontal systems disorders for medical practice and public policy. J Neuropsychiatry Clin Neurosci 6:343–347, 1994

Fogel BS: Drug therapy in neuropsychiatry, in Neuropsychiatry. Edited by Fogel BS, Schiffer RB, Rao SM. Baltimore, MD, Williams & Wilkins, 1996, pp 223–256

Fogel BS, Ratey JJ: A neuropsychiatric approach to personality and behavior, in Neuropsychiatry of Personality Disorders. Edited by Ratey JJ. Fogel BS (contributing ed). Boston, MA, Blackwell Scientific, 1995, pp 1–16

Fogel BS, Stone AB: Practical pathophysiology in neuropsychiatry: a clinical approach to depression and impulsive behavior in neurological patients, in The American Psychiatric Press Textbook of Neuropsychiatry, 2nd Edition. Edited by Yudofsky SC, Hales RE. Washington, DC, American Psychiatric Press, 1992, pp 329–344

Fogel BS, Brock D, Goldscheider F, et al: Cognitive Dysfunction and the Need for Long-Term Care: Implications for Public Policy. Washington, DC, American Association of Retired Persons, 1994

Folstein MF, Folstein SE, McHugh PR: Mini-Mental State: a practical method for grading the cognitive state of patients for the clinician. J Psychiatr Res 12: 189–198, 1975

Friedman JH: Drug-induced parkinsonism, in Drug-Induced Movement Disorders. Edited by Lang AE, Weiner WJ. Mt. Kisco, NY, Futura, 1992, pp 41–84

Goff DC, Midha KK, Brotman AW, et al: An open trial of buspirone added to neuroleptics in schizophrenic patients. J Clin Psychopharmacol 11:193–197, 1991

Goldberg RJ, Fogel BS: Integration of general hospital psychiatric services with free-standing psychiatric hospitals. Hospital and Community Psychiatry 40: 1057–1061, 1989

Hardwick SE, Pack PJ, Donohoe EA, et al: Across the States 1994. Washington, DC, American Association of Retired Persons, 1994

Heaton RK, Chelune GJ, Talley JL, et al: Wisconsin Card Sorting Test Manual, Revised and Expanded. Odessa, FL, Psychological Assessment Resources, 1993

Holohean EJ, Banks SM, Maddy BA: Patient subgroups in state psychiatric hospitals and implications for administration. Hospital and Community Psychiatry 44: 1002–1004, 1993

Laidlaw J, Richens A, Chadwick D: A Textbook of Epilepsy. Edinburgh, Churchill Livingstone, 1993

Levenson JL: Cardiovascular disease, in Psychiatric Care of the Medical Patient. Edited by Stoudemire A, Fogel BS. New York, Oxford University Press, 1993, pp 539–564

Lezak MD: Neuropsychological Assessment, 3rd Edition. New York, Oxford University Press, 1995, pp 621–625

Lombertie ER, Durelle G, Fuseau A: Use and value of the therapeutic neuroleptic-bromocriptine combination in schizophrenia (in French). Annales Medico Psychologiques (Paris) 153:531–534, 1995

Marder SR: Management of treatment-resistant patients with schizophrenia. J Clin Psychiatry 57 (suppl 9):26–30, 1996

Marin R, Fogel BS, Hawkins J, et al: Apathy: a treatable syndrome. J Neuropsychiatry Clin Neurosci 7:23–27, 1995

Munetz MR, Geller JL: The least restrictive environment in the postinstitutional era. Hospital and Community Psychiatry 44:967–973, 1993

Okin RL, Pearsall D, Athearn T: Predictions about new long-stay patients: were they valid? Am J Psychiatry 147:1596–1601, 1990

Plaa GL: Toxicology, in Antiepileptic Drugs, 3rd Edition. Edited by Levy RH, Dreifuss FE, Mattson RH, et al. New York, Raven, 1989, pp 49–58

Poewe W, Caraceni T (eds): Dopamine agonists in the treatment of Parkinson's disease. Neurology 45 (suppl 3):S1–S34, 1995

Reiss S, Levitan GW, Szyszko J: Emotional disturbance and mental retardation: diagnostic overshadowing. American Journal of Mental Deficiency 86:567–574, 1982

Richardson SA, Katz M, Koller H, et al: Some characteristics of a population of mentally retarded young adults in a British city. Journal of Mental Deficiency Research 23:275–287, 1979

Richardson SA, Koller H, Katz M, et al: A functional classification of seizures and its distribution in a mentally retarded population. American Journal of Mental Deficiency 85:446–457, 1981

Royall DR: Executive Interview Test. New York, Psychological Corporation (in press)

Royall DR, Mahurin RK, Gray K: Bedside assessment of executive impairment: the Executive Interview (EXIT). J Am Geriatr Soc 40:1221–1226, 1992

Royall DR, Mahurin RK, True J, et al: Executive impairment among the functionally dependent: comparisons between schizophrenic and elderly subjects. Am J Psychiatry 150:1813–1819, 1993

Schapel G, Chadwick D: A survey comparing lamotrigine and vigabatrin in everyday clinical practice. Seizure 5:267–270, 1996

Stip E: Memory impairment in schizophrenia: perspectives from psychopathology and pharmacotherapy. Can J Psychiatry 41 (8, suppl 2):S27–S34, 1996

Stoudemire A, Fogel BS, Gulley LR: Psychopharmacology in the medically ill: an update, in Medical-Psychiatric Practice, Vol 1. Edited by Stoudemire A, Fogel BS. Washington, DC, American Psychiatric Press, 1991, pp 29–97

Thornicroft G: Evaluation of the closure of large psychiatric hospitals in England (in French). Rev Epidemiol Sante Publique 41:292–297, 1993

Trevisol-Bittencourt PC, Becker N, Pozzi CM, et al: [Epilepsy at a psychiatric hospital.] Arq Neuropsiquiatr 48:261–269, 1990

Tune LE, Holland A, Folstein MF, et al: Association of postoperative delirium with raised serum levels of anticholinergic drugs. Lancet ii:651–652, 1981

Wilder BJ (ed): Rational polypharmacy in the treatment of epilepsy. Neurology 45 (suppl 2):S1–S38, 1995

Wilson WH: Reassessment of state hospital patients diagnosed with schizophrenia. J Neuropsychiatry Clin Neurosci 1:xx–xxx, 1989

Wolkowitz O, Pickar D: Benzodiazepines in the treatment of schizophrenia: a review and reappraisal. Am J Psychiatry 48:714–726, 1991

Wong MT, Lumsden J, Fenton GW, et al: Electroencephalography, computed tomography and violence ratings of male patients in a maximum-security mental hospital. Acta Psychiatr Scand 90:97–101, 1994

Zgola JM: Doing Things. Baltimore, MD, Johns Hopkins University Press, 1987

CHAPTER 4

Dementia in Public Mental Health Settings

Patricia Hanrahan, Ph.D.
Daniel J. Luchins, M.D.
Fred Ovsiew, M.D.

The human and social costs of dementia are enormous. Because of the chronic and impoverishing nature of the dementing disorders and because of the extensive resources necessary for the care of patients with dementia, public health institutions such as nursing homes and general and psychiatric hospitals face much of the burden of care. In this chapter, we review the epidemiology of dementia and its financial impact. We then offer a clinical approach to the differential diagnosis of dementia syndromes and a description of accompanying psychiatric symptoms. We conclude with recommendations for pharmacological and behavioral management of patients with dementia and a discussion of community and institutional services.

Incidence, Prevalence, and Survival

From a public health perspective, the striking feature of the dementias is their almost exponential increase in incidence and corresponding prevalence with age. The annual incidence of dementia doubles roughly every 5 years from age

65 to 89, from 7/1,000 in the group age 65–69 to 118/1,000 in the group age 86–89 (Bachman et al. 1993). Correspondingly, the rate of hospital admission with diagnosis of dementia also roughly doubles every 5 years starting at age 60 (Ryan 1994). Prevalence figures show a similar doubling from age 65 through age 95, with approximately one-third of individuals over 85 years (Skoog et al. 1993) and about one-half of those over 95 years having dementia (Wernicke and Reisches 1994).

Among the older population, Alzheimer's disease (AD) is usually found to be the major cause of dementia, with its incidence also doubling every 5 years, from 3.5/1,000 at ages 65–69 to 72.8/1,000 at ages 85–89, and not differing between men and women (Bachman et al. 1993). Among the very old, vascular disease may be the most prevalent cause of dementia (Skoog et al. 1993). Although dementias shorten life expectancy by approximately 50% (Martin et al. 1987; Peck at al. 1978), the 50% survival rate from onset may be longer than 8 years in Alzheimer's disease and 6 years in vascular dementia (Barclay et al. 1985).

Service Utilization and Social Costs

Nursing Homes

Half or more of nursing home patients have dementia (Strahan and Burns 1991), with some estimates as high as 60% (German et al. 1992). In a recent prospective study, the median length of stay for nursing home patients with AD was 2.75 years, which was 10 times the median length of stay for all diagnoses (Welch et al. 1992). The annual nursing home cost for an AD patient has been estimated at $38,500–$41,300 in 1991 dollars (Ernst and Hay 1994).

Psychiatric and General Hospitals

State and county mental hospitals also provide care for patients with dementia, particularly those with behavioral or psychiatric comorbidities. Policies favoring deinstitutionalization resulted in the transfer of many patients with dementia from mental hospitals to nursing homes. However, 20% of the adult patients in state hospitals are elderly, and 33% of these patients have AD or related disorders (Moak and Fisher 1990). The large majority of these patients (72%) were admitted late in life when behavioral and psychiatric problems complicated their dementia. The annual cost of mental hospitalization for AD patients was approximately $113,000 per patient in 1991 dollars

(Ernst and Hay 1994). Although findings vary, most studies report greater use of general hospitals by patients with dementia, with annual costs of about $1,200 per patient (Ernst and Hay 1994).

In a sample of institutionalized AD patients from northern California, 60% of institutional costs were covered by the patient and family (Rice et al. 1993). Public payment for institutional care came primarily from Medicaid and Medicare, which covered 34% of the cost; private insurance coverage was minimal.

Community Care

In the mild and moderate stages of dementia, most patients are likely to remain in the community if they have family support. Even in cases of severe dementia, patients with a family caregiver are most likely to die at home, although brief nursing home or hospital stays may precede death (Collins and Ogle 1994). The cost of providing community care is primarily based on the value of the family caregiver's time. Estimates of the annual cost of family caregiving range from $4,050 to $26,900 per patient (Ernst and Hay 1994). For patients with dementia who dwell in the community, the main family caregiver averaged 10 hours a day of care (Rice et al. 1993). Although most of that time involved helping the patient with activities of daily living, about a third of the time was devoted to behavior management. Caregivers for institutionalized patients provided care for an average of about 10 hours a week. Other community care costs include physician services, prescribed drugs, transportation, other home health services, case management, respite, and adult day care. Private payments by the patient and family covered 65% of the costs of community care (Rice et al. 1993).

Other Costs

Lost earnings are an important cost of disability. Ernst and Hay (1994) estimated this opportunity cost at $50,380 per patient. Also, they reported additional personal costs to family caregivers in the form of higher rates of hospitalization, physician visits, and prescription drug use, with an estimated annual cost of $153 (Ernst and Hay 1994).

Total Costs

Because a variety of studies reported a range of patient costs, Ernst and Hay (1994) used midrange estimates to develop an annual direct prevalence cost of $20.6 billion for AD in 1991. Additional indirect costs include unpaid caregiver time ($33.3 billion) and the patient's lost wages ($13.4 billion). The resulting total of direct and indirect costs was $67.3 billion. Although a MEDLINE search failed to reveal a similarly inclusive cost analysis for other dementias, costs for patients with disorders related to AD are expected to be similar.

Differential Diagnosis and Evaluation of Dementia

The now-traditional clinical approach to patients with dementia centers on ruling out reversible causes of dementia. This approach is inadequate for several reasons. First, it is intellectually unsatisfactory; we can be more precise in diagnosis. For example, AD is not a diagnosis of exclusion; AD has a characteristic clinical picture and can be diagnosed on positive criteria with satisfactory accuracy (Blacker et al. 1994), especially if the physician is prepared to make alternative diagnoses in the presence of features atypical for AD (McDaniel et al. 1993). Although today's methods do not allow curative treatment of degenerative diseases, tomorrow's may, and the choice of treatment will presumably depend on precise diagnosis. Even today, the differential diagnosis of degenerative conditions may have implications for management, such as for the use of antipsychotic drugs in dementia of the Lewy body type, as discussed below. Second, the so-called reversible dementias may not in actuality reverse despite appropriate treatment (Clarfield 1988; Cunha 1990; Rabins 1988). Yet a fixed or progressive dementia may be modified in severity by intercurrent conditions. Such factors must be sought even if the dementia is fundamentally not "reversible." Finally, even when the severity of the dementia cannot be reduced, many aspects of the patient's (and family's) situation are open to intervention: the irreversible dementias are still treatable dementias.

The first step in the management of dementia is differentiation of dementia from its imitators. Of these, *depression* is commonly mentioned, so-called pseudodementia, which is perhaps a misleading term in that depression often is accompanied by genuine cognitive dysfunction amounting to a *dementia syndrome of depression* (Folstein and McHugh 1978). Unfortunately, a depressive syndrome commonly coexists with a nondepressive dementing disorder, the latter progressing even when the former is treated (Alexopoulos et al. 1993). Consequently, the clinician's task is less to differentiate depression from dementia than to treat depression while the dementia syndrome is being investigated. The chronic defect state of *schizophrenia*—"the dementia of dementia praecox" (Johnstone et al. 1978)—can be mistaken for progressive cognitive impairment. The distinction of *delirium* from dementia rests on the recognition of a prominent disorder of attention. An acquired disorder of language, *aphasia*, may be mistaken for a global disorder of cognition, as may a restricted memory disorder, *amnesia*. *Deafness* can lead to impaired functioning suggestive of cognitive failure. *Mental retardation* can be hard to distinguish from dementia, especially when an adequate history is unavailable. Patients with mental retardation can also acquire additional cognitive impairment, notably in the case of the development of AD in individuals with Down's syndrome. The distinction of dementia, specifically AD, from *normal aging*, especially in the medically ill, can be a clinical and psychometric challenge (Caine 1993; Morris et al. 1991).

Once a dementia syndrome is identified, the next step is the differential diagnosis of its etiology. History taking and examination form the core of etiological diagnosis; batteries of laboratory tests cannot make up for cursory or inexpert clinical evaluation. Extended discussions of the clinical assessment of organic mental states are available elsewhere (Faber 1994; Hodges 1994; Ovsiew 1997; Sultzer 1994). Many clinicians (Cummings and Benson 1992; Neary 1994), but not all (Mayeux et al. 1993), utilize a division into cortical and subcortical dementia to organize their findings. Cortical dementias feature focal neuropsychological deficits, such as language impairment (aphasia) or recognition failure (agnosia); the prototype disease is AD. Subcortical dementia lacks these components and is characterized by slowness of mental processing, forgetfulness due to impaired retrieval, attentional dysfunction, apathy, and motor dysfunction (which usually occurs late, if at all, in the cortical dementias). Vascular dementia resulting from white-matter disease (subcortical arteriosclerotic encephalopathy, or Binswanger's disease) is probably the commonest cause of this syndrome in clinical practice.

History taking always requires an ancillary informant. Crucial information includes the duration and course of the dementia, the nature of observed deficits, coexisting systemic symptoms, and current pharmacotherapy. If a head injury is possibly relevant, the duration of coma and of posttraumatic amnesia are important data. A family history of dementia should be elucidated.

The examination should seek signs of concurrent systemic disease as well as neurological abnormalities such as focal signs, myoclonus, and extrapyramidal or gait disorders. Certain dementing disorders have characteristic physical findings. For example, eye signs and areflexia are still common features of neurosyphilis in the antibiotic era (Burke and Schaberg 1985), and B_{12} deficiency produces peripheral neuropathy and myelopathy (see below).

A broad assessment of the mental state should include exploring cognitive function in multiple domains (attention, memory, language, visuospatial function, executive function) as well as psychiatric symptoms such as abnormal mood and hallucinations or delusions. Bedside rating scales such as the Mini-Mental State Exam (Folstein et al. 1975), Clinical Dementia Rating Scale (Berg 1988), Cornell Scale for Depression in Dementia (Alexopoulos et al. 1988; Ott and Fogel 1992), Executive Interview Test (EXIT; Royall et al. 1992), and Neuropsychiatric Inventory (Cummings et al. 1994) can be of use.

In both the history and the examination, information about deficits in functional capacity should be sought (Lachs et al. 1990). Vision and hearing should be tested; continence should be assessed; falling should be considered an important source of morbidity. The clinician should learn whether the patient is capable of preparing a meal, driving a car, taking a bus, responding to an emergency situation, and so forth. This assessment can be profitably expanded by formal occupational therapy evaluation with measures of capacity for activities of daily living. The degree of disability owing to particular deficits depends considerably on the capacity of family or other social supports to compensate for lost function. Thus, thorough assessment of the patient's social environment, often by a social worker, is an important part of the evaluation.

The premortem differential diagnosis of the degenerative dementias is largely clinical, with laboratory tests being relatively unhelpful. The characteristic features of AD are a prolonged, gradual course with memory disorder prominent from the outset, sometimes with anomia and visuospatial deficits as well, with physical signs being absent until the disorder is well advanced. Often in the mild and moderate stages, the patient presents retained appropriate social responses but empty conversation and cognitive impairment obvious on formal examination. The characteristic pathology comprises senile plaques and neurofibrillary tangles in medial temporal lobes and association areas. Recently recognized as a relatively common degenerative dementia, though still controversial, is *dementia with Lewy bodies.* This disorder is characterized pathologically by Lewy bodies—the distinctive cytoplasmic inclusions seen in the substantia nigra in idiopathic Parkinson's disease—widespread in the cortex as well as in subcortical sites. The clinical picture comprises a fluctuating confusional state (though the cognitive impairment is at times indistinguishable from that typical of AD), mood and psychotic symptoms prominent early in the course, variable extrapyramidal findings, and a disastrous response to neuroleptics, with pronounced extrapyramidal dysfunction and even early demise (McKeith et al. 1992). Obviously, if this disorder is suspected, atypical antipsychotics should be used in lieu of traditional neuroleptics (Chacko et al. 1993).

The picture of *fronto-temporal dementia (FTD)*—prominent disinhibition or apathy early in the course, dysfluent language progressing to mutism, altered eating behavior, and relatively preserved memory and visuospatial function—is less often the result of the pathology of Pick's disease (neuronal loss, gliosis, ballooned pale neurons, intracellular inclusions) than the result of less specific histological changes involving the frontotemporal cortex ("frontal lobe degeneration") (Brun et al. 1994; Miller et al. 1991). *Normal-pressure hydrocephalus (NPH)* is characterized by the triad of dementia of subcortical type, gait disorder, and incontinence (at first with urgency and only later with indifference). Though NPH is considered a reversible dementia, the results of shunting are often disappointing when dementia is the most prominent symptom. Prominent gait disorder, a recognizable cause of the hydrocephalus (such as head trauma or subarachnoid hemorrhage), and benefit from removal of 30–40 mL of spinal fluid via lumbar puncture may predict shunt-responsiveness (Vanneste 1994). DSM-IV (American Psychiatric Association 1994) corrected the mistake of previous editions by naming *vascular dementia* as a category. The term *multi-infarct dementia* is too restrictive because several forms of cerebrovascular disease other than multiple large-artery occlusions can cause dementia (Ovsiew 1993). Its recognition by stepwise progression, focal signs, and imaging evidence of stroke or white- matter disease leads to efforts to reduce the risk of subsequent stroke, for example, by control of blood pressure or anticoagulation. In *alcoholic dementia*, memory impairment and executive dysfunction predominate, with peripheral neuropathy and gait ataxia sometimes present (Tuck and Jackson 1991).

Which laboratory investigations are indicated to evaluate the newly diagnosed patient has been controversial, more for financial reasons than because of traditional medical calculations of risk and benefit. Official recommendations for routine laboratory assessment have been offered (Table 4–1).

As each official panel indicated, clinical judgment must not be replaced by standardized batteries however constituted. Policy recommendations for reduction of expenditures by rational testing strategies assume the skill of expert clinicians. Many rare disorders can cause dementia, and laboratory strategies for their diagnosis must be guided by clinical findings (Table 4–2). Moreover, the "standard" tests must be appropriately used and interpreted. For example, B_{12} deficiency rarely causes dementia in the absence of signs of spinal cord and peripheral nerve damage (Healton et al. 1991)—although such cases have been reported (Evans et al. 1983)—so an abnormal serum B_{12} value accompanying a normal physical examination is unlikely to indicate the

TABLE 4–1.   Recommendations for screening laboratory tests in the evaluation of dementia

Canadian Consensus Conference[a]	National Institutes of Health[b]	American Academy of Neurology[c]
CBC	CBC	CBC
Glucose	Electrolytes and "screening metabolic panel"	Glucose
Electrolytes	Thyroid functions	Electrolytes
TSH	B$_{12}$	TSH, FTI
BUN/creatinine	Syphilis serology	BUN/creatinine
B$_{12}$	Chest X ray	B$_{12}$
Syphilis serology	Urinalysis	Syphilis serology
Chest X ray	Neuroimaging	Chest X ray
Urinalysis	Electrocardiogram	Urinalysis
Cranial CT	Folate	Neuroimaging
Heavy metals	HIV	Heavy metals
Folate	EEG	Folate
HIV	Lumbar puncture	HIV
Drug levels	Neuropsychometry	Toxicology screen
EEG	PET	EEG
Lumbar puncture	SPECT	Lumbar puncture
Serum NH$_3$	Biopsy	Neuropsychometry
ESR		ESR
Mammogram		PET
Cortisol		SPECT
Blood gas		
PT/PTT		

Note.   Boldface denotes standard tests considered to be indicated for all patients; other tests should be selected on the basis of clinical data.
BUN = blood urea nitrogen; CBC = complete blood cell count; CT = computed tomography; EEG = electroencephalogram; ESR = erythrocyte sedimentation rate; FTI = free thyroxine index; HIV = human immunodeficiency virus; PET = positron-emission tomography; PT/PTT = prothrombin time/partial thromboplastin time; SPECT = single photon emission computed tomography; TSH = thyroid-stimulating hormone.
[a]Clarfield 1989. [b]Consensus Development Conference 1987. [c]Quality Standards Subcommittee 1994.

cause of the dementia. On the other hand, if serum B$_{12}$ is low-normal in the presence of suggestive physical findings, the clinician may wish to measure serum homocysteine and methylmalonic acid as indicators of intracellular B$_{12}$ deficiency, which are more sensitive measures than the serum B$_{12}$ level

TABLE 4–2.   Clues to diagnosis in dementing disorders

Finding	Associated dementing illnesses
Ataxia	AzD, cerebellar degenerations, GM_2 gangliosidosis, M/T, MS, prion disease, PML, WK, WD
Dysarthria	AzD, dementia pugilistica, dialysis dementia, HS, MND, MS, PML, PSP, WD
Dystonic or choreoathetotic movements	AD, HS, HD, ICBG, PD, WD
Extrapyramidal signs	AD, ALSPDG, AzD, dementia pugilistica, DLBD, GM_1 gangliosidosis type III, HS, HD, ICBG, M/T, multiple system atrophy, neuroacanthocytosis, NPH, PD, postencephalitic parkinsonism, PSP, striatonigral degeneration, SSPE, VaD, WD
Extraocular movements	Gaucher's disease type 1, ME, MS, Niemann-Pick disease type IIc, PSP, VaD, WK
Gait disorder	AMN, ADC, AzD, dementia pugilistica, MS, NPH, PD, PSP, syphilis, VaD, WK
Neuropathy	AMN, ADC, B_{12} deficiency, MLD, porphyria, M/T, thyroid disease, uremia
Myoclonus	Dialysis dementia, HS, Kufs' disease, Lafora body disease, ME, prion disease, SSPE
Pyramidal tract signs	AMN, ADC, B_{12} deficiency, GM_2 gangliosidosis, HS, Kufs' disease, MLD, MND, MS, PML, syphilis, spinocerebellar degenerations, VaD

Note.   AD = Alzheimer's disease; ADC = AIDS dementia complex; AMN = adrenomyelo-neuropathy; ALSPDG = ALS–parkinsonism–dementia complex; AzD = Azorean disease; DLBD = diffuse Lewy body disease; HS = Hallervorden-Spatz disease; HD = Huntington's disease; ICBG = idiopathic calcification of the basal ganglia; M/T = medications/toxins; ME = mitochondrial encephalopathy; MLD = metachromatic leukodystrophy; MND = motor neuron disease; MS = multiple sclerosis; PD = Parkinson's disease; PML = progressive multifocal leukoencephalopathy; PSP = progressive supranuclear palsy; SSPE = subacute sclerosing panencephalitis; VaD = vascular dementia; WK = Wernicke-Korsakoff syndrome; WD = Wilson's disease.

Source.   Reprinted from Sandson TA, Price BH: "Diagnostic Testing and Dementia." *Neurologic Clinics* 14:45–59, 1996. Used with permission.

(Green and Kinsella 1995). The serum Venereal Disease Research Laboratory test (VDRL) is insufficiently sensitive to rule out neurosyphilis in patients with dementia; the fluorescent treponema antibody test (FTA) is more appropriate (Reeves et al. 1996). Measuring thyrotropin—thyroid-stimulating hormone (TSH)—with an ultrasensitive assay is adequate to screen for thyroid dysfunction; measuring thyroxine and triiodothyronine is not necessary unless TSH is abnormal or specific indicators exist in the history or examination. An epidemiological study suggested that elevated TSH may be surprisingly common in patients with dementia (Ganguli et al. 1996). Testing for antibodies to the human immunodeficiency virus is crucial in patients with dementia with risk factors for this infection.

Electroencephalography has specific indications but need not be part of a routine battery. In Creutzfeldt-Jakob disease, the appearance of periodic triphasic complexes is an important diagnostic feature. In the frontal dementias, changes on the electroencephalogram (EEG) occur late, much later than in AD (Neary 1994).

Cerebrospinal fluid (CSF) examination need not be performed routinely (Becker et al. 1985; Hammerstrom and Zimmer 1985) but is indicated by suggestions of infection or inflammatory disease, such as headache, fever, meningeal signs, an immunosuppressed state, a systemic autoimmune disease, or relevant laboratory abnormalities. A cancer history raising the question of meningeal carcinomatosis also indicates that a lumbar puncture should be performed. In the hydrocephalic patient, lumbar puncture is necessary for measurement of pressure, and withdrawal of CSF may be a useful predictor of response to shunting (Vanneste 1994). CSF examination may also be performed in cases of puzzling, atypical, or early-onset dementia, regardless of specific indications (Quality Standards Subcommittee 1994).

Neuroimaging is costly but has few other disadvantages. Although rational cost-containment strategies will limit the use of expensive technologies, the clinician in the public health setting will be wary of a rationale that justifies providing medical care more readily to the rich than to the poor, to the young than to the old, and to those with physical symptoms than to those with mental symptoms. The American Academy of Neurology suggested that "neuroimaging be considered in every patient with dementia" but acknowledged the lack of "consensus on the need for such studies in the evaluation of patients with the insidious onset of dementia after age 60 without focal signs or symptoms, seizures, or gait disturbances" (Quality Standards Subcommittee 1994, p. 2004). Conversely, onset before age 60, a history of head injury or cancer, headache, focal signs, gait disorder, and a rapid course are among the features that mandate imaging (Clarfield 1994). Again, expert clinical evaluation is the key to the sensible use of the laboratory. Magnetic resonance imaging (MRI) offers better visualization of white matter and of posterior fossa structures than does X-ray computed tomography (CT). However, CT may be easier for technical reasons in an agitated patient with dementia; a good CT study is better than a poor MRI. Functional neuroimaging with single photon emission computed tomography is of particular use when a diagnosis of FTD is under consideration (Miller et al. 1991).

Neuropsychological assessment has several uses. First, it may help in establishing the presence of a dementia syndrome (as opposed to, e.g., mental retardation or normal aging). Second, occasionally the profile of cognitive dysfunction is suggestive—never decisive—in establishing an etiological diagnosis, as when executive dysfunction dominates the picture and suggests Pick's disease or frontal degeneration. Usually the bedside examination is sufficient for this purpose. Third, and perhaps most important, the neuropsychological examination should be viewed as providing guidance for the provision of support in activities of daily living. The assessment of functional capacity can lead to specification of areas in which supervision is necessary or independent activity is still possible. Detailed information of this sort is often appealing to caregivers, who welcome the quantitative and objective approach the neuropsychologist provides.

Biopsy is rarely indicated. Only when definitive premortem diagnosis is required for choice of treatment will the risks of biopsy be justified; usually this is when an infection or inflammatory disease (e.g., vasculitis) is under consideration. Unfortunately, biopsy is often inconclusive (Hulette et al. 1992).

Autopsy data are invaluable (Marks et al. 1988). In public settings where long-term care is provided, the opportunity for learning from each case is enhanced by efforts to obtain permission for autopsy when a carefully observed patient dies.

The next step in management is reduction of excess disability. Correction of impaired vision and hearing, if possible, is always appropriate. Reduction of potentially psychotoxic polypharmacy and optimal treatment of potentially relevant medical conditions, such as urinary tract infection, congestive heart failure, or hypothyroidism, may be helpful even if these factors only exacerbate a progressive degenerative disorder and do not cause the dementia (Larson et al. 1984). Sleep apnea is a common phenomenon in the older population with dementia. Along with headache, snoring, and excessive daytime somnolence, cognitive impairment may be a feature of this disorder. Polysomnography can confirm the abnormality of breathing; continuous positive airway pressure at night or other interventions may bring a reduction of symptoms (Arnold and Kumar 1993).

More on the basis of functional information gathered in the assessment than on the diagnosis, a judgment must be made about the patient's needs for assistance in daily living (Steele et al. 1982). Often, driving should be prohibited (Poser 1993). Other interventions are discussed below.

Thought must be given at the initial assessment to the potential decline of the patient with progressing dementia. Writing a will, giving advance directives for resuscitation and other medical procedures, and assigning durable power of attorney for health care and financial matters may be possible in the early stages of a degenerative disease; later in the course, only guardianship will be available as a legal option. Family members should be encouraged to obtain guardianship when the patient's mental state mandates it, before the circumstances requiring its use arise. At that point the weeks of legal delay may prevent expeditious nursing home placement or other necessary procedures.

In summary, a strategy of multidisciplinary clinical assessment can lead to accurate diagnosis and functional benefit for many patients with dementia. Expert clinicians are more important to this process than laboratory tests, and public institutions caring for the population with dementia should recruit and train clinicians toward this goal.

Comorbidity: Behavioral Problems and Other Mental Disorders

Behavioral problems are common in dementia and increase with the severity of the disease. Frequently reported behavioral problems include apathy, disinhibition, wandering, agitation, aggression, and binge eating (Burns et al. 1990; Mega et al. 1996; Teri et al. 1988). These problems are pervasive in institutional settings; 65% of the patients with dementia in long-term care institutions had behavioral syndromes (Nasman et al. 1993). As the dementia progresses, apathy and disinhibited behaviors become more prevalent (Devanand et al. 1992).

Aggression is a particularly troublesome behavioral problem, reported by 33% of family caregivers who used a telephone help line (Coyne et al. 1993). In a patient registry sample, 16% of patients with dementia had been violent in the preceding year, and 5% of caregivers were violent toward the patient (Paveza et al. 1992). The serious consequences of aggression include a higher likelihood of institutionalization, either in a nursing home (C. A. Cohen et al. 1993; Haupt and Kurz 1993) or in a psychiatric hospital (Moak and Fisher 1990), and an increased risk of elder abuse on the part of the family caregiver (Pilemer and Suitor 1992).

Aggression is prevalent in institutional settings as well as in the community. In a recent survey of a geropsychiatric state hospital (Colenda and Hamer 1991), patients with dementia had higher rates of aggression than did patients without dementia. Although staff were most often unable to identify the antecedents to aggressive behavior, the most frequent triggering event that could be identified was some form of patient-staff exchange. A similar finding was reported by Bridges-Parlet et al. (1994) regarding the antecedents of physically aggressive behavior in nursing home settings. More than half of the time, aggression was directed at staff during their efforts to provide physical care (bathing, toileting, grooming). These findings, which were based on direct observation, suggest that aggression was not an expression of anger but was instead a defensive response to personal care that may have been perceived as an intrusion. Given that many of the patients in the latter study were in the end stages of dementia, they may also have experienced pain when they were moved because of complications of the disease (e.g., decubitus ulcers).

Delusions and depression were found in 40% of nursing home patients with dementia (Rovner et al. 1990). Delusions have been reported in up to 73% of patients with dementia (Wragg and Jeste 1989). Hallucinations and delusions may occur throughout the course of the dementing disorder and are likely to be associated with behavioral problems such as aggression, agitation, and wandering (Lachs et al., 1992; Teri et al. 1988). Hallucinations are present in 10%–49% of patients with dementia and may be a response to a confusional state (Burns 1992) or to a problem in visual acuity. Misidentification syndromes, of others or even of the patient's own mirror image, occasionally occur (Burns 1992).

The reported prevalence of depression varies widely, from 0% to 86%, with depressive symptoms being more prevalent than depressive syndromes (Wragg and Jeste 1989). The extreme range may be the result of variation in methods of diagnosis and in stage of disease. The use of family interviews to diagnose major depression among patients with AD produced a prevalence rate of 50%, versus 14% through direct observation (MacKenzie et al. 1989). A recent large study using stringent criteria, such as the reliance on direct observation for evidence of depressed mood, found the incidence of new cases of major depression to be low (1.3%) (Weiner et al. 1994). The study was limited, however, by the exclusion of patients with a history of depression and the underrepresentation of patients in the early stages of the disease. These limitations are important because several studies (e.g., Reding et al. 1985) suggested that depression may be most prevalent in the early stages of dementia and that late-life depression may precede the appearance of the symptoms of dementia. Other research, however, suggested a fairly constant rate of depression throughout the course of the disease (Eisdorfer et al. 1992). These inconsistencies may be the result of the varying presentation of depressive symptoms during the course of dementia. Forsell and her colleagues (1993) found that depressed patients with mild dementia had symptoms of mood disturbance, such as dysphoria and suicidal ideation. By contrast, the symptoms of depressed patients with more severe dementia included loss of interest and energy and difficulty thinking and concentrating, possibly with an organic basis.

Self-Care Deficits

The progressive deterioration in self-care skills that is typical of AD presents management problems for family and professional caregivers, particularly when urinary incontinence develops (Reisberg et al. 1982). Urinary incontinence occurred among 43% of a sample of patients with AD (Burns et al. 1990). Care of the incontinent patient is burdensome for family caregivers (Ouslander et al. 1990) and is one of several factors that may precipitate institutional placement (C. A. Cohen et al. 1993; O'Donnell et al. 1992).

Behavioral Problems and Institutional Placement

Informal care by family caregivers is crucial to maintaining individuals with dementia in the community. As indicated previously, behavioral problems are often a factor in the caregivers' decision to institutionalize relatives with dementia (C. A. Cohen et al. 1993; Haupt and Kurz 1993; O'Donnell et al. 1992). Institutional placement is also more likely when caregivers react to these problems in highly negative ways, experience poor health themselves, or feel highly burdened (C. A. Cohen et al. 1993; Zarit et al. 1986). This is an important context for our later section on psychological management of behavioral problems and the need to care for the caregiver.

Neurobiological Basis of Psychiatric Symptoms

Limited data are available to correlate behavioral disturbance in dementia with pathological alterations in the brain (Esiri 1996). Depression in AD may be related to a noradrenergic deficit resulting from cell loss in the locus ceruleus, the brainstem nucleus containing the cells of origin of noradrenergic projections to cortex (Förstl et al. 1992, 1994b).

With regard to psychotic symptoms, Zubenko et al. (1991) found a relative reduction of serotonin in the presubiculum and perhaps other regions in the brains of psychotic patients with AD. In confirmation and extension of this finding, Förstl et al. (1994a) showed that delusions and hallucinations were associated with low cell counts in the dorsal raphe, the brainstem origin of serotonergic projections, in combination with relative preservation of cell counts in the hippocampus. In contrast, delusional misidentification was associated with low cell counts in the CA1 region of the hippocampus. Cholinergic abnormalities may be particularly associated with behavioral disturbances and with psychosis in particular (Cummings and Kaufer 1996). In dementia with Lewy bodies, hallucinations may be associated with cholinergic deficits in temporal cortex (Perry et al. 1991); the same study found preservation of serotonergic activity in the cortex in hallucinating patients with degenerative dementias.

Other behavioral symptoms have been correlated with neuropathological findings as well. Apathy and communication failure in AD were found to correlate with severe tangle pathology and neuron loss (i.e., advanced disease). The Klüver-Bucy syndrome, however, was associated specifically with cell loss in parahippocampal gyrus and parietal cortex (Förstl et al. 1993). Aggressive behavior was correlated with preservation of neurons in the substantia nigra (Victoroff et al. 1996).

Psychopharmacology of Cognitive Deficit

Currently only three agents are specifically approved to treat the cognitive deficit seen in dementia. The first agent is ergoloid mesylates (Hydergine), a mixture of ergotamines initially believed to work as a vasodilator and subsequently noted to have adrenergic and other neurochemical effects (Olpe and Steinmann 1982). There have been numerous double-blind studies (Yesavage et al. 1979), many of which support the view that, especially at higher doses (4.5 mg or more daily), the drug may produce behavioral effects that include increased alertness. Most of the studies lack objective measures of cognitive function.

The second agent is tacrine, a cholinesterase inhibitor thought to partially correct the acetylcholine deficiency noted in AD. Several large, well-controlled studies found statistically significant, if modest, increases in cognitive functions with this agent (e.g., Knapp et al. 1994), with a suggestion that higher doses (up to 160 mg daily) may produce greater benefit. On the other hand, several well-designed studies failed to find significant benefit (e.g., Maltby et al. 1994) or noted modest results that were not clinically significant (Gauthier et al. 1990). The benefits of tacrine have been associated with delay in the progression of the illness by 6 months, a delay that is lost if

the medication is stopped (Winker 1994). Liver enzymes need to be moni-
tored weekly for at least the first 3 months of treatment. Elevated liver enzymes are found in more than half of the patients, with one-quarter having
values three times normal. These elevations are usually asymptomatic, and
most patients whose tacrine was initially discontinued can be safely re-
challenged (Watkins et al. 1994). The Committee on Aging of the Group for
the Advancement of Psychiatry (1994) provided a cautious endorsement of
the medication. It underscored that a relatively small percentage (7%–15%)
of patients on active medication significantly benefit and that controlled
studies were done in a select group of individuals with a minimum of
comorbid conditions.

The third agent is donepezil, a cholinesterase inhibitor that does not require monitoring of liver enzymes. Controlled studies suggest that a dose of 5
mg daily is more effective than placebo in retarding cognitive decline. Serum
drug levels correlated with various clinical measures, including the Mini-
Mental State Exam and quality-of-life scores (Rogers et al. 1996). Although
no direct comparison with tacrine has been made, donepezil probably has at
least equivalent efficacy with a minimum of side effects.

From a public health perspective, a major issue in the use of these drugs is
the cost, which is approximately $1,200 per year. Unlike clozapine, a simi-
larly expensive neuropsychiatric agent for which economic analysis showed
overall reduced costs because of reduced hospitalization (Meltzer et al.
1993), tacrine and donepezil show no evidence of cost savings.

There are several promising leads in the development of alternative treatment for dementias. These include calcium-channel blocking agents, which
are proposed to improve depression as well as cognition (Ban et al. 1990; De
Vry et al. 1997; Tollefson 1990); more specific muscarinic agents such as
xanomeline (Tollefson et al. 1994); and the selective monoamine oxidase B
inhibitor selegiline, either alone (Sano et al. 1997; Tariot et al. 1987) or with
a cholinesterase inhibitor (Schneider et al. 1993). α-Tocopherol (vitamin E)
at a dose of 1000 IU twice daily recently was shown to have a modest effect
in slowing the progression of Alzheimer's disease with minimal side effects
(Sano et al. 1997).

Psychopharmacology of Noncognitive Manifestations

Particularly when associated with behavioral disturbances, psychiatric symptoms are often the focus of pharmacological treatment. Obviously, issues that

are relevant to geriatric psychopharmacology, such as alterations in drug distribution, decreases in hepatic metabolism and renal excretion, and the increased opportunity for drug interactions because of concomitant medical illness, need to be taken into account (Montamat et al. 1989). In general, starting doses are one-half to one-third of those used in younger adults, dosage increments are smaller and at greater intervals, and therapeutic goals may need to be more modest.

Antipsychotic agents are probably the most widely used agents for the purpose of behavioral control despite frequent untoward effects (Ray et al. 1987). They may be used excessively in the United States, in comparison with their use in other countries. For example, in the early 1980s, more than 40% of a group of nursing home residents with dementia received antipsychotic medication, whereas only 20% of comparable patients in London received such treatment (Mann et al. 1984). Although many double-blind controlled studies support the efficacy of antipsychotics in comparison with placebo, the clinical benefits are modest and occur primarily in those individuals who are most disturbed (Barnes et al. 1982). A meta-analysis of placebo-controlled studies found that only 18% of patients benefit from neuroleptics (Schneider et al. 1990).

Although haloperidol is probably most frequently used in clinical practice and has been compared with other neuroleptics in at least five controlled studies, the meta-analysis found no evidence that haloperidol or any other antipsychotic was superior to another. (No atypical antipsychotic was included in these studies.) Aside from their modest benefits, the antipsychotics are prone to produce side effects in elderly persons with dementia, especially at higher doses. Devanand et al. (1989), reporting on a small sample of AD patients who were administered 1–5 mg of haloperidol daily for 4 weeks, noted both significant extrapyramidal side effects and decreases in cognition that only partially abated during a 4-week posttreatment placebo period. Furthermore, none of the patients could tolerate the full 5 mg; the mean dose was approximately 2.5 mg. Fortunately, trials with lower doses of antipsychotics (i.e., 7 mg of fluphenazine decanoate monthly) reported fewer side effects (Gottlieb et al. 1988). It is possible that newer antipsychotics, such as risperidone, that produce less parkinsonism without significant intrinsic anticholinergic effects will be useful in the older population with dementia (Meco et al. 1994).

The use of antipsychotic medication to treat behavioral and psychiatric problems in patients in nursing homes must conform to congressional guidelines established by the Omnibus Budget Reconciliation Act of 1987 (OBRA 87). Currently, psychotropic drug use is limited to specific indications, such as for dementia with psychotic symptoms or extremely agitated behavior, which must be documented in the patient's chart (Semla et al. 1994). This documentation must 1) include quantitative and objective information, 2) demonstrate that the condition is not caused by preventable factors, and 3) indicate that the problem is causing the resident to be a danger to herself or himself or to others and either to have a very high frequency of agitated behavior that causes functional impairment or to experience other psychotic or behavioral symptoms that cause distress or functional impairment to the resident.

OBRA 87 guidelines consider antipsychotics inappropriate for problems such as wandering, restlessness, insomnia, agitation that is not a danger, anxiety, withdrawal, and poor self-care. As-needed antipsychotic use is restricted to five doses in 7 days for appropriate conditions. After antipsychotic drugs are prescribed, a gradual reduction in dosage is required. A revision of this requirement has developed as the regulatory pendulum has begun to swing toward greater attention to the appropriate use of antipsychotics. Dosage reduction is no longer required if there have been two previous efforts to reduce dosage in the past year with a subsequent return of symptoms.

A recent study suggested that OBRA guidelines have functioned to reduce the use of antipsychotics (Semla et al. 1994). However, the discontinuation of antipsychotics was greatest among residents with a dementia-only diagnosis and among residents who had no justifiable target symptoms. For those with a psychiatric diagnosis, the dosage of antipsychotics tended to increase. This suggests that problem symptoms returned after reduction or discontinuation.

Another group of medicines frequently used in this population is the benzodiazepines, which controlled studies have indicated are probably better than placebo, but which have even less clinical efficacy than the antipsychotics (Coccaro et al. 1990; Risse and Barnes 1986). Aside from problems with sedation and confusion, long-term use of benzodiazepines raises issues of tolerance, dependency, and withdrawal (Salzman 1991).

Several other agents have been used to treat behavioral disturbance in dementia. For most of these agents, there are many studies, including double-blind controlled trials, of populations other than patients with dementia but few in patients with dementia (Schneider and Sobin 1992). Probably the most benign agents are the serotonergic agents. Case reports suggested efficacy of trazodone (Pinner and Rich 1988; Simpson and Foster 1986), buspirone (Herrmann and Eryavec 1993), and selective serotonin reuptake inhibitors (Sobin et al. 1989). Valproate (Mazure et al. 1992) and β-blockers (Jenike 1983) have also been used. A nonrandomized, placebo-controlled crossover study of carbamazepine in 25 patients with dementia showed significant reductions on both the Brief Psychiatric Rating Scale (Overall and Gorham 1962) and measures of behavioral disturbance during the 5 weeks of active treatment with carbamazepine (modal dose 300 mg/day) (Tariot el al. 1994). Treatment of apathy with dopaminergic drugs such as bromocriptine is an emerging strategy (Marin et al. 1995). With increased concern about chronic antipsychotic medication, especially preliminary data suggesting that neuroleptics may accelerate cognitive decline (McShane et al. 1997), further exploration of these alternatives is warranted. However, we are unaware of systematic studies examining the capacity of alternative agents to replace or reduce use of antipsychotics in patients with dementia, although such was demonstrated in patients with mental retardation (Luchins et al. 1993).

Psychological Management

Psychological management of behavioral problems is complicated by the patient's inability to retain insight or information because of memory problems and other facets of cognitive decline. The treatment focus must shift to training family and professional caregivers in behavioral principles and to careful structuring of the patient's environment. Procedures for helping patients with problems such as depression and urinary incontinence provide examples of behavioral therapy for this population (Engel et al. 1990; Teri and Uomoto 1991). Modifying the patient's environment is important in managing problems such as wandering (Grossberg et al. 1990).

Assessment

The assessment of behavioral problems can combine the use of structured caregiver questionnaires, such as the Memory and Behavior Problem Checklist (Zarit et al. 1986), direct observation, and information gathered from the diagnostic interview with the patient. The effect of disturbed behavior, as well as the dementia itself, on the patient's family is also an important area for assessment and treatment. The behavioral problems that often accompany dementia are frequently troublesome to caregivers, yet individuals vary considerably in their responses to specific behaviors (Donaldson et al. 1997). This means that it is important to assess caregivers' responses to specific behavioral difficulties. The Memory and Behavior Problem Checklist provides a section in which caregivers can indicate how troublesome they find specific behaviors (Zarit et al. 1986). An assessment of the patient's and family's service needs is also important. A wide array of services has developed through the Older Americans Act and the Administration on Aging. Effective linkage with social services can increase patients' quality of life while providing respite and support for family caregivers.

Behavioral Management

Behavioral management includes the use of appropriate cues, such as a prompt for scheduled toileting, social and tangible reinforcement for specific adaptive behaviors, and attention to structuring the environment for safety and adequate stimulation. Several resources provide extensive discussions of behavioral procedures for geriatric populations (Burgio and Bourgeois 1992; Fisher and Carstensen 1990; Pinkston and Linsk 1984; Rabins 1989). It is also important to plan for the reinforcement of family and staff caregivers who bear the burden of implementing these procedures (Engel et al. 1990; Pinkston and Linsk 1984).

Caring for the Caregivers

Both clinical reports and subsequent large studies indicate that family caregivers are themselves at risk for psychiatric disorders, particularly depression (Gallagher et al. 1989; Goldman and Luchins 1984; Pruchno and Resch 1989). In a large registry study, nearly half of all wives who were caregivers scored over the cutoff score for clinical severity on the Center for Epidemiological Studies Depression Index (D. Cohen et al. 1990; Radloff 1977). Among other family caregivers, about a quarter of husbands, a fifth of daughters, and a seventh of sons scored above the cutoff. Daughters-in-law, who frequently provided care, also had significant depressive symptoms.

Research on negative expressed emotion (EE) suggests a way to identify family caregivers who are vulnerable to depression (G. W. Brown et al. 1962; Leff and Vaughn 1985). The term *negative EE* refers to families that are highly critical, overinvolved, or hostile toward the patient. High EE among families tends to predict relapse or deterioration among patients with a range of psychiatric problems including schizophrenia and eating disorders (Fischmann-Havstad and Marston, 1993; Leff and Vaughn 1985). High EE caregivers of patients with dementia are themselves vulnerable to negative outcomes, including depression, burden, and physical illness (Bledin et al. 1990; Luchins et al. 1990; Vitaliano et al. 1989).

In addition to counseling and pharmacotherapy for depression, these families could benefit from psychoeducation and may need respite care (Leff 1989). Family psychoeducation includes information about the disease and medication as well as skills training (Falloon et al. 1982, 1985; Hogarty et al. 1986, 1991). Skills training for families of impaired elders involves the delineation of problems that families are having with their impaired relative, followed by instruction, role play, and task assignments based on behavioral therapies (Pinkston and Linsk 1984).

Competing demands on the caregiver's time is another issue that complicates family efforts to care for impaired elders. The National Long-Term Care and Informal Caregivers Survey found that 21% of family caregivers also had child care responsibilities, and 29% reported work-related problems (Stone et al. 1987). As expected, families were found to be the primary source of community care for the older population. Fewer than 10% used formal services and then only as a last resort when the patient's deterioration became too difficult to manage.

As dementia progresses, the burden of caregiving increases; families become more in need of interventions and service linkage. Family burden is a strong predictor of institutional placement and should be evaluated as part of the assessment of the patient with dementia (L. J. Brown et al. 1990; C. A. Cohen et al. 1993). The Memory and Behavior Problem Checklist, developed by Zarit and colleagues (1986), includes information about the extent to which specific problems cause distress to the family caregiver; this checklist may be supplemented by the Family Burden Interview (Zarit et al. 1980) for a broader assessment of sources of strain such as financial and health problems. Given its high incidence among caregivers, depression should also be assessed.

Services for Patients With Dementia and Their Families

The prevalence of depression and burden among family caregivers highlights the importance of linkage to public services. Many states have case management systems that can provide information and referral services. Controlled studies of case-managed community care for impaired elders documented positive outcomes, such as reductions in unmet service needs and problems with the environment, with accompanying gains for families, such as reduced limitations on privacy and social life, greater overall life satisfaction, and less worry about obtaining sufficient help (Kemper 1988). Advocacy groups, notably the Alzheimer's Association, are another source of referrals, education, and support groups for the family caregiver (Alzheimer's Association, Central Office, 919 N. Michigan Avenue, Suite 1000, Chicago, IL, 60611; phone: 312-335-8700; http://www.alz.org).

Family caregivers are most likely to need and use respite services, although respite may not be readily available (Caserta et al. 1987; Shope et al. 1993). Those who use respite services spend most of their respite time on paid employment (Berry et al. 1991). In a controlled study of respite, institutional placement was delayed and family satisfaction with care was greater than among controls, although burden and family caregiver depression did not decrease (Lawton et al. 1989). However, many control group families received respite services despite the experimental design. A recent analysis provided further support for the role of respite in delaying nursing home placement (Kosloski and Montgomery 1995).

In the mild and moderate stages of dementia, service options include adult day care (Conrad et al. 1993), home health care (Hughes et al. 1990, 1992; Zimmer et al. 1985), and brief inpatient care (Mintzer et al. 1993; Zubenko et al. 1992). As the disease progresses, additional services may become appropriate, such as special care units in nursing homes (Sloane et al. 1995). Although nursing home placement is an important alternative, many families choose to continue caring for their relatives with dementia at home (Collins and Ogle 1994). During the terminal phase of dementia, hospice programs can provide palliative care and support to patients either at home or in the nursing home (Hanrahan and Luchins 1995; Luchins and Hanrahan 1993a, 1993b; Luchins et al. 1997).

In a controlled study of adult day care and homemaker services, both services improved the quality of life of impaired elders (Wan et al. 1980). However, the kind of services provided through adult day care varies considerably. In a survey of 774 adult day care centers, six types of adult day care programs were identified, with considerable variability on measures of program quality (Conrad et al. 1993). Clinicians should assess specific program referrals or suggest that family caregivers visit programs to assess them (Linsk et al. 1991).

Research on institutional respite has usually found benefits to families, but patients with dementia have not always faired as well, with some temporary declines in self-care and behavior (e.g., Hirsch et al. 1993). On the other hand, two uncontrolled studies of brief institutional care that focused on resolving patient problems had positive findings (Mintzer et al. 1993; Zubenko et al. 1992). These preliminary findings suggest the utility of a hospitalization focused on specific behavioral complications and the need to evaluate special reimbursement status under Medicare rates for Diagnosis-Related Group (DRG)–exempt units.

As dementia progresses, family members may need to consider nursing home placement. Special care units (SCUs) in nursing homes have been developed for patients with dementia. The number of patients in SCUs has doubled from 3% of the nursing home population in 1987 to 6% in 1990 (Leon et al. 1990). Although the development of programs specifically designed for patients with dementia has conceptual appeal, evaluations of this approach have been mixed (Sloane et al. 1995). On the positive side, uncontrolled and quasi-experimental studies have reported reduced disruptive behaviors (Greene et al. 1985), fewer catastrophic reactions and more socialization (Swanson et al. 1993, 1994), and reduced discomfort and cost (L. Volicer et al. 1994). However, no differences in patient status were reported in one small study with randomized controls (Wells and Jorm 1987). These mixed findings may be partly the result of variability in the kinds of programs being evaluated (Sloane et al. 1995). At present, there is no consensus as to what an SCU should be like. Judgments as to the adequacy of a referral to an SCU must be made on an individual basis.

Care of patients in the end stage of dementia is a significant clinical problem. Because the terminal care preferences of patients with impaired decision making are frequently unknown (High 1988; Sachs et al. 1989; Steiber 1987), families and professional caregivers must often make surrogate judgments as to what kind of terminal care the patient should receive (Myers and Grodin 1991; President's Commission 1983). In a recent study, we sought to determine what kind of care was viewed as appropriate for patients with end-stage dementia (Luchins and Hanrahan 1993). We surveyed more than 1,400 families of patients with dementia, physicians who cared for elders, and gerontologists. The clear majority favored palliative care, with its focus on pain relief and easing dying, rather than aggressive efforts to prolong life. Ninety percent viewed hospice as an appropriate alternative to conventional care for end-stage dementia. Yet most were not aware of hospice programs that served patients with dementia.

To determine the extent to which patients who are dying of their dementia have access to hospice programs, we conducted a national survey of all hospices known to the National Hospice Organization (Hanrahan and Luchins 1995a). Fewer than 1% of hospice patients had a primary diagnosis of end-stage dementia. For 80% of the hospices, the major problem in serving patients with dementia was the difficulty in predicting their survival time. As a condition of enrollment, many hospices require a physician to certify that the patient is likely to die within 6 months. Because survival times are highly variable in AD and related disorders, predicting survival time is difficult even when patients are severely demented.

In a pilot study of home-based hospice, we developed criteria for the enrollment of patients with end-stage dementia that predicted a mean survival time of 6.6 months (Hanrahan and Luchins 1995b). The enrollment criteria included the characteristics of advanced dementia (stage 7, Reisberg et al. 1982) and a history of medical complications related to the functional impairments typical of severe dementia (e.g., aspiration pneumonia resulting from problems with swallowing). Preliminary findings from a replication study in progress indicated a similar pattern with a mean survival time of 6.9 months (Luchins et al., in press). Related research by L. Volicer and his colleagues (1986, 1994) supported the feasibility of providing palliative care to patients with dementia in an institutional setting. Specific components of palliative care, such as whether or not to treat fevers in patients with severe dementia, also affect survival time (B. J. Volicer et al. 1993). These findings should form the basis for empirically based standards for enrolling patients with dementia in hospices.

In summary, promising new kinds of programs have emerged, yet gaps in the service delivery system remain, particularly adequate respite for family caregivers and hospice for patients with end-stage dementia. Inconsistent findings about the adequacy of institutional respite and SCU programs are a concern. Variability as to the kind and quality of care provided in social and health services is a recurrent theme in program research (Conrad and Roberts-Gray 1988). There is a need for empirically based standards for quality of care in services for patients with dementia and for research to determine the validity of existing standards. Although community services are important, family caregivers play an essential role in maintaining patients with dementia in the community.

References

Alexopoulos GS, Abrams RC, Young RC, et al: Cornell Scale for Depression in Dementia. Biol Psychiatry 23:271–284, 1988

Alexopoulos GS, Meyers BS, Young RC, et al: The course of geriatric depression with "reversible dementia": a controlled study. Am J Psychiatry 150:1693–1699, 1993

American Psychiatric Association: Diagnostic and Statistical Manual of Mental Disorders, 4th Edition. Washington, DC, American Psychiatric Association, 1994

Arnold SE, Kumar A: Reversible dementias. Med Clin North Am 77:215–230, 1993

Bachman DL, Wolf PA, Linn RT, et al: Incidence of dementia and probable Alzheimer's disease in a general population. Neurology 43:515–519, 1993

Ban TA, Morey L, Aguglia E, et al: Nimodipine in the treatment of old age dementias. Prog Neuropsychopharmacol Biol Psychiatry 14:525–551, 1990

Barclay LL, Zemcor A, Blass JP, et al: Survival in Alzheimer's disease and vascular dementias. Neurology 35:834–840, 1985

Barnes R, Veith R, Okimoto J, et al: Efficacy of antipsychotic medication in behaviorally disturbed dementia patients. Am J Psychiatry 139:1170–1174, 1982

Becker PM, Feussner JR, Mulrow CD, et al: The role of lumbar puncture in the evaluation of dementia: the Durham Veterans Administration/Duke University study. J Am Geriatr Soc 33:392–396, 1985

Berg L: Clinical Dementia Rating. Psychopharmacol Bull 24:637–639, 1988

Berry GL, Zarit SH, Rabatin VX: Caregiver activity on respite and nonrespite days: a comparison of two service approaches. Gerontology 31:830–835, 1991

Blacker D, Albert MS, Bassett SS, et al: Reliability and validity of NINCDS-ADRDA criteria for Alzheimer's disease. Arch Neurol 51:1198–1204, 1994

Bledin KD, MacCarthy B, Kuipers L, et al: Daughters of people with dementia: expressed emotion, strain and coping. Br J Psychiatry 157:221–227, 1990

Bridges-Parlet S, Knopman D, Thompson T: A descriptive study of physically aggressive behavior in dementia by direct observation. J Am Geriatr Soc 42:192–197, 1994

Brown GW, Monck EM, Carstairs GM, et al: Influence of family life on the course of schizophrenic illness. British Journal of Preventative and Social Medicine 16: 55–68, 1962

Brown LJ, Potter JF, Foster BG: Caregiver burden should be evaluated during geriatric assessment. J Am Geriatr Soc 38:455–460, 1990

Brun A, Englund B, Gustafson L, et al: Clinical and neuropathological criteria for frontotemporal dementia. J Neurol Neurosurg Psychiatry 57:416–418, 1994

Burgio LD, Bourgeois M: Treating severe behavioral disorders in geriatric residential settings. Behav Residential Treatment 7:145–168, 1992

Burke JM, Schaberg DR: Neurosyphilis in the antibiotic era. Neurology 35: 1368–1371, 1985

Burns A: Psychiatric phenomena in dementia of the Alzheimer's type. Int Psychogeriatr 4:43–54, 1992

Burns A, Jacoby R, Levy R: Psychiatric phenomena in Alzheimer's disease, IV: disorders of behavior. Br J Psychiatry 157:86–94, 1990

Caine ED: Should aging-associated cognitive decline be included in DSM-IV? J Neuropsychiatry Clin Neurosci 5:1–5, 1993

Caserta MS, Lund DA, Wright SD, et al: Caregivers to dementia patients: the utilization of community services. Gerontology 27:209–214, 1987

Chacko RC, Hurley RA, Jankovic J: Clozapine use in diffuse Lewy body disease. J Neuropsychiatry Clin Neurosci 5:206–208, 1993

Clarfield AM: The reversible dementias: do they reverse? Ann Intern Med 109: 476–486, 1988

Clarfield AM: Canadian Consensus Conference on the Assessment of Dementia, Montréal, Canadian Consensus Conference on the Assessment of Dementia, 1989

Clarfield AM: Diagnostic procedures for dementia, II: reversible dementias from gross structural lesions, in Dementia: Presentations, Differential Diagnosis, and Nosology. Edited by Emery VOB, Oxman TE. Baltimore, MD, Johns Hopkins University Press, 1994, pp 64–76

Coccaro E, Kramer E, Zemishlany Z, et al: Pharmacologic treatment of noncognitive behavioral disturbances in elderly demented patients. Am J Psychiatry 147: 1640–1645, 1990

Cohen CA, Gold DP, Shulman KJ, et al: Factors determining the decision to institutionalize dementing individuals: a prospective study. Gerontologist 33:714–720, 1993

Cohen D, Luchins DJ, Eisdorfer C: Caring for relatives with Alzheimer's disease: the mental health risks to spouses, adult children and other family caregivers. Behavior, Health and Aging 1:171–182, 1990

Colenda CC, Hamer RM: Antecedents and interventions for aggressive behavior of patients at a geropsychiatric state hospital. Hospital and Community Psychiatry 42:287–292, 1991

Collins C, Ogle K: Patterns of predeath service use by dementia patients with a family caregiver. J Am Geriatr Soc 42:719–722, 1994

Committee on Aging of the Group for the Advancement of Psychiatry: Impact of tacrine in the care of patients with Alzheimer's disease. J Am Geriatr Soc 2:285–289, 1994

Conrad KJ, Roberts-Gray C (eds): Evaluating Program Environments. San Francisco, CA, Jossey-Bass, 1988

Conrad KJ, Hughes SL, Hanrahan P, et al: Classification of adult day care: a cluster analysis of services and activities. J Gerontol 48:S112–S122, 1993

Consensus Development Conference: Differential diagnosis of dementing diseases. JAMA 258:3411–3416, 1987

Coyne AC, Reichman WE, Berthig LJ: The relationship between dementia and elder abuse. Am J Psychiatry 150:643–646, 1993

Cummings JL, Benson DF: Dementia: A Clinical Approach, 2nd Edition. Boston, MA, Butterworth-Heinemann, 1992

Cummings JL, Kaufer D: Neuropsychiatric aspects of Alzheimer's disease: the cholinergic hypothesis revisited. Neurology 47:876–883, 1996

Cummings JL, Mega M, Gray K, et al: The Neuropsychiatric Inventory: comprehensive assessment of psychopathology in dementia. Neurology 44:2308–2314, 1994

Cunha UGV: An investigation of dementia among elderly outpatients. Acta Psychiatr Scand 82:261–263, 1990

Devanand DP, Sackein HA, Brown RP, et al: A pilot study of haloperidol treatment of psychosis and behavioral disturbance in Alzheimer's disease. Arch Neurol 46:854–857, 1989

Devanand DP, Brockington CD, Moody BJ: Behavioral syndromes in Alzheimer's disease. Int Psychogeriatr 4:16–18, 1992

De Vry J, Fritze J, Post RM: The management of coexisting depression in patients with dementia: potential of calcium channel antagonists. Clin Neuropharmacol 20:22–35, 1997

Donaldson C, Rarrier N, Burns A: The impact of the symptoms of dementia on caregivers. Br J Psychiatry 170:62–68, 1997

Eisdorfer C, Cohen D, Paveza G: An empirical evaluation of the Global Deterioration Scale for staging Alzheimer's disease. Am J Psychiatry 149:195–198, 1992

Engel BT, Burgio LD, McCormick KS: Behavioral treatment of incontinence in the long-term care setting. J Am Geriatr Soc 38:361–363, 1990

Ernst RL, Hay JW: The U.S. economic and social costs of Alzheimer's disease revisited. Am J Public Health 84:1261–1264, 1994

Esiri MM: The basis for behavioural disturbances in dementia. J Neurol Neurosurg Psychiatry 61:127–130, 1996

Evans DL, Edelsohn GA, Golden RN: Organic psychosis without anemia or spinal cord symptoms in patients with vitamin B_{12} deficiency. Am J Psychiatry 140: 218–221, 1983

Faber R: Neuropsychiatric assessment, in American Psychiatric Press Textbook of Geriatric Neuropsychiatry. Edited by Coffey CE, Cummings JL. Washington, DC, American Psychiatric Press, 1994, pp 99–109

Falloon IRH, Boyd JL, McGill CW, et al: Family management in the prevention of exacerbations of schizophrenia: a controlled study. N Engl J Med 306:1437–1440, 1982

Falloon IRH, Boyd JL, McGill CW, et al: Family management in the prevention of morbidity of schizophrenia: clinical outcome of a two-year longitudinal study. Arch Gen Psychiatry 42:887–896, 1985

Fischmann-Havstad L, Marston AR: Weight loss and maintenance as an aspect of family emotion and process. Br J Clin Psychol 23:265–271, 1993

Fisher JE, Carstensen LL: Behavior management of the dementias. Clin Psychol Rev 10:611–629, 1990

Folstein MF, McHugh PR: Dementia syndrome of depression, in Alzheimer's Disease, Senile Dementia and Related Disorders. Edited by Katzman R, Terry RD, Bick KL. New York, Raven, 1978, pp 87–93

Folstein MF, Folstein SE, McHugh PR: Mini-Mental State: a practical method for grading the cognitive state of patients for the clinician. J Psychiatr Res 12: 189–198, 1975

Forsell Y, Jorm AF, Fratiglioni L: Application of DSM-III-R criteria for major depressive episode to elderly subjects with and without dementia. Am J Psychiatry 150:1199–1202, 1993

Förstl H, Burns A, Luthert P, et al: Clinical and neuropathological correlates of depression in Alzheimer's disease. Psychol Med 22:877–884, 1992

Förstl H, Burns A, Levy R, et al: Neuropathological correlates of behavioral disturbances in confirmed Alzheimer's disease. Br J Psychiatry 163:364–368, 1993

Förstl H, Burns A, Levy R, et al: Neuropathological correlates of psychotic phenomena in confirmed Alzheimer's disease. Br J Psychiatry 165:53–59, 1994a

Förstl H, Levy R, Burns A, et al: Disproportionate loss of noradrenergic and cholinergic neurons as cause of depression in Alzheimer's disease. Pharmacopsychiatry 27:11–15, 1994b

Gallagher D, Rose J, Rivera P, et al: Prevalence of depression in family caregivers. Gerontologist 24:449–456, 1989

Ganguli M, Burmeister LA, Seaberg EC, et al: Association between dementia and elevated TSH: a community-based study. Biol Psychiatry 40:714–725, 1996

Gauthier S, Bouchard R, Lamantagne A, et al: Tetrahydroamineacridine-lecithin combination treatment in patients with intermediate-stage Alzheimer's disease. Results of a Canadian double-blind, crossover, multicenter study. N Engl J Med 322:1272–1276, 1990

German PS, Rovner BW, Burton LC: The role of mental morbidity in the nursing home experience. Gerontologist 32:152–158, 1992

Goldman LS, Luchins DJ: Depression in the spouses of demented patients. Am J Psychiatry 141:1467–1468, 1984

Gottlieb GL, McAllister TW, Gur RC: Depot neuroleptics in the treatment of behavioral disorders in patients with Alzheimer's disease. J Am Geriatr Soc 36:619–621, 1988

Green R, Kinsella LJ: Current concepts in the diagnosis of cobalamin deficiency (editorial). Neurology 45:1435–1440, 1995

Greene JA, Asp J, Crane N: Specialized management of the Alzheimer's disease patient: does it make a difference? a preliminary progress report. Journal of the Tennessee Medical Association 78:559–563, 1985

Grossberg GT, Hassan R, Szwabo P, et al: Psychiatric problems in the nursing home: St. Louis Geriatric Grand Rounds. J Am Geriatr Soc 38:907–917, 1990

Hammerstrom DC, Zimmer B: The role of lumbar puncture in the evaluation of dementia: the University of Pittsburgh study. J Am Geriatr Soc 33:397–401, 1985

Hanrahan P, Luchins DJ: Access to hospice care for end-stage dementia patients: a national survey of hospice programs. J Am Geriatr Soc 43:56–59, 1995a

Hanrahan P, Luchins DJ: Feasible criteria for enrolling end-stage dementia patients in home hospice care. Hosp J 10:47–54, 1995b

Haupt M, Kurz A: Predictors of nursing home placement in patients with Alzheimer's disease. Int J Geriatr Psychiatry 8:741–748, 1993

Healton EB, Savage DG, Brust JCM, et al: Neurologic aspects of cobalamin deficiency. Medicine 70:229–245, 1991

Herrmann N, Eryavec G: Buspirone in the management of agitation and aggression associated with dementia. Am J Geriatr Psychiatry 1:249–253, 1993

High DM: All in the family: extended autonomy and expectations in surrogate health care decision-making. Gerontologist 28:46–51, 1988

Hirsch CH, Davies HD, Boatwright F, et al: Effects of a nursing-home respite admission on veterans with advanced dementia. Gerontologist 33:523–528, 1993

Hodges JR: Cognitive Assessment for Clinicians. Oxford, UK, Oxford University Press, 1994

Hogarty GE, Anderson CM, Reiss DJ, et al: Family psychoeducation, social skills training, and maintenance chemotherapy in the after-care of schizophrenia, I: one-year effects of a controlled study on relapse and expressed emotion. Arch Gen Psychiatry 43:633–642, 1986

Hogarty GE, Anderson CM, Reiss DJ, et al: Family psychoeducation, social skills training, and maintenance chemotherapy in the after-care of schizophrenia, II: two-year effects of a controlled study on relapse and adjustment. Arch Gen Psychiatry 48:340–347, 1991

Hughes SL, Cummings J, Weaver F, et al: A randomized trial of Veterans Administration home care for severely disabled veterans. Med Care 28:135–145, 1990

Hughes SL, Cummings J, Weaver F, et al: A randomized trial of the cost effectiveness of VA hospital-based home care for the terminally ill. Health Serv Res 26: 801–817, 1992

Hulette CM, Earl NL, Crain BJ: Evaluation of cerebral biopsies for the diagnosis of dementia. Arch Neurol 49:28–31, 1992

Jenike MA: Treating the violent elderly patient with propranolol. Geriatrics 38: 29–31, 1983

Johnstone EC, Crow TJ, Frith CD, et al: The dementia of dementia praecox. Acta Psychiatr Scand 57:305–324, 1978

Kemper P: The evaluation of the National Long Term Care Demonstration. Overview of the findings. Health Serv Res 23:161–174, 1988

Knapp MJ, Knopman DS, Solomon PR, et al: The Tacrine Study Group: a 30-week randomized controlled trial of high dose tacrine in patients with Alzheimer's disease. JAMA 271:985–991, 1994

Kosloski K, Montgomery RJV: The impact of respite use on nursing home placement. Gerontologist 35:67–74, 1995

Lachs MS, Feinstein AR, Cooney LM, et al: A simple procedure for general screening for functional disability in elderly patients. Ann Intern Med 112:699–706, 1990

Lachs MS, Becker M, Siegal AP, et al: Delusions and behavioral disturbances in cognitively impaired elderly persons. J Am Geriatr Soc 40:768–773, 1992

Larson EB, Reifler BV, Featherstone HJ, et al: Dementia in elderly outpatients: a prospective study. Ann Intern Med 100:417–423, 1984

Lawton MP, Brody EM, Saperstein AR: A controlled study of respite services for caregivers of Alzheimer's patients. Gerontologist 29:8–16, 1989

Leff J: Family factors in schizophrenia. Psychiatric Annals 19:542–545, 1989

Leff J, Vaughn C: Expressed Emotion in Families: Its Significance for Mental Illness. New York, Guilford, 1985

Leon JD, Potter D, Cunningham P: Current and projected availability of special nursing home programs for Alzheimer's disease patients (DHHS Publ No PHS 90-3463). National Medical Expenditure Survey Data Summary 1; Agency for Health Care Policy and Research. Rockville, MD, U.S. Public Health Service, 1990

Linsk N, Hanrahan P, Pinkston EM: Teaching older people and their families to use community resources, in Clinical Behavior Therapy for the Elderly Client. Edited by Wisocki PA. New York, Plenum, 1991, pp 479–504

Luchins DJ, Hanrahan P: What is the appropriate level of health care for end-stage dementia patients? J Am Geriatr Soc 41:25–30, 1993

Luchins DJ, Hanrahan P, Mathews MD, et al: Negative expressed emotion among families of dementia patients compared to families of schizophrenics. Paper presented at the annual meeting of the American Psychiatric Association, New York, 1990

Luchins DJ, Dojka DM, Hanrahan P: Factors associated with reduction in antipsychotic medication dosage in mentally retarded adults. Am J Ment Retard 98:165–172, 1993

Luchins DJ, Hanrahan P, Murphy K: Criteria for enrolling dementia patients in hospice. J Am Geriatr Soc 45:1054–1059, 1997

MacKenzie TB, Robiner WN, Knopman DS: Differences between patient and family assessments of depression in Alzheimer's disease. Am J Psychiatry 146:1174–1178, 1989

Maltby N, Broco HA, Creasey H, et al: Efficacy of tacrine and lecithin in mild to moderate Alzheimer's disease: double-blind trial. BMJ 308:879–883, 1994

Mann AH, Jenkins R, Cross PS, et al: A comparison of the prescriptions received by the elderly in long-term care in New York and London. Psychiatr Med 14:891–897, 1984

Marin RS, Fogel BS, Hawkins J, et al: Apathy: a treatable syndrome. J Neuropsychiatry Clin Neurosci 7:23–30, 1995

Marks WA, Shuman RM, Leech RW, et al: Cerebral degenerations producing dementia: importance of neuropathologic confirmation of clinical diagnoses. J Geriatr Psychiatry Neurol 1:187–198, 1988

Martin DC, Miller JK, Kapoor W, et al: A controlled study of survival with dementia. Arch Neurol 44:1122–1126, 1987

Mayeux R, Foster NL, Rossor M, et al: The clinical evaluation of patients with dementia, in Dementia. Edited by Whitehouse PJ. Philadelphia, PA, FA Davis, 1993, pp 92–129

Mazure CM, Druss BG, Cellar JS: Valproate treatment of older psychotic patients with organic mental syndromes and behavioral dyscontrol. J Am Geriatr Soc 40:914–916, 1992

McDaniel LD, Lukovits T, McDaniel KD: Alzheimer's disease: the problem of incorrect clinical diagnosis. J Geriatr Psychiatry Neurol 6:230–234, 1993

McKeith IG, Perry RH, Fairbairn AF, et al: Operational criteria for senile dementia of Lewy body type (SDLT). Psychol Med 22:911–922, 1992

McShane R, Keene J, Gedling K, et al: Do neuroleptic drugs hasten cognitive decline in dementia? prospective study with necropsy follow up. BMJ 314:266–270, 1997

Meco G, Alessandria A, Bonifati V, et al: Risperidone for hallucinations in levo-dopa treated Parkinson's disease patients. Lancet 343:1320–1371, 1994

Mega MS, Cummings JL, Fiorello T, et al: The spectrum of behavioral changes in Alzheimer's disease. Neurology 46:130–135, 1996

Meltzer HY, Cola P, Way L, et al: Cost effectiveness of clozapine in neuroleptic resistant schizophrenia. Am J Psychiatry 150:1630–1638, 1993

Miller BL, Cummings JL, Villanueva-Meyer J, et al: Frontal lobe degeneration: clinical, neuropsychological, and SPECT characteristics. Neurology 41:1374–1382, 1991

Mintzer JE, Lewis L, Pennypaker L, et al: Behavioral Intensive Care Unit (BICU): a new concept in the management of acute agitated behavior in elderly demented patients. Gerontologist 33:801–806, 1993

Moak GS, Fisher WH: Alzheimer's disease and related disorders in state mental hospitals: data from a nationwide survey. Gerontologist 30:798–802, 1990

Montamat SC, Cusack B, Vestal RE: Management of drug therapy in the elderly. N Engl J Med 321:303–309, 1989

Morris JC, McKeel DW, Storandt M, et al: Very mild Alzheimer's disease: informant-based clinical, psychometric, and pathologic distinction from normal aging. Neurology 41:469–478, 1991

Myers RM, Grodin MA: Decision making regarding the initiation of tube feedings in the severely demented elderly: a review. J Am Geriatr Soc 39:526–531, 1991

Nasman F, Bucht G, Eriksson S: Behavioural symptoms in the institutionalized elderly: relationship to dementia. Int J Geriatr Psychiatry 8:843–849, 1993

Neary D: Classification of the dementias. Reviews in Clinical Gerontology 4: 131–140, 1994

O'Donnell BF, Drachman DA, Barnes HJ, et al: Incontinence and troublesome behaviors predict institutionalization in dementia. J Geriatr Psychiatry Neurol 5:45–52, 1992

Olpe HR, Steinmann MW: The effects of vincamine, Hydergine and piracetam on the firing rate of locus coeruleus neurons. J Neural Transm 55:101–109, 1982

Ott BR, Fogel BS: Measurement of depression in dementia: self vs clinician rating. Int J Geriatr Psychiatry 7:899–904, 1992

Ouslander JG, Zarit SH, Orr NK, et al: Incontinence among elderly community-dwelling patients: characteristics, management and impact on caregivers. J Am Geriatr Soc 38:440–445, 1990

Overall JE, Gorham DR: The Brief Psychiatric Rating Scale. Psychol Rep 10: 799–812, 1962

Ovsiew F: Neuropsychiatric sequelae of brain injury of vascular and traumatic origin. Current Opinion in Psychiatry 6:101–108, 1993

Ovsiew F: Bedside neuropsychiatry: eliciting the clinical phenomena of neuropsychiatric illness, in American Psychiatric Press Textbook of Neuropsychiatry, 3rd Edition. Edited by Yudofsky SC, Hales RE. Washington, DC, American Psychiatric Press, 1997, pp 121–163

Paveza GJ, Cohen D, Eisdorfer S, et al: Severe family violence and Alzheimer's disease: prevalence and risk factors. Gerontologist 32:493–497, 1992

Peck A, Walloch L, Rodstein M: Mortality of the aged with chronic brain syndrome. J Am Geriatr Soc 26:170–174, 1978

Perry EK, McKeith I, Thompson P, et al: Topography, extent, and clinical relevance of neurochemical deficits in dementia of Lewy body type, Parkinson's disease, and Alzheimer's disease. Ann N Y Acad Sci 640:197–202, 1991

Pilemer K, Suitor JJ: Violence and violent feelings: what causes them among family caregivers? J Gerontol 47:S165–S172, 1992

Pinkston EM, Linsk N: Care of the elderly: a family approach. New York, Pergamon, 1984

Pinner E, Rich CL: Effects of trazodone on aggressive behavior in seven patients with organic mental disorders. Am J Psychiatry 145:1295–1296, 1988

Poser CM: Automobile driving fitness and neurological impairment. J Neuropsychiatry Clin Neurosci 5:342–348, 1993

President's Commission for the Study of Ethical Principles in Medicine and Biomedical and Behavioral Research: Deciding to Forego Life-Sustaining Treatment. Washington, DC, U.S. Government Printing Office, 1983

Pruchno RA, Resch NL: Husbands and wives as caregivers: antecedents of depression and burden. Gerontologist 29:159–165, 1989

Quality Standards Subcommittee of the American Academy of Neurology: Practice parameter for diagnosis and evaluation of dementia. Neurology 44:2203–2206, 1994

Rabins PV: Does reversible dementia exist and is it reversible? Arch Intern Med 148:1905, 1988

Rabins PV: Behavior problems in the demented, in Alzheimer's Disease Treatment and Family Stress: Directions for Research. Edited by Light E, Lebowitz BD. Rockville, MD, U.S. Department of Health and Human Services, 1989, pp 322–339

Radloff LS: The CES-D Scale: a self-report depression scale for research in the general population. Applied Psychological Measurement 1:385–401, 1977

Ray WA, Griffin MR, Schaffner W, et al: Psychotropic drug use and the risk of hip fracture. N Engl J Med 316:363–369, 1987

Reding M, Haycox J, Blass J: Depression in patients referred to a dementia clinic: a three-year prospective study. Arch Neurol 42:894–896, 1985

Reeves RR, Pinkofsky HB, Kennedy KK: Unreliability of current screening tests for syphilis in chronic psychiatric patients. Am J Psychiatry 153:1487–1488, 1996

Reisberg B, Ferris SH, De Leon MJ, et al: The Global Deterioration Scale for assessment of primary degenerative dementia. Am J Psychiatry 139:1136–1139, 1982

Rice DP, Fox PJ, Max W: The economic burden of Alzheimer's disease care. Health Aff (Millwood) 12:164–176, 1993

Risse SC, Barnes R: Pharmacological treatment of agitation associated with dementia. J Am Geriatr Soc 34:368–371, 1986

Rogers SL, Friedhoff LT, and the Donepezil Study Group: The efficacy and safety of donepezil in patients with Alzheimer's disease: results of a U.S. multicentre, randomized, double-blind, placebo-controlled trial. Dementia 7:293–303, 1996

Rovner BW, German PS, Broadhead J: The prevalence and management of dementia and other psychiatric disorders in nursing homes. Int Psychogeriatr 2:13–24, 1990

Royall DR, Mahurin RK, Gray K: Bedside assessment of executive impairment: the Executive Interview (EXIT). J Am Geriatr Soc 40:1221–1226, 1992

Ryan DH: Age-specific hospital incidence rates in dementia. A record linkage study of first admission rates to Scottish hospitals (1968–1987). Dementia 5:29–35, 1994

Sachs G, Stocking C, Miles S: Empowerment of the elderly: increasing advance directives? Gerontologist 29:190(A), 1989

Salzman C: The APA Task Force Report on benzodiazepine dependence, toxicity and abuse. Am J Psychiatry 148:151–152, 1991

Sandson TA, Price BH: Diagnostic testing and dementia. Neurol Clin 14:45–59, 1996

Sano M, Ernesto C, Thomas RG, et al: A controlled trial of selegiline, alpha-tocopherol, or both as treatment for Alzheimer's disease. N Engl J Med 336:1216–1222, 1997

Schneider LS, Sobin PB: Non-neuroleptic treatment of behavioral symptoms and agitation in Alzheimer's disease and other dementia. Psychopharmacol Bull 28:71–79, 1992

Schneider LS, Pollack VE, Lyness SA: A metaanalysis of controlled trials of neuroleptic treatment in dementia. J Am Geriatr Soc 38:553–563, 1990

Schneider LS, Olin JT, Pawluczyk S: A double-blind crossover pilot study of L-deprenyl (selegiline) combined with cholinesterase inhibitor in Alzheimer's disease. Am J Psychiatry 150:321–323, 1993

Semla TP, Palla K, Poddig B, et al: Effect of the Omnibus Reconciliation Act 1987 on antipsychotic prescribing in nursing home residents. J Am Geriatr Soc 42:648–652, 1994

Shope JT, Holmes SB, Sharpe PA, et al: Services for persons with dementia and their families: a survey of information and referral agencies in Michigan. Gerontologist 33:529–533, 1993

Simpson DM, Foster D: Improvement in organically disturbed behavior with trazodone treatment. J Clin Psychiatry 47:191–193, 1986

Skoog I, Nielson L, Palmertz B, et al: A population based study of dementia in 85 year olds. N Engl J Med 328:153–158, 1993

Sloane PD, Lindeman DA, Phillips C, et al: Evaluating Alzheimer's special care units: reviewing the evidence and identifying potential sources of study bias. Gerontologist 35:103–111, 1995

Sobin P, Schneider L, McDermott H: Fluoxetine in the treatment of agitated dementia (letter). Am J Psychiatry 146:1636, 1989

Steele C, Lucas MJ, Tune LE: An approach to the management of dementia syndromes. Johns Hopkins Medical Journal 151:362–368, 1982

Steiber SR: Right to die: public balks at deciding for others. Hospitals 61:72, 1987

Stone R, Cafferata GL, Sangl J: Caregivers of the frail elderly: a national profile. Gerontologist 27:616–626, 1987

Strahan G, Burns BJ: Mental Illness in Nursing Homes: United States, 1985. Hyattsville, MD, U.S. Department of Health and Human Services, 1991

Sultzer DL: Mental status examination, in American Psychiatric Press Textbook of Geriatric Neuropsychiatry. Edited by Coffey CE, Cummings JL. Washington, DC, American Psychiatric Press, 1994, pp 111–127

Swanson EA, Maas ML, Buchwalter KC: Catastrophic reactions and other behaviors of Alzheimer's residents: special units compared with traditional units. Arch Psychiatr Nurs 5:292–299, 1993

Swanson EA, Maas ML, Buchwalter KC: Alzheimer's residents' cognitive and functional measures: special and traditional unit comparison. Clinical Nursing Research 3:27–41, 1994

Tariot PN, Cohen RM, Sunderland T, et al: L-deprenyl in Alzheimer's disease: preliminary evidence for behavioral change with monoamine oxidase B inhibition. Arch Gen Psychiatry 44:427–433, 1987

Tariot PN, Erb R, Leibovici A, et al: Carbamazepine treatment of agitation in nursing home patients with dementia: a preliminary study. J Am Geriatr Soc 42:1160–1166, 1994

Teri L, Uomoto, JM: Reducing excess disability in dementia patients: training caregivers to manage patient depression. Clinical Gerontologist 10:49–63, 1991

Teri L, Larson EB, Reifler BV: Behavioral disturbance in dementia of the Alzheimer's type. J Am Geriatr Soc 36:1–6, 1988

Tollefson GD: Short-term effects of the calcium channel blocker nimodipine (Bay-e-9726) in the management of primary degenerative dementia. Biol Psychiatry 27:1133–1142, 1990

Tollefson GD, Bodick NC, Shannon HC, et al: Xanomeline: a potent and specific M_1 agonist in the treatment of Alzheimer's disease. American College of Neuropsychopharmacology, San Juan, Puerto Rico, 1994, p 31

Tuck RR, Jackson M: Social, neurological and cognitive disorders in alcoholics. Med J Aust 155:225–229, 1991

Vanneste JAL: Three decades of normal pressure hydrocephalus: are we wiser now? J Neurol Neurosurg Psychiatry 57:1021–1025, 1994

Victoroff J, Zarow C, Mack WJ, et al: Physical aggression is associated with preservation of substantia nigra pars compacta in Alzheimer disease. Arch Neurol 53: 428–434, 1996

Vitaliano PP, Becker J, Fusso J, et al: Expressed emotion in spouse caregivers of patients with Alzheimer's disease. Journal of Applied Social Science 131:215–250, 1989

Volicer BJ, Hurley A, Fabiszewski KJ, et al: Predicting short-term survival for patients with advanced Alzheimer's disease. J Am Geriatr Soc 41:535–540, 1993

Volicer L, Rheaume Y, Brown J, et al: Hospice approach to the treatment of patients with advanced dementia of the Alzheimer type. JAMA 256:2210–2213, 1986

Volicer L, Collard A, Hurley A, et al: Impact of special care unit for patients with advanced Alzheimer's disease on patients' discomfort and costs. J Am Geriatr Soc 42:597–603, 1994

Wan TTH, Weissert WG, Livierators BB: Geriatric day care and homemaker services: an experimental study. J Gerontol 35:256–274, 1980

Watkins PB, Zimmerman HJ, Knapp MJ, et al: Hepatotoxic effects of tacrine administration in patients with Alzheimer's disease. JAMA 271:992–998, 1994

Weiner MF, Edland SD, Luszczynska H: Prevalence and incidence of major depression in Alzheimer's disease. Am J Psychiatry 151:1006–1009, 1994

Welch HG, Walsh JS, Larson EB: The cost of institutional care in Alzheimer's disease: nursing home and hospital use in a prospective cohort. J Am Geriatr Soc 40:221–224, 1992

Wells Y, Jorm AF: Evaluation of a special nursing home unit for dementia sufferers: a randomized controlled comparison with community care. Aust N Z J Psychiatry 21:524–531, 1987

Wernicke TF, Reisches FM: Prevalence of dementia in old age: clinical diagnoses in subjects ages 95 years and older. Neurology 44:250–253, 1994

Winker A: Tacrine for Alzheimer's disease. Which patient? Which dose? JAMA 271:1023–1024, 1994

Wragg RE, Jeste DV: Overview of depression and psychosis in Alzheimer's disease. Am J Psychiatry 146:577–587, 1989

Yesavage JA, Tinklenberg JR, Hollister LE, et al: Vasodilators in senile dementias: a review of the literature. Arch Gen Psychiatry 31:220–223, 1979

Zarit SH, Reever KE, Bach-Peterson J: Relatives of the impaired elderly: correlates of feelings of burden. Gerontologist 20:649–655, 1980

Zarit SH, Todd PA, Zarit JM: Subjective burden of husbands and wives as caregivers: a longitudinal study. Gerontologist 26:260–266, 1986

Zimmer JG, Groth-Juncker A, McCusker J: A randomized controlled study of a home health care team. Am J Public Health 75:134–141, 1985

Zubenko GS, Moossy J, Martinez AJ, et al: Neuropathologic and neurochemical correlates of psychosis in primary dementia. Arch Neurol 48:619–624, 1991

Zubenko GS, Rosen J, Sweet RA, et al: Impact of psychiatric hospitalization on behavioral complications of Alzheimer's disease. Am J Psychiatry 149:1484–1491, 1992

CHAPTER 5

Neuropsychiatry of Substance Abuse

E. Jane Marshall, M.R.C.P.(I), M.R.C.Psych.

Substance abuse is a major public health problem worldwide. The total economic cost of alcohol abuse to the United States in 1990 was estimated to be more than $100 billion, mostly related to health care expenses, morbidity, and mortality (Rice 1993). However, the economic cost is only the tip of the iceberg.

Evidence of an association between substance abuse and neuropsychiatric problems is accumulating. However, neuropsychiatric problems are not routinely assessed in substance-abusing populations; their relevance to outcome is poorly understood, and their contribution to the economic, social, and human cost of substance abuse has not been documented. With such gaps in our knowledge, it is not surprising that neuropsychiatric problems do not influence public health policies.

In this chapter, I describe the epidemiology of substance abuse and review the associated neuropsychiatric syndromes. I discuss the implications of these syndromes in the assessment and treatment of psychiatric patients in public health settings, with a focus on the clinical and institutional requirements for appropriate treatment.

Epidemiology of Substance Abuse

Alcohol Abuse/Dependence

In the United States, the five-site Epidemiologic Catchment Area (ECA) study estimated a 13.8% lifetime prevalence for alcohol abuse/dependence (Helzer et al. 1991) as defined in DSM-III (American Psychiatric Association 1980). Lifetime prevalence rates were higher for men (23.8%) than for women (4.6%) and were highest in the 18- to 29-year and 30- to 44-year age groups for both sexes. Male-to-female ratios were lower in the younger age groups, suggesting convergence. Ethnic differences emerged, with Hispanics having a higher lifetime prevalence (16.7%) than whites (13.6%) or African Americans (13.8%). Hispanic men had the highest lifetime prevalence and Hispanic women the lowest lifetime prevalence compared with whites and African Americans. One-year prevalence rates were 6.8% for all respondents, 11.9% for men and 2.2% for women.

In 1988 a national survey on alcoholism was included in the Annual Nationwide Household Survey, and the 1-year prevalence of alcohol abuse/dependence, as defined in DSM-III-R (American Psychiatric Association 1987), was estimated at 13.4% of all males and 4.4% of all females (B. F. Grant et al. 1992). This study supported convergence in prevalence among men and women.

In Great Britain, no epidemiologic data exist on alcohol abuse/dependence comparable to the ECA data. A recent national survey indicated that 27% of men and 11% of women were drinking above the recommended sensible levels of 21 U/week for men and 14 U/week for women (Office of Population Censuses and Surveys 1990, 1995).

Chronic alcohol abuse is associated with a range of neuropsychiatric impairments. It is estimated that general cerebral impairment associated with long-term use of alcohol accounts for approximately 10% of adult dementia (Oscar-Berman 1990b), though this is likely to be an underestimate. Autopsy studies suggest that Korsakoff's syndrome occurs in 1.7%–2.8% of alcoholic patients (Victor et al. 1989). This diagnosis, however, is often missed. Neuropsychological deficits associated with chronic alcohol consumption may be more common than is generally realized. Polysubstance abuse is frequent among younger alcoholic patients and is likely to affect neuropsychiatric function. The co-use of alcohol and cocaine is a problem that occurs more commonly than would be expected by chance.

Drug Abuse/Dependence

The ECA study estimated a 6.2% lifetime prevalence of an abuse/dependence syndrome, as defined in DSM-III, involving illicit drugs (Anthony and Helzer

1991). Prevalence levels were 7.7% for men and 4.8% for women, concentrated in the 18- to 29-year and 30- to 44-year age groups. Cannabis abuse/dependence was the most commonly diagnosed drug disorder, affecting an estimated 4.4% of the adult population. Lifetime prevalence estimates were under 1% for opioid abuse/dependence (0.7%), hallucinogen abuse (0.4%), and cocaine abuse (0.2%). The prevalence levels for abuse/dependence of sedatives and stimulants were 1.2% and 1.7%, respectively. Ethnicity was related to drug abuse/dependence, with whites having the highest rates; Hispanics, the lowest; and African Americans, intermediate rates.

Since these data were collected in the early 1980s, important changes have taken place in drug use prevalence in the United States (Kandel 1992). The use of all classes of illicit drugs has been declining. Cocaine use in the population peaked in 1986, several years later than for most other illicit drugs. The annual number of cocaine-related emergency room admissions increased fourfold between 1985 and 1988, from 10,248 to 42,512 (Harrison 1992). The number of cocaine-related deaths over the same period also increased, from 717 to 2,252. Admissions and deaths stabilized in 1989 and fell thereafter. This increase in cocaine-related admissions and deaths could possibly be explained by a trend toward more dangerous routes of administration, especially freebasing and smoking crack cocaine.

In Great Britain, no reliable figures exist for drug abuse/dependence. Population surveys suggest that the drugs most commonly used are cannabis and volatile substances such as glue or butane gas (Institute for the Study of Drug Dependence 1994). Recent surveys indicate a trend for more young people to sample amphetamines, lysergic acid diethylamide (LSD), and 3,4-methylenedioxymethamphetamine (MDMA, or ecstasy). The rise in use of LSD and ecstasy has paralleled the emergence of a new youth culture centered on "rave" and dance music. Among 16- to 19-year-olds, 11% have used amphetamines, 9% ecstasy, and 8% LSD (Mott and Mirrlees-Black 1993). Among population samples, fewer than 1% report ever using heroin, cocaine, or crack. Rates may be higher in deprived urban areas, where samples of 16- to 25-year-olds indicate that 1% have used crack cocaine and 2% and 4% have used heroin and cocaine, respectively. The prevalence of dependent illicit drug use is less than 1%, as is the proportion of the British population that has injected.

Neuropsychiatric Effects of Alcohol Abuse/Dependence

The mechanisms underlying neuropsychiatric complications in individuals abusing or dependent on alcohol are complex. Poor nutrition and diminished vitamin reserves predispose to thiamine and nicotinic acid depletion. Alcohol has a direct neurotoxic action and produces neuronal death in animals (Freund 1973; Melgaard 1983) and possibly in the human brain. Acetaldehyde, the main metabolite of alcohol, is a highly reactive and toxic substance and may have a similar effect. Metabolic factors, such as hypoxia, electrolyte imbalance, and hypoglycemia, which result from acute or chronic intoxication and withdrawal, are also important. Recurrent alcohol withdrawal has been hypothesized to have a kindling effect (Ballenger and Post 1978; Becker and Hale 1993). "Kindling" means that each episode of alcohol withdrawal plays a role in the progression of the disorder by producing more severe withdrawal symptoms and causing neurodegeneration, perhaps via excitotoxicity. If this is true, withdrawal symptoms should be treated aggressively to prevent progression of alcohol-related brain damage.

During alcohol withdrawal, N-methyl-D-aspartate (NMDA) function increases, and it is postulated that this leads to increased neuronal excitability and to glutamate-induced neurotoxicity (Grant et al. 1990; Little 1991; Michaelis and Michaelis 1980; Tsai et al. 1995). Evidence also points to a marked activation of the hypothalamic-pituitary-adrenal axis (HPA) during withdrawal (Hawley et al. 1985). In particular, plasma cortisol concentrations are raised during withdrawal (Adinoff et al. 1991) and may contribute to alcohol-related cognitive impairment. Neuropsychiatric syndromes can develop as a result of other alcohol-induced physical complications, including alcohol withdrawal seizures, hepatic encephalopathy, subarachnoid hemorrhage, and stroke. Head injuries are common in this group and may cause subdural hematomata and posttraumatic epilepsy.

Intoxication States

After an initial excitatory action on the cerebral cortex, alcohol depresses both cortical and subcortical structures. Neuropsychiatric complications include memory blackouts, pathological intoxication, seizures, sedation, and coma.

Memory blackouts are acute episodes of alcohol-induced memory loss that are most closely related to early onset of drinking, high peak levels of alcohol, and a history of head trauma (Kopelman 1991). Memory blackouts are not predictive of long-term cognitive impairment (Tarter and Schneider 1976).

Pathological intoxication (mania à potu) describes acute episodes of aggression and often violent behavior, which occur soon after drinking small amounts of alcohol and are followed by a prolonged sleep and amnesia for events (Coid 1979; World Health Organization 1992). An association with abnormalities on the electroencephalogram (EEG) and other signs of organic brain damage, particularly frontal lobe dysfunction, is a possibility.

Seizures have been reported during acute intoxication, when blood alcohol levels are high, but they are rare, and the concept of acute intoxication as a cause of seizures remains controversial (Hauser et al. 1988).

The clinical features of *alcohol intoxication* are related to blood alcohol concentrations. Severe intoxication with stupor, hypoglycemia, and seizures is seen at levels of 300–500 mg/100 mL. *Coma* ensues at concentrations over 500 mg/100 mL. Alcohol-dependent individuals have higher blood alcohol concentrations for a given clinical picture because of their increased tolerance.

When the presentation is one of severe intoxication or coma, other causes must be ruled out and treated, including hypoglycemia, head injury (and subdural hematoma), systemic injection, and accidental or intentional overdose with licit or illicit drugs (Peters 1996).

Withdrawal Syndrome

Severe alcohol syndromes are relatively rare and include withdrawal seizures and delirium tremens.

Withdrawal seizures are generalized (grand mal) seizures that occur between 12 and 48 hours after cessation of drinking in about 5%–15% of alcohol-dependent individuals (Brennan and Lyttle 1987). During a particular withdrawal period, the patient may have only one seizure, but more commonly there will be three to four seizures over a couple of days. Status epilepticus is rare. Predisposing factors include hypokalemia, hypomagnesemia, a history of withdrawal seizures, and concurrent epilepsy. The EEG is generally unhelpful (Victor and Brausch 1967), but computed tomography (CT) may help to rule out underlying intracranial lesions (Earnest et al. 1988). Alcohol-dependent individuals who have experienced withdrawal seizures are prone to developing further seizures in future withdrawal episodes. Therefore, detoxification should be carried out in an inpatient setting.

Delirium tremens is a toxic confusional state that occurs as a result of alcohol reduction in chronically alcohol-dependent individuals. Symptoms typically occur from about 24 to 150 hours after the last drink and peak between 72 and 96 hours (Naranjo and Sellers 1986). Onset is usually at night and is accompanied by restlessness, insomnia, and fear (Lishman 1998). The classic triad of symptoms includes clouding of consciousness and confusion, vivid hallucinations affecting any sensory modality, and marked tremor. Delusions, agitation, sleeplessness, and autonomic activity (tachycardia, marked elevation in blood pressure, increased respiratory rate, and pyrexia) are often present (Nordstrum and Bergland 1988).

Predisposing factors include severe medical problems, recent surgery, pyrexia, hypoglycemia, hypokalemia, and hypocalcemia. The condition usually lasts for 3–5 days with gradual resolution. The mortality rate is approximately 5% of admissions (Cushman 1987).

Organic Brain Syndrome

Chronic heavy use of alcohol is associated with a variety of organic syndromes that arise as a result of alcohol-related vitamin deficiencies, the chronic toxic effect of alcohol, trauma, and metabolic disturbance. These problems usually occur in combination, albeit to differing degrees.

Wernicke-Korsakoff syndrome, caused by thiamine depletion, has long been regarded as the classic form of brain damage in alcoholism. Wernicke's encephalopathy, the acute component, consists of the triad of ophthalmoplegia, gait ataxia, and abnormal mental state (acute confusion, impairment of consciousness). The Korsakoff syndrome, the chronic component, is characterized by profound anterograde and retrograde amnesia, disorientation in time and place, and lack of insight (Jacobson et al. 1990). Associated neurological abnormalities include polyneuropathy, nystagmus, and ataxia, the latter two signs being related to earlier episodes of Wernicke's syndrome.

If treated promptly with parenteral thiamine, Wernicke's encephalopathy does not progress to chronic Korsakoff's syndrome. However, the diagnosis is often missed in life because clinical signs are atypical or absent (Cravioto et al. 1961; Harper 1983; Harper et al. 1986; Reuler et al. 1985; Victor et al. 1971). Thiamine-dependent brain damage may exist in many alcoholic patients long before it is suspected, developing either insidiously or in a stepwise fashion during repeated subclinical episodes of Wernicke's syndrome. This hypothesis would explain why the amnesic symptom of Korsakoff's syndrome does not generally improve after the administration of thiamine.

Although Wernicke's and Korsakoff's syndromes are distinguishable clinically, the underlying neuropathological lesions are the same and are located in the paraventricular and periaqueductal gray matter, the walls of the third ventricle, the floor of the fourth ventricle, and the cerebellum (Harper 1983; Victor et al. 1971). The circuit involving the mammillary bodies, the mammillothalamic tract, and the anterior thalamus is now thought to be particularly critical in the formation of new memories (Kopelman 1995). Cortical abnormalities (selective neuronal loss in the frontal lobes and generalized neuronal shrinkage) and loss of white matter (Harper et al. 1985, 1987a) are also reported. It has been hypothesized that these cortical abnormalities could be a remote effect of lesions within diencephalic structures that project to the frontal cortex. Frontal lobe dysfunction could explain the apathy, lack of initiative and insight, and the retrograde amnesia displayed by patients with Korsakoff's syndrome.

CT confirms the presence of cortical and subcortical damage in patients with Wernicke-Korsakoff syndrome (Jacobson 1989; Jacobson and Lishman 1987; Shimamura et al. 1988), and low-density lesions in the diencephalon of patients with acute Wernicke's encephalopathy have been reported (McDowell and LeBlanc 1984; Mensing et al. 1984; Shimamura et al. 1988).

Magnetic resonance imaging (MRI) can identify small lesions in patients with acute Wernicke's encephalopathy that would be missed by CT (Gallucci et al. 1990). Chronic lesions are not as easily identified because they may have resolved, either fully or partially (Donnal et al. 1990). MRI studies indicate reduced mammillary body volume (Charness and De La Paz 1987; Squire et al. 1990) and widespread cortical and subcortical gray matter loss, particularly in the anterior diencephalon and mesial temporal and orbitofrontal regions, in patients with Korsakoff's syndrome (Jernigan et al. 1991b).

Cerebral blood flow is reduced in both the cerebral cortex and subcortical white matter in acute Wernicke's encephalopathy, returning to normal after thiamine replacement (Meyer et al. 1985). Frontal cortical blood flow has been reported as impaired in Korsakoff's syndrome (Hunter et al. 1989). In a positron-emission tomography (PET) study of nine patients with Korsakoff's syndrome, Joyce (1994) found a relative reduction in glucose utilization in medial hemispheric areas corresponding to anterior cingulate cortex and the precuneate region, even when analysis allowed for cortical shrinkage.

In vivo CT and MRI investigations complement autopsy studies of the alcoholic brain, confirming *brain shrinkage*, particularly in the frontal cortex, and ventricular enlargement, compared with brains of age-matched control subjects (H. Bergman et al. 1980a; Cala et al. 1980; Carlen et al. 1978, 1981; Harper and Kril, 1985, 1988; Harper et al. 1984, 1985; Ron 1983; Ron et al. 1980, 1982). These changes are evident in young "social drinkers" (Cala et al. 1983) but are more prominent in older age groups (Cala et al. 1978), and women seem to be particularly susceptible. Abstinence leads to reversibility of brain shrinkage, but this is more likely to occur in younger individuals and in women (Carlen and Wilkinson 1987; Jacobson 1986). Many abstinent alcoholic patients continue to have enlarged ventricles (Carlen and Wilkinson 1980).

CT studies also have revealed altered absorption densities in the brains of alcoholic patients (Cala 1982; Carlen and Wilkinson 1987; Golden et al. 1981; Gurling et al. 1986; Lishman et al. 1987). These findings are not fully understood but "may reflect some enduring abnormality in the brains of alcoholics that serves as a marker of their past addiction" (Lishman 1990, p. 638).

MRI studies confirm cortical atrophy and mild ventricular enlargement (Jernigan et al. 1991a; Pfefferbaum et al. 1992). Volume reductions in localized cortical and subcortical cerebral structures have also been reported, particularly in the diencephalon, caudate nucleus, dorsolateral frontal and parietal cortex, and mesial temporal lobe structures (Jernigan et al. 1991a). These structural changes did not correlate with lifetime alcohol intake, and it is thought that the vulnerability to such abnormalities may increase with age (Pfefferbaum et al. 1992).

Functional neuroimaging (PET) studies of alcoholic patients without Korsakoff's syndrome have revealed a relative decrease in glucose utilization within the medial frontal cortex (Gilman et al. 1990; Samson et al. 1986).

Brain shrinkage in alcoholic patients is related to a selective loss of white matter in the cerebral hemispheres (Harper et al. 1985; Jensen and Pakkenberg 1993). Harper's group (Harper and Kril 1989; Harper et al. 1987a, 1987b; Kril and Harper 1989) reported selective neuronal loss in the superior frontal cortex of alcoholic patients, but Jensen and Pakkenberg (1993) did not find any loss of total neocortical neurons in the brains of 11 chronic alcoholic men compared with a matched control group. However, animal research suggests that alcohol has a direct neurotoxic effect (Riley and Walker 1978; Walker et al. 1980; West et al. 1982), and abstinence in a rat model was followed by an increase in the dendritic arborization of hippocampal pyramidal neurons (McMullen et al. 1984).

Regarding *neuropsychological deficits*, many individuals with a history of chronic alcohol abuse have mild-to-moderate impairment in short- and long-term memory, learning, visuoperceptual abstraction, visuospatial organization, the maintenance of cognitive set, and impulse control (Oscar-Berman 1990a). This tendency for alcoholic patients to show proportionally greater visuospatial than language-related functional impairments suggested that alcohol might have a selective effect on the right hemisphere: the "right hemisphere hypothesis" (Oscar-Berman and Ellis 1987). However, right hemisphere functions also decline with aging, and the current view is that the functional lateralities of alcoholic patients and aging individuals are similar to those of normal control subjects (Ellis and Oscar-Berman 1989). Neuropsychological performance improves with abstinence, but impairments are still detectable after 5 years of abstinence (Brandt et al. 1983). Performance on cognitive tests has generally been poorly correlated with CT scan changes (Carlen et al. 1981; Ron 1983).

Alcoholic cerebellar degeneration usually develops insidiously and is characterized by ataxic gait and uncoordinated legs (Victor et al. 1959). Nystagmus and dysarthria occur rarely. Alcoholic cerebellar degeneration is thought to be the result of thiamine deficiency, but alcohol neurotoxicity may also play a part. Pathological lesions occur mainly in the midline cerebellar structures, particularly the vermis and to a lesser degree the anterior lobe. Significant loss of Purkinje cells (Phillips et al. 1987; Torvik and Torp 1986) and shrinkage of the molecular and granular layers occur.

Cerebellum degeneration may be asymptomatic in chronically alcohol-dependent individuals. Haubeck and Lee (1979), in their CT study, reported atrophy of the anterior and superior parts of the cerebellar vermis in the absence of clinical signs. A PET study found that patients with clinical evidence of alcoholic cerebellar degeneration had reduced glucose utilization in the superior cerebellar vermis and in the medial frontal cortex bilaterally (Gilman et al. 1990).

Alcoholic pellagra encephalopathy is caused by deficiency of nicotinic acid and of its precursor, tryptophan (Serdaru et al. 1988). Clinical features include a fluctuating confusional state with global memory loss, visual hallucinations, and restlessness alternating with apathy and other physical signs, including myoclonic jerks and hyperreflexia.

Vitamin B_{12} deficiency should always be considered in the differential diagnosis of an organic brain syndrome in someone with an alcohol problem. Malnutrition and malabsorption of vitamin B_{12} are the two main mechanisms underlying this deficiency in alcoholic patients. The psychiatric disturbance associated with vitamin B_{12} deficiency includes affective disorder, schizophrenia, paranoid states, episodes of disorientation and delirium, and progressive dementia (Lishman 1998). Neurological disturbances include subacute combined degeneration of the cord and a peripheral neuropathy.

Marchiafava-Bignami disease is a rare disorder of the corpus callosum and adjacent subcortical white matter that is not confined to alcoholic patients. The etiology is unknown, but a nutritional deficiency or a contaminant of alcohol has been postulated. Marchiafava-Bignami disease may present insidiously, with dementia, spasticity, dysarthria, and inability to walk, or acutely, with agitation, apathy, hallucinations, epilepsy, and coma. Lesions can be seen on CT and MRI scans (Kawamura et al. 1985).

Central pontine myelinolysis (CPM), first described by Adams et al. (1959), is a neurological disorder caused by the rapid correction of hyponatremia (Laureno and Karp 1988). Extrapontine lesions affecting the thalamus, internal capsule, cerebellum, lower levels of the cerebral cortex, and adjacent white matter occur in approximately 10% of patients (Wright et al. 1979). The clinical disorder has a range of presentations, from coma, quadriplegia, and pseudobulbar palsy, to behavioral changes (Price and Mesulam 1987). Pontine and extrapontine myelinolysis have been described in patients with hyponatremia from a variety of causes, including alcoholism, chronic renal disease, and malignancy (Lundborn et al. 1993). Lesions can be visualized on CT and MRI scans. MRI is more sensitive, and the commonest finding is an area of decreased T1 signal and an increased T2 signal within the basal pons. Lesions seen on MRI may resolve with recovery (Charness 1993).

The prevalence of *head injury* in alcoholic patients is two to four times higher than in the general population (Hillbom and Holm 1986), but alcoholic patients are liable to forget about head injuries, which then go unrecognized. Experimental evidence suggests that alcohol potentiates central nervous system (CNS) trauma (Flamm et al. 1977). Therefore, minor injuries in alcoholic patients are likely to result in more severe complications and residual neuropsychological deficits than minor injuries in the general population (Grant et al. 1984). A history of head injury is a significant factor contributing to poor treatment outcome.

Head injury has been found to be more common in alcoholic patients with a positive family history of alcohol problems (Alterman and Tarter 1985). It is hypothesized that antecedent conditions such as attention-deficit disorder or adult antisocial personality disorder increase the risk for coincidental trauma (Tarter et al. 1985).

The majority of *subdural hematomas* follow head injury (Lishman 1998). Alcoholic patients are at higher risk of developing these problems, and the situation may be complicated by intoxication and withdrawal states. Subdural hematoma may present acutely with coma or a fluctuating confusion. Hemiparesis and ocular signs may be present, but neurological signs may be minimal.

Chronic subdural hematomas may be difficult to uncover. The head injury may have been trivial, and often there is a latent period of days to months. Presenting features include headache of insidious onset, impaired concentration, memory lapses, a fluctuating level of consciousness, and variable mental state. The picture is usually of few and nonspecific neurological signs—unequal pupils and an upgoing plantar response (Lishman 1998). Skull X ray and EEG may reveal a shift of midline structures, but a CT or MRI scan will usually provide the diagnosis. Lumbar puncture is contraindicated.

Psychosis

Alcoholic hallucinosis is a term used to describe auditory or visual hallucinations that occur either during or after a period of heavy alcohol consumption. The hallucinations are vivid and of acute onset and occur in clear consciousness. Delusional misinterpretation may follow. Primary alcoholic patients who consume large quantities of drugs and/or alcohol might be at an increased risk for developing alcoholic hallucinosis (Tsuang et al. 1994). Alcoholic hallucinosis usually resolves over a period of weeks but occasionally persists for months. Little evidence supports the view that alcoholic hallucinosis is a form of latent schizophrenia.

Alcohol-induced psychotic disorder with delusions affects approximately 1%–9% of individuals with alcohol dependence. These patients develop paranoid or grandiose delusions in the context of heavy drinking but do not have any clouding of consciousness. There appears to be no association with schizophrenia, and the prognosis is thought to be good.

Fetal Alcohol Syndrome

In 1973, Jones and Smith introduced the term *fetal alcohol syndrome* (FAS) to describe a constellation of birth defects (growth retardation, craniofacial abnormalities, and CNS impairment) observed in children exposed to alcohol in utero. The estimated incidence of FAS is 0.33/1,000 live births (Abel and Sokol 1991), but this figure may be an underestimate because the disorder is not always obvious at birth. The incidence of FAS increases with maternal age, and this may be the result of age-related changes in maternal alcohol metabolism and physiology (J. L. Jacobson et al. 1996).

Craniofacial abnormalities include microcephaly, shortened eyelids, an underdeveloped upper lip, and flattened, wide nose. CNS abnormalities range from subtle cognitive dysfunction to severe mental retardation (Spohr et al. 1993). Cognitive deficits, together with concentration, attention, and behavioral problems, may make education or employment impossible. In vivo brain magnetic resonance imaging confirms callosal abnormalities and abnormalities in the anterior vermal region of the cerebellum (E. P. Riley et al. 1995; Sowell et al. 1996).

Moderate-to-heavy alcohol consumption in pregnancy, at levels below those associated with FAS, have now been shown to have long-term effects on the psychomotor development of children (Larrogue et al. 1995).

Clinical Significance of Alcohol-Related Brain Damage

Individuals with alcohol-related brain damage (ARBD) are often seen in emergency departments of general medical and psychiatric hospitals. The more obvious deficits associated with Wernicke-Korsakoff syndrome will usually be picked up, but subtle neuropsychological impairments in individuals who seem to be cognitively intact can be overlooked. Frontal lobe deficits in problem solving, organization, and abstraction are the most insidious aspect of alcohol-induced decline (Clifford and Maddocks 1988). Careful assessment will usually show that individuals with ARBD have difficulty at the level of day-to-day living (Price et al. 1988a). Although abstinence should be the negotiated treatment goal, these patients have little motivation, and often a vicious cycle of continuing alcohol abuse and further cognitive deterioration ensues.

Further research is needed to clarify the relationship of brain damage to treatment outcome (Glass 1991). Neuropsychological test scores do not predict outcome (Alterman et al. 1990; Leenane 1988). Leenane (1986, 1988) followed 104 patients (83 men, 11 women; mean age 53.8 years) with alcohol-related brain damage for a mean of 16 months after discharge from a specialist unit in Australia. Paradoxically, those shown to be more severely brain damaged on neuropsychological testing had a better outcome than those shown to be less severely brain damaged because the former were more willing to accept their situation, did better in a structured inpatient program, and were happy to live in a sheltered environment where they were less likely to drink.

Alterman et al. (1990) reported 1- and 6-month outcomes for 87 alcohol-dependent men (mean age 42 years) attending a 30-day hospital rehabilitation program. Greater baseline alcohol problems and poorer complex cognitive functioning (as measured by the Category test, the Symbol Digit Paired-Associate Learning task, and Trails B) (De Fillippis and McCampbell 1979; Kapur and Butters 1977; Reitan 1958) were most consistently related to improved alcohol-related outcome. Other cognitive measures were not significantly associated with treatment outcome.

It is likely that cognitive deficits represent only one of a number of possible factors contributing to treatment outcome in the early stages of rehabilitation. Alcohol-related cognitive dysfunction is not a unitary phenomenon. Cognitive deficits may retard learning in treatment (Wilkinson and Sanchez-Craig 1981) and influence treatment effectiveness. This is a difficult area to investigate because the degree of impairment is usually related to chronicity of drinking and therefore age.

Clinicians and drug and alcohol workers should be familiar with the risk factors and early signs of brain damage in their clients. The pattern of neuropsychological impairment and changes on MRI, together with an assessment of behavior and daily living skills, will help the clinician to tailor an appropriate treatment program. Objective feedback about neuropsychological and brain scans may motivate the patient to abstinence. Patients with moderate to severe brain damage who appear to be cognitively "intact" are not likely to respond to standard treatment such as motivational interviewing, relapse prevention, cognitive-behavioral therapy, group therapy, psychotherapy, or family therapy. Their initial needs are more basic, for instance, improved nutrition, parenteral and oral thiamine, and admission to institute abstinence and discharge to a supervised setting. Leenane (1988) described a rehabilitation program for patients with ARBD that included group and individual reorientation, the use of prominent labels for ward areas, display of ward timetables, a memory aid book to record a personal timetable, and a structured day. The repetitive structure and routine of Alcoholics Anonymous was well suited to those with mild-to-moderate brain damage.

Neuropsychiatric Effects of Drug Abuse/Dependence

In this section, the neuropsychiatric effects of benzodiazepines, stimulants, opioids and prescription analgesics, cannabis, hallucinogens and related drugs, inhalants, and nicotine are considered.

The illegality of drugs contributes to violence and trauma, and thus indirectly to neuropsychiatric effects. Polydrug abuse is common in the drug-abusing population, and combinations of drugs—for example, alcohol and cocaine—may have more serious effects than do these drugs individually.

Neuropsychiatric complications can occur following acute or chronic use of drugs and are also related to the route of administration, particularly injecting. Injecting drugs causes neuropsychiatric effects directly and indirectly. The sharing of injecting equipment is a risk factor for the transmission of the human immunodeficiency virus (HIV) and hepatitis B and C. Injecting also increases the risk of endocarditis, septicemia, meningitis, brain abscess, and stroke. Cocaine is an immunosuppressant, and intravenous users are at particular risk of endocarditis (Brust 1992). The many complications of HIV infection are further discussed in Chapter 8.

Benzodiazepines

Benzodiazepines are among the most commonly prescribed drugs worldwide. Their abuse liability is at a lower level than that for heroin or cocaine, but individuals with a history of alcohol or other drug problems have an increased risk for the development of benzodiazepine abuse. Polydrug users take benzodiazepines to self-medicate the withdrawal effects of stimulant drugs and the anxiety associated with opiate withdrawal and also to enhance the "buzz" from heroin and alcohol. Benzodiazepines are commonly used by individuals in methadone maintenance programs (Perera et al. 1987). The most common neuropsychiatric effects are toxic overdose, withdrawal states, and long-term memory impairment as well as fetal effects.

Overdose.   A toxic reaction develops over a period of a few hours, usually in the context of an overdose (deliberate or otherwise) and usually when other drugs, for example, alcohol, have also been taken. Patients can present in a confusional state, stupor, or coma with respiratory depression and low blood pressure. The specific benzodiazepine receptor antagonist flumazenil is effective in treating overdose.

Elderly individuals and those with brain damage are very sensitive to benzodiazepines and are at risk of developing a toxic confusional state, even with low doses.

Withdrawal syndrome.   The symptoms of the benzodiazepine withdrawal syndrome are well described (Greenblatt et al. 1990; Petursson and Lader 1981). Although withdrawal symptoms are usually mild in degree, there are well-documented case reports of severe withdrawal syndromes with delirium and seizures (Greenblatt et al. 1990; Hollister et al. 1961; Preskorn and Denner 1977). The withdrawal syndrome occurs soon after discontinuation, and the time course depends on the pharmacokinetics of the drug in question. Secondary abstinence syndromes of lesser severity may continue for months. Benzodiazepines with a short half-life appear to be associated with withdrawal syndromes of rapid onset and greatest severity. Auditory hallucinations and paranoid delusions have been reported during withdrawal from high doses of benzodiazepines (Fraser and Ingram 1985; Preskorn and Denner 1977). These mostly resolve within 2 days to 2 weeks.

Neuropsychological deficits.   Reports suggest that benzodiazepine use, abuse, and dependence are associated with neuropsychological impairment. Acute use of benzodiazepines can result in mild anterograde memory and attention impairment, but access to information in long-term memory is spared (Mac et al. 1985; Scharf et al. 1983; Wolkowitz et al. 1987). Triazolam, lorazepam, and alprazolam, which have the highest affinity to the benzodiazepine receptor, fewer lipophilic properties, and lower volumes of distribution, have shown the greatest amnestic potential.

Temazepam, diazepam, and clorazepate have lower benzodiazepine receptor affinities and show the least amnestic potential (Mohler and Okada 1978). The amnestic effects are mediated via the benzodiazepine receptor and can be blocked by specific benzodiazepine antagonists. The older population may be more susceptible to memory deficits when taking benzodiazepines. Little is known about differential amnestic properties with chronic administration (Scharf et al. 1988). A series of 55 consecutively admitted patients with a history of chronic exclusive sedative or hypnotic abuse had lower neuropsychological performance levels and a higher prevalence of intellectual impairment compared with a matched control group from the general population (H. Bergman et al. 1980b). A study by Kumar et al. (1987) suggested that neither lorazepam nor alprazolam used chronically (5 days) had any effect on immediate recall of word lists. The amnestic effects of benzodiazepines may be dose-related, and further work is needed to clarify this matter.

Fetal effects. In 1987, a Swedish study reported developmental abnormalities, including dysmorphism and mental retardation, similar to features of FAS, in seven infants whose mothers had taken high doses of diazepam or oxazepam during pregnancy (Laegreid 1987). To test this putative association, the records of 104,000 inpatient deliveries between 1980 and 1983 in a United States Medicaid database were investigated (U. Bergman et al. 1992). This study indicated that the earlier findings were likely to be confounded by maternal alcohol problems.

Stimulants

Cocaine

Cocaine is an alkaloid prepared from the leaves of the coca bush, *Erythroxylon coca*, which grows in the mountainous regions of Central and South America. It can be taken by almost any route, but mostly it is injected intravenously or ingested intranasally ("snorted"). When the cocaine alkaloid is separated from its hydrochloride base, its melting point is lowered to 98°C, and it can be smoked. The use of crack cocaine as a form of freebase cocaine is widespread. The acute effects of cocaine are dependent on the strength of the dose and the route of administration; thus, higher concentrations of injected cocaine hydrochloride and smoked crack cocaine are associated with higher toxicity and more frequent and severe complications.

Cocaine is a potent CNS stimulant and also has actions on the peripheral nervous and cardiovascular systems. It causes euphoria; increases energy, wakefulness, pulse rate, blood pressure, and temperature; and dilates pupils. At higher concentrations, dysphoria, anxiety, agitation, and suspiciousness occur. Toxic levels lead to autonomic instability, hyperthermia, catatonic excitement, seizures, and death.

Intoxication state. Neuropsychiatric complications of the intoxication state include mood disorder, hallucinosis, psychotic disorder, and neurological sequelae.

Mood disorder symptoms of cocaine intoxication mimic the full range of affective disorders and include manic-like symptoms, dysthymia, and periods of mood elevation, followed by depressive swings. Mood elevation is associated with binges or "runs" of cocaine, and the depressive symptoms are associated with the subsequent "crash" (Gawin and Ellinwood 1988).

Hallucinations can appear in several modalities—auditory, visual (e.g., lights sparkling at the edge of the visual field), and tactile (e.g., insects felt under the skin, also known as formication and "cocaine bugs").

Prolonged, repeated, high-dose use can lead to a *toxic psychosis*, which usually resolves within hours to days but may be prolonged after a long binge. Cocaine-induced *paranoid psychoses* may resemble any of the psychotic disorders, from delusional disorders to schizophrenia-like illness (Mendoza et al. 1992).

Cocaine-induced *delirium* usually presents dramatically with paranoia, which is followed by extremely violent and bizarre behavior (Mendoza et al. 1992). There is diminished alertness and attention, with evidence of disorientation and cognitive impairment. Hyperthermia, mydriasis, autonomic instability, and seizures have also been described.

The *seizures* associated with cocaine intoxication are typically generalized, although focal seizures have also been reported (Mody et al. 1988). Seizures can occur even in the absence of any other signs of toxicity (Pascual-Leone et al. 1990). Cocaine-induced status epilepticus is a rare complication of cocaine abuse.

Abstinence syndrome. The cocaine abstinence syndrome follows three phases: crash, withdrawal, and abstinence. Neuropsychiatric symptoms are evident during the first two phases (see Gawin and Kleber 1986 for review).

Symptoms during the crash, or first phase of cocaine withdrawal, include intense depression, agitation, anxiety, cocaine craving, and sometimes suicidal and paranoid ideation. These symptoms disappear over a period of 1–4 hours after cessation of cocaine administration and are followed by a period of hypersomnolence with intermittent awakenings and hyperphagia that lasts for 8–50 hours. Mood usually returns to normal after 3–4 days, although some dysphoria may remain (Gawin and Kleber 1986). The length of the crash is proportional to the length and intensity of cocaine use.

After the crash, the second phase of withdrawal sets in and lasts for between 1 and 10 weeks. Symptoms include anhedonia, fluctuating mild dysphoria, and anergia.

Psychosis.   Chronic cocaine abuse is associated with delusions of parasitosis and a psychotic disorder characterized by a more deteriorated presentation with delusions, hallucinations, incoherence, loosening of associations, catatonic behavior, and flat or inappropriate affect (Mendoza et al. 1992). The differential diagnosis should include brief reactive psychosis (if a stressor is reported), schizophreniform disorder, or schizophrenia.

Neurological complications.   Neurological complications of cocaine abuse such as seizures, stroke, and vasculitis increased in the mid-1980s in the United States as users switched to the crack form of cocaine (Mendoza et al. 1992).

The recent epidemic of cocaine abuse in the United States has led to a growing number of *cocaine-induced strokes* in young healthy individuals, many of whom are first-time abusers (Miller et al. 1992). The association between cocaine use and stroke is particularly strong for crack cocaine and remains even when stroke risk factors are taken into account (Kaku and Lowenstein 1990). Cocaine hydrochloride predisposes to hemorrhagic stroke, and at least 50% of patients in this category are found to have an underlying abnormality of their cerebral blood vessels, particularly arteriovenous malformations and cerebral aneurysms (Miller et al. 1992). The etiology of cocaine-induced hemorrhagic stroke is not understood but may be related to cocaine-induced hypertension or cerebral vasculitis. Cerebral vasculitis has been confirmed by cerebral biopsy in some reports (Fredericks et al. 1991; Krendel et al. 1990). Transient ischemic attacks and ischemic stroke are associated with the use of crack cocaine (Levine et al. 1991) and the simultaneous use of cocaine and alcohol (Miller et al. 1992). The etiology is not known, but the toxic cocaine-alcohol metabolite cocaethylene (Hearn et al. 1991) and accelerated atherosclerosis may be factors.

Cocaine may precipitate a granulomatous angiitis, which persists for months after cocaine has been stopped. Transient vasculitis may be more common than previously suspected and may explain the persistence of psychiatric symptoms long after cessation of cocaine use (Krendel et al. 1990).

Daras et al. (1994) reported acute dyskinesias following use of crack cocaine in seven patients. The movement disorders included choreoathetosis, akathisia, and parkinsonism with tremor. Although the incidence of these disorders is not high, the fact that street names exist suggests that the incidence is higher than is recognized. The condition is benign, but it may recur in individuals who continue to abuse cocaine.

Organic brain syndrome.   Chronic cocaine use may be associated with diffuse *cerebral atrophy*, but few controlled studies have been carried out. One CT study reported an association between cerebral atrophy and duration of habitual cocaine use (Pascual-Leone et al. 1991), and a second found that a negative correlation between severity of cocaine use and sulcal width disappeared when the age of the subjects was partialed out (Cascella et al. 1991). Severity of alcohol use showed a tendency for association with ventricular brain ratio (VBR) even after age was controlled.

A small number of functional imaging studies suggest perfusion deficits in cocaine users. PET studies by Volkow and colleagues (1988, 1991) revealed lower relative cerebral blood flow (CBF) values in the prefrontal cortex both before and after detoxification and in the second week following cocaine withdrawal. Single photon emission computed tomography studies have reported scalloping of cerebral perfusion in the periventricular region (Mena et al. 1990) and multifocal, mostly frontotemporal, perfusion deficits (Tumeh et al. 1990).

Little is known about the long-term *neuropsychological effects* of chronic cocaine abuse. Impairments in memory, concentration, psychomotor speed, problem solving, and abstraction abilities have been reported in the acute withdrawal phase (Ardila et al. 1991; O'Malley and Gawin 1990) and after 2 weeks of abstinence (Berry et al. 1993). However, few studies have been carried out, and more controlled studies with retesting after abstinence are needed. A vascular dementia can occur with chronic use, but prospective neuropsychological and imaging studies are needed to investigate this further.

In utero exposure to cocaine predisposes infants to a variety of *fetal effects* such as stillbirth, low birth weight, microcephaly, tremor, irritability, hemorrhagic and ischemic stroke, and neurobehavioral deficits (Chasnoff et al. 1985). Similar problems are seen following in utero exposure to amphetamines. The long-term effects of fetal exposure to cocaine are still largely unknown.

Amphetamines and Related Agents

Amphetamine, dextroamphetamine, methamphetamine, phenmetrazine, methylphenidate, and diethylpropion all produce subjective effects similar to those of cocaine. Amphetamines increase synaptic dopamine mainly by stimulating presynaptic release, rather than by blockade, as occurs with cocaine (O'Brien 1996). The acute intoxication states induced by amphetamines (mood disorder, hallucinosis, psychotic disorder, delirium, neurological complications) are similar to those induced by cocaine.

Amphetamine psychosis, which mimics acute schizophrenia or mania, usually develops gradually with chronic abuse (Connell 1958), but it has been seen acutely after a large dose. It has also been reproduced in healthy volunteers. Characteristic features include paranoid delusions, auditory or tactile hallucinations, visual hallucinations or delusions, and labile mood (Schuckit 1995). Subjects have little or no insight into the paranoid delusions. The psychosis usually clears within days to a week. Physical examination may reveal severe weight loss, skin lesions (from scratching at tactile hallucinations), needle marks, hypertension, tachycardia, and raised temperature (Schuckit 1995). It has been reported that a proportion of patients presenting with an amphetamine psychosis have residual symptoms for up to 1 year or more (Schuckit 1995). This may reflect an uncovering of vulnerability to a psychotic disorder such as schizophrenia.

Neurological complications of amphetamine intoxication include seizures (with possible death); cerebral infarcts; intracranial, intraventricular, and subarachnoid hemorrhage (Cahill et al. 1981; Delaney and Estes 1980; D'Souza and Shraberg 1981); and cerebral vasculitis and angiitis (Bostwick 1981; Matick et al. 1983). Cerebral vasculitis has been confirmed by cerebral biopsy. Methamphetamine use has also been linked with cerebral infarct (Rothrock et al. 1988), intracerebral and subarachnoid hemorrhage, and cerebral angiitis (Weiss et al. 1970; Yu et al. 1983). Reports also indicate that over-the-counter agents such as phenylpropanolamine can cause cerebral vasculitis (Forman et al. 1989; Glick et al. 1987).

Opioids and Prescription Analgesics

Opioid drugs, used primarily for their analgesic properties, also induce euphoria and thus have an abuse liability. Of this group, opium, morphine, and codeine are natural substances, obtained from the opium poppy, *Papaver somniferum*. Semisynthetic compounds include heroin, hydromorphone, and oxycodone. Synthetic analgesics include propoxyphene and meperidine. The analgesic effect of these drugs is largely mediated through μ-receptors, which are also implicated in the development of dependence. Opioids are variably absorbed from the gastrointestinal tract (heroin is poorly absorbed; dextropropoxyphene is well absorbed) but are readily absorbed after subcutaneous or intramuscular administration. The effect of a given dose is less after oral than after parenteral administration because of variable first-pass metabolism in the liver.

Opioid analgesics produce symptomatic pain relief and are the treatment of choice for chronic pain associated with malignant disease or terminal illness. Oral dosing is usually effective.

The abuse of prescription analgesics is not well documented. Long-term treatment is not recommended in chronic, non–life-threatening disorders such as backache, chronic headache, and abdominal pain. High rates of abuse have been reported in health care professionals who have easy access to these drugs (McAuliffe et al. 1986).

Intoxication state.   Acute opioid toxicity can occur from overdose, either accidental or planned, and is a significant cause of mortality. Coma, pinpoint pupil, depressed respiration, and evidence of needle marks suggest opioid poisoning.

Withdrawal syndrome.   Although the opioid withdrawal syndrome is unpleasant, it is not associated with any major neuropsychiatric symptoms and is not further discussed here.

Organic brain syndrome.   Organic brain syndromes are not usually seen in connection with opioid abuse apart from toxic overdose. An agitated confusional state has been reported following meperidine use (Eisendrath et al. 1987).

Heroin, like other opiates, lowers the seizure threshold, and heroin users have a higher risk of seizures independent of other risk factors (Brust 1992). Hemorrhagic stroke has been reported in association with heroin use and is thought to be mediated by a heroin-induced vasculitis (Brust and Richter 1976).

Neuropsychological impairment and CT abnormalities have been reported in a case-control study of seven long-term heroin addicts who injected prescribed pharmaceutical heroin over a 20-year period using a clean injecting technique (Strang and Gurling 1989).

Postmortem examinations of heroin addicts reveal neuropathological abnormalities, which include transverse myelitis, central pontine myelinolysis, neuronal depletion in the globus pallidus, and delayed postanoxic encephalopathy (Strang and Gurling 1989), but these changes could be technique-related rather than substance-specific and may also reflect the lack of systematic research. The presence of neuropsychiatric syndromes in HIV disease has prompted research into the chronic effects of opiates on the brain.

Cannabis

Cannabis, the most widely used drug after nicotine and alcohol, is obtained from the Indian hemp plant, *Cannabis sativa*. This plant contains many psychoactive substances called cannabinoids, of which the principal one is delta-9-tetrahydrocannabinol (THC). Various preparations of cannabis are available including bhang, marijuana, ganja, hashish (cannabis resin), and liquid cannabis (hashish oil), the potency of which is related to their THC content (Ghodse 1989). Cannabis can be ingested, smoked, or administered intravenously (rare). The pharmacological effects of THC vary with the dose, route of administration, experience of the user, vulnerability to psychoactive effects, and setting of use (O'Brien 1996). THC is readily absorbed across the lung mucosa, and peak plasma concentrations are reached after 10–30 minutes. The effects of a single cigarette emerge within minutes and last for 2–3 hours. The onset of action for ingested cannabis is slower, and the effects last longer. The rate of clearance of THC and its metabolites is slow because of their lipid solubility. Chronic use of cannabis leads to tolerance, but this is uncommon in Western countries. Cannabis dependence is a recognized entity in DSM-IV (American Psychiatric Association 1994), but the question of a dependence syndrome is still considered controversial by some.

Intoxication. Cannabis intoxication is characterized by a variety of psychological and behavioral effects, including euphoria, relaxation, sleepiness, self-confidence, a sense of well-being, the perception that time is passing slowly, and impairment of concentration, performance skills, and short-term memory (Chesher et al. 1990; Heishman et al. 1990; Stillman et al. 1976). Social withdrawal, anxiety, tension, and confusion have also been described. These effects occur in association with physical effects such as dry mouth, increased appetite, conjunctival infection, and tachycardia. A fluctuating and marked disturbance of consciousness associated with a change in cognition should raise the possibility of cannabis intoxication delirium, which usually settles over a period of hours or days. Higher doses of THC are associated with suspiciousness and paranoia, distortions in visual and auditory perceptions, hallucinations, and depersonalization (Mathew et al. 1993).

Psychosis.   A cannabis-induced psychosis can develop during intoxication with high doses of THC. Although uncommon in Western countries, it is well recognized in India, the Caribbean, and other countries where heavy consumption of cannabis is common. Cannabis-induced psychosis is characterized by a sudden onset of confusion, persecutory delusions, and hallucinations. Depersonalization, marked anxiety, emotional lability, and amnesia for the episode are also described. It is a short-lived state, usually remitting within hours to days.

The existence of an acute cannabis-induced psychosis in clear consciousness has been a matter of considerable debate and investigation. Mathers and Ghodse (1992) reported evidence for such an entity and found that it was more likely to occur against a background of major psychotic disorder. The current view is that cannabis abuse can precipitate relapse in patients with schizophrenia and related disorders and that it may also act as a premorbid precipitant in vulnerable individuals (Chaudry et al. 1991; Linzen et al. 1994; Mathers and Ghodse 1992; Negrete 1989). This effect can be explained by the putative action of THC as a dopaminergic agonist in the projections of the medial forebrains of patients (Linzen et al. 1994).

There is, however, little evidence to support the existence of the *amotivational syndrome*, a condition of chronic apathy associated with long-term, heavy cannabis abuse.

Organic brain syndrome.   Regarding *neuropsychological effects*, the clinical impression that chronic cannabis use is associated with cognitive impairment has not been borne out by research (Deahl 1991). Early studies were methodologically flawed. Specific tests of memory were not employed, and the samples included either college students who were occasional and light users (Culver and King 1974; I. Grant et al. 1973; Mendelson et al. 1984; Rochford et al. 1977) or extremely heavy users. Control groups were absent or poorly matched, particularly in terms of premorbid intellectual functioning. A more recent case-control study of 26 long-term heavy cannabis users reported significant impairments in short-term memory and perceptuomotor function after 12 weeks of abstinence (Varma et al. 1988). Problems with short-term memory have been documented in a sample of 10 cannabis-dependent adolescents compared with carefully matched control groups after 6 weeks of abstinence (Schwartz et al. 1989). Block and Ghoneim (1993) compared 144 cannabis users with 72 nonusers matched on intellectual functioning before the onset of drug use. The researchers found that "heavy use" was associated with deficits in mathematical skills and selective impairments in memory retrieval processes.

Cannabis smoking has been reported to increase CBF, cerebral metabolism, and cerebral blood velocity in experienced smokers (Mathew et al. 1992a, 1992b), and it is thought that this increase in CBF may underlie brain arousal associated with cannabis-induced euphoria.

Hallucinogens and Related Drugs

Lysergic Acid Diethylamide

Lysergic acid diethylamide (LSD), an indolealkylamine, is a potent hallucinogen, even at doses as low as 25–50 μg. It is available in a variety of forms (powder, solution, capsule, and pill) and, although usually taken orally, can be administered subcutaneously or intravenously or smoked with tobacco. Effects set in at 40–60 minutes following oral administration, peak at 2–4 hours, and diminish over 6–8 hours (O'Brien 1996).

Intoxication state. Doses of 100 μg produce perceptual distortions, hallucinations, mood changes (elation, paranoia, depression), and anxiety. Depersonalization and confusion have also been described. Physical signs include palpitations, raised blood pressure, perspiration, pupillary dilation, and hyperreflexia. Colors seem more intense. No withdrawal syndrome is associated with hallucinogens.

Psychosis. LSD induces a psychotic reaction that lasts approximately 2 days. Symptoms may be complicated by other drug use and are variable. Uncontrolled hallucinations and paranoid ideation are usually seen, together with depressed mood and panic. Use of LSD may predispose to schizophrenic illness in vulnerable individuals.

Hallucinogen persisting perception disorder (flashbacks). It is estimated that 15%–30% of LSD users have at some time experienced episodic visual disturbances resembling the experiences of "bad trips." Symptoms include false fleeting perceptions in the peripheral fields, flashes of color, geometric pseudohallucinations, and positive afterimages (Abraham and Aldridge 1993). Precipitants include stress, fatigue, marijuana, neuroleptics, and anxiety states. This syndrome is now included in DSM-IV as hallucinogen persisting perceptual disorder.

3,4-Methylenedioxymethamphetamine (Ecstasy)

3,4-Methylenedioxymethamphetamine (MDMA, or ecstasy) is a ring-substituted amphetamine derivative that has both stimulant and mild hallucinogenic properties. Reports of recreational use have soared in the past decade (Steele et al. 1994), and this is a matter of concern because MDMA has been shown to be toxic to serotonin neurons in the animal brain (Ricaurte et al. 1985; Schmidt et al. 1986; Stone et al. 1986). Two studies have used cerebrospinal fluid 5-hydroxyindoleacetic acid to screen for possible MDMA neurotoxicity in humans; one reported a reduction in levels (Ricaurte et al. 1990), whereas the other did not (Peroutka et al. 1987). Another study suggested that MDMA users may have altered serotonin-dependent neuroendocrine function (L. H. Price et al. 1988b).

In the United States MDMA is taken when the user is alone or at parties, whereas in Britain recreational use typically occurs in the setting of large organized dance parties known as *raves*. Doses range from 70 to 150 mg, with a booster of between 50 and 100 mg several hours later (Steele et al. 1994). The average total dose taken during an all-night rave is not known.

Intoxication. Acute neuropsychiatric effects occurring within 24 hours of ingestion include altered consciousness, transient gait disturbance, trismus, flashbacks, anxiety, insomnia, panic attacks, and psychosis. Hallucinations are not reported at typical doses. In Britain, several deaths and adverse reactions have followed the use of MDMA as a "dance drug" (Henry 1992). Seizures, collapse, hyperpyrexia, disseminated intravascular coagulation, rhabdomyolysis, and acute renal failure can follow ingestion.

Subacute effects occur between 24 hours and 1 month after ingestion and include drowsiness, depression, anxiety, and irritability.

Chronic syndromes. Chronic syndromes occur after 1 month and include panic disorder, psychosis (McGuire and Fahy 1991), flashbacks, major depressive disorder, and memory disturbance (McCann and Ricaurte 1991). Neuropsychiatric effects may be dose-related and occur in individuals with particular susceptibility.

Phencyclidine

Phencyclidine (PCP), a cyclohexylamine anesthetic that induces a state of dissociative anesthesia, was developed in the 1950s but was later abandoned because of high levels of postoperative delirium and hallucinations (O'Brien 1996). Ketamine, a phencyclidine hydrochloride derivative, is still used as a dissociative anesthetic (Krystal et al. 1994).

PCP has been recognized as a drug of abuse since the 1970s. It can be taken as a pill, snorted, smoked, or injected intravenously, but the most common routes of administration are smoking and oral ingestion (Garey et al. 1987). PCP is a crystalline, water-soluble, lipophilic substance that penetrates fat stores and has a long half-life. Both PCP and ketamine are noncompetitive NMDA antagonists, binding to a site distinct from NMDA within the ion channel and acting as open channel blockers (Tsai et al. 1995). PCP is also thought to act at some types of opiate receptors and nicotinic and muscarinic cholinergic receptors (Schuckit 1995). It has cholinergic effects at some doses and anticholinergic effects at other levels.

Intoxication.   Acute toxic reactions are characterized by sympathetic overactivity and changes in cholinergic function ranging from overactivity to anticholinergic effects. Symptoms can emerge at oral doses of 5–10 mg and worsen with higher doses. The lipophilic nature of the drug means that it can be repeatedly released from fat stores; thus blood levels are an unreliable guide.

Low doses lead to confusion. Moderate doses (>10 mg) can cause catalepsy, coma, and stupor. Doses over 25–50 mg usually result in coma and seizures. PCP coma may last 7–10 days (O'Brien 1996) and may take 2–6 weeks to clear, progressing via an organic brain syndrome, with or without psychotic symptoms, which slowly recede. A toxic reaction to PCP can be life-threatening and tends to resolve slowly. The combination of a comalike state, open eyes, nystagmus, and increased deep-tendon reflexes, with temporary periods of excitation, should suggest PCP intoxication (Schuckit 1995). Acute PCP intoxication is a medical emergency.

Psychosis.   A psychotic picture can be seen with moderate intoxication. The level and duration of psychotic features are proportional to the amount of drug ingested, with such features lasting from 24 hours to 1 month (Yesavage and Freman 1978). Hallucinations and/or delusions, usually in the context of a clouded sensorium, are evident during the resolution of a severe toxic reaction. Psychotic features include paranoid ideation, manic behavior, grandiosity, hyperactivity, and rapid thoughts and speech (Schuckit 1995; Slavney et al. 1977; Yesavage and Freman 1978).

Inhalant Abuse (Glues, Solvents, Aerosols)

Inhalants, volatile substances used for altering mental states, are rarely administered by routes other than inhalation (Sharp 1992). A variety of readily available substances are abused: toluene and xylenes (adhesives), butane and halons (aerosols), trichloroethylene and tetrachloroethylene (dry cleaning fluids), n-butane and isobutane (cigarette lighter fluids), and trichloroethane (typewriter correction fluid and thinner), among others. These volatile solvents are highly lipophilic and are therefore well distributed in the brain.

Acute exposure induces short-acting effects on brain function, most of which are reversible. The initial effect is an excitatory action on the central nervous system that results in euphoria. This is followed by confusion, perceptual distortions, hallucinations, and delusions (Ashton 1990). Larger doses cause central nervous system depression with ataxia, nystagmus, dysarthria, drowsiness, coma, and occasionally seizures and even sudden death.

Chronic toxicity may cause irreversible damage to the brain. Clinical effects include a cerebellar syndrome, peripheral neuropathy, neuropsychological deficits, and psychiatric disorder (Ron 1986).

Cerebellar disease is associated particularly with toluene abuse. Ataxia, dysarthria, tremor, and nystagmus are the main symptoms. The presence and severity of toluene-related cerebellar signs correlated significantly with the width of cerebellar sulci and superior cerebellar cisterns in a CT scan study of toluene abusers (Fornazzari et al. 1983). The natural history of the cerebellar abnormalities is unclear.

Chronic inhalation of toluene produces an irreversible multifocal central nervous system syndrome characterized by dementia, cerebellar ataxia, spasticity, and brainstem dysfunction (Hormes et al. 1986).

Peripheral neuropathy occurs mainly as a result of n-hexane and methyl butyl ketone (MBK). Clinical signs develop 2–3 months after abuse. The clinical picture is a symmetrical and mainly distal motor neuropathy leading to paralysis and muscle atrophy in the legs and sometimes the arms. These signs generally improve after a few weeks of abstinence.

Neuropsychological impairments were reported in schoolchildren who abuse solvents (Chadwick et al. 1989). Psychiatric morbidity is high among volatile substance abusers, but there is little evidence to support a causal relationship.

Further research is needed to increase our understanding of the long-term neuropsychiatric sequelae of volatile substance abuse.

Nicotine

Nicotine is a natural liquid alkaloid that is present in tobacco and has a significant propensity for dependence. Nicotine is readily absorbed from the respiratory tract, buccal membranes, and skin. The average cigarette contains 8–9 mg of nicotine (Benowitz et al. 1983) and delivers 1 mg systemically to the smoker. Nicotine activates the nucleus accumbens, causing release of endogenous opioids and glucocorticoids.

Toxic reactions. Stimulation of the CNS is followed by depression, and death can result from failure of respiration resulting from central paralysis and peripheral blockade of muscles of respiration (Taylor 1996).

Withdrawal syndrome. Sudden cessation of nicotine leads to a well-characterized withdrawal syndrome with irritability, impatience, frustration, anxiety, dysphoria and depressed mood, difficulty concentrating, restlessness, disturbed sleep, decreased heart rate, increased appetite, and weight gain (Jaffe 1990). Depressed mood, which is associated with nicotine dependence, increases during the withdrawal syndrome.

Organic brain syndrome. Nicotine does not cause a confusional state, except in toxic doses. However, confusion is associated with chronic obstructive lung disease, or emphysema, which arises as a result of smoking.

Dual Diagnosis

High rates of alcohol and drug disorders have been reported in people with major mental illness such as schizophrenia (Regier et al. 1990) and psychosis (Menezes et al. 1996). Substance abuse in this group leads to poorer clinical and social outcomes than in patients with mental illness alone (Lehman et al. 1993). Further problems include homelessness, heavy use of inpatient services (Bartels et al. 1993), behavioral problems, abnormal involuntary movements, and violence (Swanson et al. 1990).

Conventional services have great difficulty in engaging patients with dual diagnoses, but some innovative programs have been developed successfully (Drake et al. 1993; Jerrell et al. 1994). Alcohol, benzodiazepines, cannabis, cocaine, and amphetamines are the most commonly used drugs, but hallucinogen use is also reported. Some studies have attempted to determine the onset of psychosis and substance abuse and whether drugs (particularly cannabis, stimulants, and hallucinogens) were implicated in the genesis of psychosis. It is possible that dual-diagnosis patients would have developed a psychotic illness even in the absence of drug use. Substance abuse may serve to uncover psychosis in vulnerable individuals. It clearly interferes with resolution and is a risk factor for chronicity.

Clinical Implications of Neuropsychiatric Problems in Substance Abuse

There is overwhelming evidence that substance abuse/dependence is associated with a variety of neuropsychiatric syndromes. Many of these syndromes are readily diagnosed and treated, but a proportion—in particular, subtle cases of alcohol-related cognitive impairment and subclinical episodes of Wernicke-Korsakoff' syndrome—may be overlooked in clinical settings, and this can result in deterioration, chronicity, and ultimately an inability to benefit from standard treatment programs.

Neuropsychiatric syndromes cannot be divorced from psychosocial factors that may influence neuropsychiatric status indirectly. Such factors include poverty, unemployment, homelessness, poor nutrition, physical illness, complications of intravenous drug use, psychiatric comorbidity, prostitution, and criminality. Problem severity must, therefore, be assessed across a range of areas. Substance-abusing individuals who present to the public mental health setting tend to have complex chronic problems, chaotic lifestyles, and little social support, and they often present to the clinical services in crisis. The need to assess the dominant problem may be so pressing that other, more subtle issues, such as neuropsychiatric status, are ignored.

Individuals with substance abuse/dependence present to a variety of public health care settings, and clinical staff in these settings should be aware of the risk factors predisposing to neuropsychiatric complications.

Emergency department.   Individuals with overt neuropsychiatric complications of substance abuse/dependence such as acute intoxication or withdrawal states typically present to emergency departments in public hospitals. If they are confused, violent, comatose, psychotic, or just unhelpful, it may be difficult to obtain a full history and carry out a physical and mental state examination. Physical assessment for evidence of needle track marks, poor nutritional status, and a breath alcohol level can support clinical judgment, which can be supported with confirmatory urinary drug screens, blood alcohol levels, and serum biochemistry.

In the 1980s, cocaine became the leading cause of drug-related presentations to emergency departments in the United States. Schrank (1992) reviewed four surveys of cocaine-related problems in urban emergency departments. The 555 patients were young (average age 30 years), and most were male. Concurrent use of other drugs, especially alcohol, was common.

The presenting complaints were largely neuropsychiatric, but only 10%–20% of patients were admitted. None of the patients in these surveys presented with ischemic stroke or intracranial hemorrhage.

Medical ambulatory care and inpatient settings. A substantial proportion of individuals with substance abuse/dependence are seen in medical ambulatory and inpatient settings. Gastroenterologists and orthopedic specialists frequently see patients whose medical problems are associated with high alcohol consumption. Maternal abuse of or dependence on alcohol, cocaine, and opiates causes fetal effects. Ideally, abuse should be noticed in the prenatal clinic, but often the first indication of a drug problem manifests itself postnatally in the baby. Intravenous drug users with, or at risk for, HIV and hepatitis B and C will be attending other medical services. In these settings, it is possible that drug and alcohol problems will be uncovered only if they are obvious. Subtle neuropsychiatric problems such as alcohol-related cognitive impairment or subclinical Wernicke-Korsakoff's syndrome will be overlooked.

Despite economic constraints, it should be policy in public health hospitals to screen for alcohol and drug problems. Once these problems come to light, risk factors for neuropsychiatric complications, history, and physical examination should point to those individuals who need further neuropsychological screening. Neuropsychological assessment should be carried out after the acute withdrawal period; therefore, such patients should be admitted.

For many patients, particularly the urban poor, the public health services are the only ones available; therefore, any opportunity to treat them must not be missed. Inpatient admission can offer a period of abstinence; improved nutrition; thiamine and other vitamin therapy; assessment of hepatitis B, hepatitis C, and HIV status; help with psychosocial factors; and referral to psychiatric and/or specialist services. This is good practice and, in itself, a form of harm minimization. Unfortunately, individuals with substance misuse/dependence may prove to be so chaotic and difficult that they are likely to be discharged as soon as possible or to discharge themselves against medical advice, only to resume the lifestyle that led to their admission in the first place. Many will get caught in the revolving door of hospital–community–prison and do not remain in contact with the services long enough to undergo a careful assessment. Public services are so stretched and underfunded that, in reality, admission for assessment is a luxury that for many is not an option.

Psychiatric and specialist substance abuse services. Individuals with drug and alcohol abuse are not readily attracted into treatment programs

(Kosten 1991). They may select programs that are not appropriate to their needs or, more commonly, have to accept what is there. Valid and reliable assessment indicators must be developed to match clients to the appropriate treatment (McLellan and Alterman 1991). Individuals with cognitive impairment are unlikely to respond to the usual treatment modalities. The therapeutic process is often lengthy and the rate of progression extremely slow. A long period of abstinence may be needed before a realistic program tailored to their needs can be attempted. Unfortunately, illicit drug abuse and alcohol consumption often continue in treatment. This, together with low retention rates and high relapse rates, does not augur well for the patient. For patients with neuropsychiatric problems, the goal must go beyond abstinence. These patients rarely have a single disorder; medical, psychiatric, family, housing, and employment problems all need to be addressed.

Enhanced diagnostic and clinical skills are needed to tackle complex issues such as multidrug abuse and psychiatric comorbidity. Most current multidrug use involves cocaine, alcohol, opiates, benzodiazepines, and combinations of drugs. Opiate and cocaine users, the two main risk groups for HIV, have high rates of multidrug use (Woody et al. 1991).

Patients with major mental disorders such as schizophrenia have a high rate of alcohol and drug abuse/dependence (Regier et al. 1990). These patients are also likely to have neuropsychiatric problems, which in turn lead to poorer outcomes for both substance abuse and psychotic illness. The numbers of dually diagnosed patients are rising (Cuffel 1992), and more are being seen in alcohol and drug abuse treatment programs. However, there is often an absence of professional input and guidance in these programs, and psychiatric comorbidity is not addressed. Innovative programs targeting this group have succeeded in engaging these patients in treatment (Drake et al. 1993) by integrating substance abuse programs with mental health programs.

The acquired immunodeficiency syndrome (AIDS) epidemic has challenged drug treatment services and significantly stimulated a shift from a goal of abstinence toward harm minimization with methadone maintenance, needle exchanges, and so forth. Patients using drugs intravenously and showing evidence of promiscuous behavior are at risk of HIV. They should be offered HIV testing, and every attempt should be made to retain them in drug treatment programs. Evidence shows that effective methadone maintenance treatment has resulted in a reduced incidence of new cases of infectious diseases, such as hepatitis B and HIV infection, transmitted by use of contaminated needles (Kreek 1991).

Program issues are important for patients with neuropsychiatric problems of substance abuse. Drug and alcohol treatment programs in the public health setting vary in quality, but most have difficulty meeting the demands made of them. They find it difficult to attract and retain qualified staff because of low salaries, large caseloads, difficult patients, poor support and training, and unattractive and possibly dangerous work surroundings. Staff turnover is high; good staff leave after gaining skills, and morale is low.

The public health care system is now challenged by a crack epidemic, AIDS, homelessness, and psychiatric comorbidity. Patients are becoming more difficult, many having multidrug abuse and psychiatric comorbidity. Patients with a poor prognosis are filtering down from the private into the public health setting. Reassessment of the way in which public health services reach individuals with substance abuse and neuropsychiatric problems is urgently needed. General psychiatric, neuropsychiatric, and substance abuse services should work together to offer an integrated service.

References

Abel EL, Sokol RJ: A revised conservative estimate of the incidence of FAS and its economic impact. Alcohol Clin Exp Res 15:514–524, 1991

Abraham HD, Aldridge AM: Adverse consequences of lysergic acid diethylamine. Addiction 88:1327–1334, 1993

Adams RD, Victor M, Mancall EL: Central pontine myelinolysis. A hitherto undescribed disease occurring in alcoholic and malnourished patients. Arch Neurol 81:154–172, 1959

Adinoff B, Risher-Flowers D, De Jong J, et al: Disturbances of hypothalamic-pituitary-adrenal axis functioning during alcohol withdrawal in six men. Am J Psychiatry 148:1023–1025, 1991

Alterman AI, Tarter RE: Relationship between familial alcoholism and head injury. J Stud Alcohol 46:256–258, 1985

Alterman AI, Kushner H, Holahan JM: Cognitive functioning and treatment outcome in alcoholics. J Nerv Ment Dis 178:494–499, 1990

American Psychiatric Association: Diagnostic and Statistical Manual of Mental Disorders, 3rd Edition. Washington, DC, American Psychiatric Association, 1980

American Psychiatric Association: Diagnostic and Statistical Manual of Mental Disorders, 3rd Edition, Revised. Washington, DC, American Psychiatric Association, 1987

American Psychiatric Association: Diagnostic and Statistical Manual of Mental Disorders, 4th Edition. Washington, DC, American Psychiatric Association, 1994

Anthony JC, Helzer JE: Syndromes of drug abuse and dependence, in Psychiatric Disorders in America: The Epidemiologic Catchment Area Study. Edited by Robins LN, Region DA. New York, Free Press, 1991, pp 116–154

Ardila A, Rosselli M, Strumwasser S: Neuropsychological deficits in chronic cocaine abusers. Int J Neurosci 57:73–79, 1991

Ashton CH: Solvent abuse. BMJ 300:135–136, 1990

Ballenger JC, Post RM: Kindling as a model for alcohol withdrawal syndromes. Br J Psychiatry 133:1–14, 1978

Bartels SJ, Teague GB, Drake RE, et al: Service utilization and costs associated with substance use disorder among severely mentally ill patients. J Nerv Ment Dis 181:227–232, 1993

Becker HC, Hale RL: Repeated episodes of ethanol withdrawal potentiate the severity of subsequent withdrawal seizures: an animal model of alcohol withdrawal "kindling." Alcohol Clin Exp Res 17:94–98, 1993

Benowitz NL, Hall SM, Herning RI, et al: Smokers of low yield cigarettes do not consume less nicotine. N Engl J Med 309:139–142, 1983

Bergman H, Borg S, Hindmarsh T, et al: Computed tomography of the brain and neuropsychological assessment of male alcoholic patients in a random sample from the general male population. Acta Psychiatr Scand Suppl 286:47–56, 1980a

Bergman H, Borg S, Holm L: Neuropsychological impairment and exclusive abuse of sedatives or hypnotics. Am J Psychiatry 137:215–217, 1980b

Bergman U, Rosa FW, Baum C, et al: Effects of exposure to benzodiazepine during fetal life. Lancet 340:694–696, 1992

Berry J, van Gorp WG, Herzberg DS: Neuropsychological deficits in abstinent cocaine abusers: preliminary findings after two weeks of abstinence. Drug Alcohol Depend 32:231–237, 1993

Block RI, Ghoneim MM: Effects of chronic marijuana use on human cognition. Psychopharmacology (Berl) 110:219–228, 1993

Bostwick DG: Amphetamine-induced cerebral vasculitis. Hum Pathol 12:1031–1033, 1981

Brandt J, Butters N, Ryan C, et al: Cognitive loss and recovery in long term alcohol abusers. Arch Gen Psychiatry 40:435–442, 1983

Brennan FN, Lyttle JA: Alcohol and seizures: a review. J R Soc Med 80:571–573, 1987

Brust JCM: Neurological complications of substance abuse, in Addictive States. Edited by O'Brien CP, Jaffe JH. New York, Raven, 1992, pp 193–203

Brust JCM, Richter RW: Stroke associated with addiction to heroin. J Neurol Neurosurg Psychiatry 39:194, 1976

Cahill DW, Knipp H, Mosser J: Intracranial haemorrhage with amphetamine abuse. Neurology 31:1058–1059, 1981

Cala LA: CAT scan measurement of brain density changes due to alcohol ingestion. Australian Drug and Alcohol Review 1:62–64, 1982

Cala LA, Jones B, Mastaglia FL, et al: Brain atrophy and intellectual impairment in heavy drinkers—a clinical, psychometric and computed tomography study. Aust N Z J Med 8:147–153, 1978

Cala LA, Jones B, Wiley B, et al: A computerised axial tomography (CAT) study of alcohol induced cerebral atrophy; in conjunction with other correlates. Acta Psychiatr Scand Suppl 286:31–40, 1980

Cala LA, Jones B, Burns P, et al: Results of computerised tomography, psychometric testing and dietary studies in social drinkers, with emphasis on reversibility after abstinence. Med J Aust 2:264–269, 1983

Carlen PL, Wilkinson DA: Alcoholic brain damage and reversible deficits. Acta Psychiatr Scand Suppl 286:103–118, 1980

Carlen PL, Wilkinson DA: Reversibility of alcohol-related brain damage: clinical and experimental observations. Acta Medica Scandinavica Supplementum 717: 19–26, 1987

Carlen PL, Wortzman G, Holgate RC, et al: Reversible cerebral atrophy in recently abstinent chronic alcoholics measured by computed tomography scans. Science 200:1076–1078, 1978

Carlen PL, Wilkinson DA, Wortzman G, et al: Cerebral atrophy and functional deficits in alcoholics without clinically apparent liver disease. Neurology 31:377–385, 1981

Cascella NG, Pearlson G, Wong DF, et al: Effects of substance abuse on ventricular and sulcal measures assessed by computerized tomography. Br J Psychiatry 159: 217–221, 1991

Chadwick O, Anderson R, Bland M, et al: Neuropsychological consequences of volatile substance abuse: a population based study of secondary school pupils. BMJ 298:1679–1684, 1989

Charness ME: Brain lesions in alcoholics. Alcohol Clin Exp Res 17:2–11, 1993

Charness ME, De La Paz RL: Mammillary body atrophy in Wernicke's encephalopathy: antemortem identification using magnetic resonance imaging. Ann Neurol 22:595–600, 1987

Chasnoff IJ, Burns WJ, Schnoll SH, et al: Cocaine use in pregnancy. N Engl J Med 313:666–669, 1985

Chaudry HR, Moss HB, Bashir A, et al: Cannabis psychosis following bhang ingestion. British Journal of Addiction 86:1075–1081, 1991

Chesher GB, Bird KD, Jackson DM, et al: The effects of orally administered delta-9 tetrahydrocannabinol in man on mood and performance measures: a dose-response study. Pharmacol Biochem Behav 35:861–864, 1990

Clifford CA, Maddocks D: Alcohol-related brain damage: the neuropsychological deficits and their implication for independent living. Australian Drug and Alcohol Review 7:79–81, 1988

Coid J: "Mania à potu": a critical review of pathological intoxication. Psychol Med 9:709–719, 1979

Connell PH: Amphetamine Psychosis. Maudsley Monograph 5. London, Oxford University Press, 1958

Cravioto H, Korein J, Silberman J: Wernicke's encephalopathy. A clinical and pathological study of 28 autopsied cases. Arch Neurol 4:510–519, 1961

Cuffel BJ: Prevalence estimates of substance abuse in schizophrenia and their correlates. J Nerv Ment Dis 180:589–592, 1992

Culver CM, King FW: Neuropsychological assessment of under-graduate marihuana and LSD users. Arch Gen Psychiatry 31:707–711, 1974

Cushman P: Delirium tremens. Postgrad Med 82:117–122, 1987

Daras M, Koppel BS, Akos-Radzion E: Cocaine-induced choreoathetoid movements ("crack dancing"). Neurology 44:751–752, 1994

Deahl M: Cannabis and memory loss. British Journal of Addiction 86:249–252, 1991

De Fillippis WA, McCampbell E: Manual for the Booklet Category Test research and clinical form. Odessa, FL, Psychological Assessment Resources, 1979

Delaney P, Estes M: Intracranial hemorrhage with amphetamine abuse. Neurology 30:1125–1128, 1980

Donnal J, Heinz E, Burger P: MR of reversible thalamic lesions in Wernicke syndrome. American Journal of Neuroradiology 11:893–894, 1990

Drake RE, McHugo GJ, Noordsy DL: Treatment of alcoholism among schizophrenic patients: 4 year outcomes. Am J Psychiatry 150:328–329, 1993

D'Souza T, Shraberg D: Intracranial hemorrhage associated with amphetamine use. Neurology 31:922–923, 1981

Earnest MP, Feldman H, Marx JA, et al: Intracranial lesions shown by CT scans in 259 cases of first alcohol-related seizures. Neurology 38:1561–1565, 1988

Eisendrath SJ, Goldman B, Douglas J, et al: Meperidine-induced delirium. Am J Psychiatry 144:1062–1065, 1987

Ellis RJ, Oscar-Berman M: Alcoholism, aging, and functional cerebral asymmetries. Psychol Bull 106:128–147, 1989

Flamm ES, Demopoulos HB, Seligman ML, et al: Ethanol potentiation of central nervous system trauma. J Neurosurg 46:328–335, 1977

Forman HP, Levin S, Stewart B, et al: Cerebral vasculitis and hemorrhage in an adolescent taking diet pills containing phenylpropranolamine: case report and review of literature. Pediatrics 83:737–741, 1989

Fornazzari L, Wilkinson DA, Kapur BM, et al: Cerebellar, cortical and functional impairment in toluene abusers. Acta Neurol Scand 67:319–329, 1983

Fraser AA, Ingram IM: Lorazepam dependence and chronic psychosis (letter). Br J Psychiatry 147:211, 1985

Fredericks RK, Lefkowitz DS, Challa VR, et al: Cerebral vasculitis associated with cocaine abuse. Stroke 22:1437–1439, 1991

Freund G: Chronic nervous system toxicity of alcohol. Annual Review of Pharmacology 13:217–227, 1973

Gallucci M, Bozzao A, Spendiani A, et al: Wernicke encephalopathy: MR findings in five patients. American Journal of Neuroradiology 11:887–892, 1990

Garey RE, Daul GC, Samuels MS, et al: PCP abuse in New Orleans: a six-year study. Am J Drug Alcohol Abuse 13:135–144, 1987

Gawin FH, Ellinwood EH: Cocaine and other stimulants. Actions, abuse and treatment. N Engl J Med 318:1173–1182, 1988

Gawin FH, Kleber HD: Abstinence symptomatology and psychiatric diagnosis in cocaine abusers. Arch Gen Psychiatry 43:107–113, 1986

Ghodse HA: Drugs and Addictive Behaviour. Oxford, UK, Blackwell Scientific, 1989

Gilman S, Adams K, Koeppe R, et al: Cerebellar and frontal hypometabolism in alcoholic cerebellar degeneration studied with position emission tomography. Ann Neurol 28:775–785, 1990

Glass IB: Alcoholic brain damage: what does it mean to patients? British Journal of Addiction 86:819–821, 1991

Glick R, Hoying J, Cerullo L, et al: Phenylpropanolamine: an over-the-counter drug causing central nervous system vasculitis and intracerebral hemorrhage: case report and review. Neurosurgery 20:969–974, 1987

Golden CJ, Grabler B, Blose I, et al: Difference in brain densities between chronic alcoholics and normal control patients. Science 211:508–510, 1981

Grant BF, Harford TC, Chou P, et al: Prevalence of DSM-III-R alcohol abuse and dependence. Alcohol Health Res World 15:91–96, 1992

Grant I, Rochford J, Fleming T, et al: A neuropsychological assessment of the effects of moderate marihuana use. J Nerv Ment Dis 156:278–280, 1973

Grant I, Adams KM, Reed R: Aging, abstinence, and medical risk factors in the prediction of neuropsychological deficit among long-term alcoholics. Arch Gen Psychiatry 41:710–718, 1984

Grant KA, Valverius P, Hudspith M, et al: Ethanol withdrawal seizures and the NMDA receptor complex. Eur J Pharmacol 176:289–296, 1990

Greenblatt DJ, Miller LG, Shader RI: Benzodiazepine discontinuation syndromes. J Psychiatr Res 24:73–79, 1990

Gurling HMD, Murray RM, Ron MA: Increased brain radiodensity in alcoholism. A co-twin control study. Arch Gen Psychiatry 43:764–767, 1986

Harper CG: The incidence of Wernicke's encephalopathy in Australia—a neuropathological study of 131 cases. J Neurol Neurosurg Psychiatry 46:593–598, 1983

Harper CG, Kril J: Brain atrophy in chronic alcoholic patients—a quantitative pathological study. J Neurol Neurosurg Psychiatry 48:211–217, 1985

Harper CG, Kril JJ: Corpus callosal thickness in alcoholics. British Journal of Addiction 83:577–580, 1988

Harper CG, Kril J: Patterns of neuronal loss in the cerebral cortex in chronic alcoholic patients. J Neurol Sci 92:81–89, 1989

Harper CG, Kril J, Raven D, et al: Intracranial cavity volumes: a new method and its potential applications. Neuropathol Appl Neurobiol 10:25–32, 1984

Harper CG, Kril JJ, Holloway RL: Brain shrinkage in chronic alcoholics: a pathological study. BMJ 290:510–514, 1985

Harper CG, Giles M, Finlay-Jones R: Clinical signs in the Wernicke-Korsakoff complex. A retrospective analysis of 131 cases diagnosed at necropsy. J Neurol Neurosurg Psychiatry 49:341–345, 1986

Harper CG, Kril J, Daly J: Are we drinking our neurones away? BMJ 294:534–536, 1987a

Harper CG, Kril JJ, Daly JM: The specific gravity of the brains of alcoholic and control patients: a pathological study. British Journal of Addiction 82:1349–1354, 1987b

Harrison LD: Trends in illicit drug use in the United States: conflicting secrets from national surveys. Int J Addict 27:817–842, 1992

Haubeck A, Lee K: Computed tomography in alcoholic cerebellar atrophy. Neuroradiology 18:77–79, 1979

Hauser WA, Ng SKC, Brust JCM: Alcohol, seizures and epilepsy. Epilepsia 29 (suppl 2):66–78, 1988

Hawley RJ, Major LF, Schulman E, et al: Cerebrospinal fluid 3-methoxy-4-hydroxyphenylglycol and norepinephrine levels in alcohol withdrawal. Arch Gen Psychiatry 42:1056–1062, 1985

Hearn WL, Flynn DD, Hime GW, et al: Cocaethylene: a unique cocaine metabolite displays high affinity for the dopamine transporter. J Neurochem 56:698–701, 1991

Heishman SJ, Huestis MA, Henningfield JE, et al: Acute and residual effects of marijuahna: profiles of plasma THC levels, physiological, subjective and performance measures. Pharmacol Biochem Behav 37:561–565, 1990

Helzer JE, Burnam A, McEvoy L: Alcohol abuse and dependence, in Psychiatric Disorders in America: The Epidemiological Catchment Area Study. Edited by Robins LN, Regier DA. New York, Free Press, 1991, pp 81–115

Henry JA: Ecstasy and the dance of death. BMJ 305:5–6, 1992

Hillbom M, Holm L: Contribution of traumatic head injury to neuropsychological deficits in alcoholics. J Neurol Neurosurg Psychiatry 49:1348–1353, 1986

Hollister LE, Motzenbecker FP, Degan RO: Withdrawal reactions from chlordiazepoxide. Psychopharmacology 2:63–68, 1961

Hormes JT, Filley CM, Rosenberg NL: Neurologic sequelae of chronic solvent vapor abuse. Neurology 36:698–702, 1986

Hunter R, McLuskie R, Wyper D, et al: The pattern of function-related regional cerebral blood flow investigated by single photon emission tomography with ^{99m}Tc-HMPAO in patients with presenile Alzheimer's disease and Korsakoff's psychosis. Psychol Med 19:847–855, 1989

Institute for the Study of Drug Dependence: Drug Misuse in Britain. London, Institute for the Study of Drug Dependence, 1994

Jacobson JL, Jacobson SW, Sokol RJ: Increased vulnerability to alcohol-related birth defects in the offspring of mothers over 30. Alcohol Clin Exp Res 20:359–363, 1996

Jacobson RR: Female alcoholics—a controlled CT brain scan and clinical study. British Journal of Addiction 81:661–669, 1986

Jacobson RR: Alcoholism, Korsakoff's syndrome and the frontal lobes. Behaviour Neurology 2:25–38, 1989

Jacobson RR, Lishman WA: Selective memory loss and global intellectual deficits in alcoholic Korsakoff's syndrome. Psychol Med 17:649–655, 1987

Jacobson RR, Acker CF, Lishman WA: Patterns of neuropsychological deficit in alcoholic Korsakoff's syndrome. Psychol Med 20:321–334, 1990

Jaffe JH: Tobacco smoking and nicotine dependence, in Nicotine Psychopharmacology. Edited by Wonnacott S, Russell MAH, Stolerman IP. Oxford, UK, Oxford University Press, 1990, pp 1–37

Jensen GB, Pakkenberg B: Do alcoholics drink their neurons away? Lancet 342: 1201–1204, 1993

Jernigan TL, Butters N, Di Traglia G: Reduced cerebral gray matter observed in alcoholics using magnetic resonance imaging. Alcohol Clin Exp Res 15:418–427, 1991a

Jernigan T, Schafer K, Butters N, et al: Magnetic resonance imaging of alcoholic Korsakoff patients. Neuropsychopharmacology 4:175–186, 1991b

Jerrell JM, Hu T, Ridgely MS: Cost-effectiveness of substance disorder interventions for the severely mentally ill. Journal of Mental Health Administration 21: 281–295, 1994

Jones KL, Smith DW: Recognition of the fetal alcohol syndrome in early infancy. Lancet 2:999–1001, 1973

Joyce EM: Aetiology of alcoholic brain damage: alcoholic neurotoxicity or thiamine malnutrition? Br Med Bull 50:99–114, 1994

Kaku DA, Lowenstein DH: Emergence of recreational drug abuse as a major risk factor for stroke in young adults. Ann Intern Med 113:821–827, 1990

Kandel DB: Epidemiological trends and implications for understanding the nature of addiction, in Addictive States. Edited by O'Brien CP, Jaffe JH. New York, Raven, 1992, pp 23–40

Kapur N, Butters N: An analysis of visuoperceptual deficits in Korsakoff's and long-term alcoholics. J Stud Alcohol 38:1718–1729, 1977

Kawamura M, Shiota J, Yagishita T, et al: Computed tomographic scan and magnetic resonance imaging. Ann Neurol 18:103–104, 1985

Kopelman MD: Alcoholic brain damage, in The International Handbook of Addiction Behaviour. Edited by Glass IB. London, Routledge, 1991, pp 141–151

Kopelman MD: The Korsakoff syndrome. Br J Psychiatry 166:154–173, 1995

Kosten TR: Client issues in drug abuse treatment: assessing multiple drug use. NIDA Res Monogr 106:136–151, 1991

Kreek MJ: Using methadone effectively: achieving goals by application of laboratory, clinical and evaluative research and by development of innovative programs. NIDA Res Monogr 106:245–266, 1991

Krendel DA, Ditter SM, Frankel MR, et al: Biopsy proven cerebral vasculitis associated with cocaine abuse. Neurology 40:1092–1094, 1990

Kril JJ, Harper CG: Neuronal counts from four cortical regions in alcoholic brains. Acta Neuropathol (Berl) 79:200–204, 1989

Krystal JH, Karper LP, Seibyl JP, et al: Sub-anaesthetic effects of the non-competitive NMDA antagonist, ketamine, in humans. Arch Gen Psychiatry 51: 199–214, 1994

Kumar R, Mac DS, Gabrielli WF, et al: Anxiolytics and memory: a comparison of lorazepam and alprazolam. J Clin Psychiatry 48:158–160, 1987

Laegreid L: Abnormalities in children exposed to benzodiazepines in utero. Lancet 1:108–109, 1987

Larrogue B, Kaminski M, Dehaene P, et al: Moderate prenatal alcohol exposure and psychomotor development at preschool age. Am J Public Health 85:1654–1661, 1995

Laureno R, Karp BI: Pontine and extrapontine myelinolysis following rapid correction of hyponatraemia. Lancet 1:1439–1441, 1988

Leenane KJ: Management of moderate to severe alcohol-related brain damage. Med J Aust 145:136–139, 1986

Leenane KJ: Patients with alcohol-related brain damage: therapy and outcome. Australian Drug and Alcohol Review 7:89–92, 1988

Lehman AF, Myers CP, Thompson JW, et al: Implications of mental health and substance use disorders: a comparison of single and dual diagnosis patients. J Nerv Ment Dis 181:365–370, 1993

Levine SR, Brust JCM, Futrell N, et al: A comparative study of the cerebrovascular complications of cocaine: alkaloidal versus hydrochloride—a review. Neurology 41:1173–1177, 1991

Linzen DH, Dingemans PM, Lenior ME: Cannabis abuse and the course of recent-onset schizophrenic disorders. Arch Gen Psychiatry 51:273–279, 1994

Lishman WA: Organic Psychiatry, 3rd Edition. Oxford, UK, Blackwell, 1998

Lishman WA: Alcohol and the brain. Br J Psychiatry 156:635–644, 1990

Lishman WA, Jacobson RR, Acker C: Brain damage in alcoholism: current concepts. Acta Medica Scandinavica Supplementum 717:5–17, 1987

Little HJ: The role of neuronal calcium channels in dependence of ethanol and other sedative/hypnotics. Pharmacol Ther 50:347–365, 1991

Lovinger DM, White G, Weight FF: Ethanol inhibits NMDA activated ion currents in hippocampal neurones. Science 243:1721–1724, 1989

Lundborn N, Laurila O, Laurila S: Central pontine myelinolysis after correction of chronic hyponatraemia. Lancet 342:247–248, 1993

Mac DS, Kumar R, Goodwin D: Anterograde amnesia with oral lorazepam. J Clin Psychiatry 46:137–138, 1985

Mathers DC, Ghodse AH: Cannabis and psychotic illness. Br J Psychiatry 161: 648–653, 1992

Mathew RJ, Wilson WH, Humphreys DF, et al: Changes in middle cerebral artery velocity after marijuana. Biol Psychiatry 32:164–169, 1992a

Mathew RJ, Wilson WH, Humphreys DF, et al: Regional cerebral blood flow after marijuana smoking. J Cereb Blood Flow Metab 12:750–758, 1992b

Mathew RJ, Wilson WH, Humphreys DF, et al: Depersonalisation after marijuana smoking. Biol Psychiatry 33:431–441, 1993

Matick H, Anderson D, Brumlik J: Cerebral vasculitis associated with oral amphetamine overdose. Arch Neurol 40:253–254, 1983

McAuliffe WE, Rohman M, Santangelo S, et al: Psychoactive drug use among practising physicians and medical students. N Engl J Med 315:805–810, 1986

McCann VD, Ricaurte GA: Lasting neuropsychiatric sequelae of (+)methylenedioxyamphetamine ("ecstasy") in recreational users. J Clin Psychopharmacol 11:302–305, 1991

McDowell JR, LeBlanc HJ: Computed tomographic findings in Wernicke-Korsakoff syndrome. Arch Neurol 41:453–454, 1984

McGuire P, Fahy T: Chronic paranoid psychosis after misuse of MDMA ("ecstasy"). BMJ 302:697, 1991

McLellan AT, Alterman AI: Patient treatment matching: a conceptual and methodological review with suggestions for further research. NIDA Res Monogr 106: 114–135, 1991

McMullen PA, Saint-Cyr JA, Carlen PL: Morphological alterations in rat CA1 hippocampal pyramidal cell dendrites resulting from chronic ethanol consumption and withdrawal. J Comp Neurol 225:111–118, 1984

Melgaard B: The neurotoxicity of ethanol. Acta Neurol Scand 67:131–142, 1983

Mena I, Giombetti R, Mody CK, et al: Acute cerebral blood flow changes with cocaine intoxication. Neurology 40:179, 1990

Mendelson JH, Ellingboe J, Mello N: Acute effects of natural and synthetic cannabis compounds on prolactin levels in human males. Pharmacol Biochem Behav 20: 103–106, 1984

Mendoza RP, Miller BL, Mena I: Emergency room evaluation of cocaine-associated neuropsychiatric disorders, in Recent Developments in Alcoholism, Vol 10: Alcohol and Cocaine. Edited by Galanter M. New York, Plenum, 1992, pp 73–87

Menezes PR, Johnson S, Thornicroft G, et al: Drug and alcohol problems among individuals with severe mental illness in South London. Br J Psychiatry 168:612–619, 1996

Mensing JWA, Hoogland PH, Slooff JL: Computed tomography in the diagnosis of Wernicke's encephalopathy: a radiological-neuropathological correlation. Ann Neurol 16:363–365, 1984

Meyer J, Tanahashi N, Ishikawa Y, et al: Cerebral atrophy and hypoperfusion improve during treatment of Wernicke-Korsakoff syndrome. J Cereb Blood Flow Metab 5:376–385, 1985

Michaelis EK, Michaelis ML: Ethanol interaction with brain synaptic membrane glutamate receptors and with model membranes. Drug Alcohol Depend 6:68–75, 1980

Miller BL, Chiang F, McGill L, et al: Cardiovascular complications from cocaine: possible long-term sequelae. Current methods of treatment. NIDA Res Monogr 123:129–145, 1992

Mody CK, Miller BL, McIntyre HB, et al: Neurological complications of cocaine abuse. Neurology 38:1189–1193, 1988

Mohler H, Okada T: Biochemical identification of the site of action of benzodiazepines in human brain by ³H-diazepam binding. Life Sci 22:985–995, 1978

Mott J, Mirrlees-Black C: Self-Reported Drug Misuse in England and Wales: Main Findings From the 1992 British Crime Survey. London, Home Office Research and Statistics Department, 1993

Naranjo CA, Sellers EM: Clinical assessment and pharmacotherapy of the alcohol withdrawal syndrome, in Recent Developments in Alcoholism, Vol 4. Edited by Galanter M. New York, Plenum, 1986, pp 265–281

Negrete JC: Cannabis and schizophrenia. British Journal of Addiction 84:349–351, 1989

Nordstrum G, Bergland M: Delirium tremens. J Stud Alcohol 49:178–185, 1988

O'Brien CP: Drug addiction and drug abuse, in Goodman and Gilman's The Pharmacological Basis of Therapeutics, 9th Edition. Edited by Hardman JG, Limbird LE, eds-in-chief. New York, McGraw-Hill, 1996, pp 557–577

Office of Population Censuses and Surveys: Drinking Habits in England and Wales During the 1980s. London, Office of Population Censuses and Surveys, 1990

Office of Population Censuses and Surveys: General Household Survey 1992 (Series CHS No 23). London, Office of Population Censuses and Surveys, 1995

O'Malley SS, Gawin FH: Abstinence symptomatology and neuropsychological impairment in chronic cocaine abusers. NIDA Res Monogr 101:179–190, 1990

Oscar-Berman M: Learning and memory deficits in detoxified alcoholics. NIDA Res Monogr 101:136–155, 1990a

Oscar-Berman M: Severe brain dysfunction: alcoholic Korsakoff's syndrome. Alcohol Health Res World 14:120–129, 1990b

Oscar-Berman M, Ellis RJ: Cognitive deficits related to memory impairments in alcoholism, in Recent Developments in Alcoholism. Edited by Galanter M. New York, Plenum, 1987, pp 59–80

Pascual-Leone A, Dhuna A, Altafullah I, et al: Cocaine-induced seizures. Neurology 40:404–407, 1990

Pascual-Leone A, Dhuna A, Anderson DC: Cerebral atrophy in habitual cocaine abusers: a planimetric CT study. Neurology 41:34–38, 1991

Perera KMH, Tulley M, Jenner FA: The use of benzodiazepines among drug addicts. British Journal of Addiction 82:511–515, 1987

Peroutka ST, Pasco N, Faull KF: Monoamine metabolites in the cerebrospinal fluid of recreational users of 3,4-methylene dioxymethamphetamine (MDMA: "ecstasy"). Research Communications in Substance Abuse 8:125–138, 1987

Peters TJ: Physical complications of alcohol misuse, in Oxford Textbook of Medicine, 3rd Edition. Edited by Weatherall DJ, Ledingham JGG, Warrell DA. Oxford, UK, Oxford University Press, 1996, pp 4276–4278

Petursson H, Lader MH: Withdrawal from long-term benzodiazepine treatment. BMJ 283:643–649, 1981

Pfefferbaum KO, Lim RB, Zipursky DH, et al: Brain gray and white matter volume loss accelerates with aging in chronic alcoholics: a quantitative MRI study. Alcohol Clin Exp Res 16:1078–1089, 1992

Phillips SC, Harper CG, Kril J: A quantitative histological study of the cerebellar vermis in alcoholic patients. Brain 110:301–314, 1987

Preskorn SH, Denner LJ: Benzodiazepines and withdrawal psychosis. JAMA 237:36–38, 1977

Price BH, Mesulam MM: Behavioural manifestations of central pontine myelinolysis. Arch Neurol 44:671–673, 1987

Price J, Mitchell S, Wiltshire B, et al: A follow-up study of patients with alcohol-related brain damage in the community. Australian Drug and Alcohol Review 7:83–87, 1988a

Price LH, Ricaurte GA, Krystal J, et al: Neuroendocrine and mood responses to intravenous L-tryptophan in (+)3,4-methylenedioxy methamphetamine (MDMA) users. Arch Gen Psychiatry 46:20–22, 1988b

Regier DA, Farmer ME, Rae LS, et al: Comorbidity of mental disorders with alcohol and other substances: results from the Epidemiological Catchment Area Study. JAMA 264:2511–2518, 1990

Reitan R: Validity of the Trail Making Test as an indicator of organic brain damage. Percept Mot Skills 8:271–276, 1958

Reuler JB, Girard DE, Cooney TG: Current concepts—Wernicke's encephalopathy. N Engl J Med 312:1035–1039, 1985

Ricaurte G, Bryan G, Strauss L, et al: Hallucinogenic amphetamine selectively destroys brain serotonin nerve terminals. Science 229:986–988, 1985

Ricaurte GA, Finnegan KT, Irwin I, et al: Aminergic metabolites in cerebrospinal fluid of humans previously exposed to MDMA: preliminary observations. Ann N Y Acad Sci 600:699–710, 1990

Rice RD: The economic cost of alcohol abuse and alcohol dependence. Alcohol Health Res World 17:10–18, 1993

Riley EP, Mattson SN, Sowell ER, et al: Abnormalities of the corpus callosum in children prenatally exposed to alcohol. Alcohol Clin Exp Res 19:1198–1202, 1995

Riley JN, Walker DW: Morphological alterations in hippocampus after long-term alcohol consumption in mice. Science 201:646–648, 1978

Rochford J, Grant I, LaVigne G: Medical students and drugs: further neuropsychological and use pattern considerations. Int J Addict 12:1057–1065, 1977

Ron MA: The Alcoholic Brain: CT Scan and Psychological Findings. Psychological Medicine Monograph 3. Cambridge, UK, Cambridge University Press, 1983

Ron MA: Volatile substance abuse: a review of possible long-term neurological, intellectual and psychiatric sequelae. Br J Psychiatry 148:235–246, 1986

Ron MA, Acker W, Lishman WA: Morphological abnormalities in the brains of chronic alcoholics: a clinical, psychological and computerised axial tomography study. Acta Psychiatr Scand Suppl 286:31–49, 1980

Ron MA, Acker W, Shaw GK, et al: Computerised tomography of the brain in chronic alcoholics. A survey and follow up study. Brain 105:497–514, 1982

Rothrock JF, Rubenstein R, Lyden PD: Ischaemic stroke associated with methamphetamine inhalation. Neurology 38:589–595, 1988

Samson Y, Baron J-C, Feline A: Local cerebral glucose utilisation in chronic alcoholics: a positron tomographic study. J Neurol Neurosurg Psychiatry 49:1165–1170, 1986

Scharf MB, Khosla N, Lysaght R, et al: Anterograde amnesia with oral lorazepam. J Clin Psychiatry 44:362–364, 1983

Scharf M, Fletcher K, Graham JP: Comparative amnestic effects of benzodiazepine hypnotic agents. J Clin Psychiatry 49:134–137, 1988

Schmidt CJ, Wu L, Lovenberg W: Methylenedioxymethamphetamine: a potentially neurotoxic amphetamine analog. Eur J Pharmacol 124:175–178, 1986

Schrank KS: Cocaine-related emergency department presentations in acute cocaine intoxication. Current methods of treatment. NIDA Res Monogr 123:110–128, 1992

Schuckit MA: Drug and Alcohol Abuse: A Clinical Guide to Diagnosis and Treatment, 4th Edition. New York, Plenum, 1995

Schwartz RH, Gruenewald PJ, Klitzner M, et al: Short-term memory impairment in cannabis-dependent adolescents. American Journal of Diseases of Children 143:1214–1219, 1989

Serdaru M, Hausser-Haw C, Laplane D, et al: The clinical spectrum of alcoholic pellagra encephalopathy. Brain 111:829–842, 1988

Sharp CW: Introduction to inhalant abuse. NIDA Res Monogr 129:1–11, 1992

Shimamura AP, Jernigan TL, Squire LR: Korsakoff's syndrome: radiological (CT) findings and neuropsychological correlates. J Neurosci 8:4400–4410, 1988

Slavney PR, Rich GB, Pearlson GD, et al: Phencyclidine abuse and symptomatic mania. Biol Psychiatry 12:697–700, 1977

Sowell ER, Jernigan TL, Mattson SN, et al: Abnormal development of the cerebellar vermes in children prenatally exposed to alcohol: size reduction in lobules I—V. Alcohol Clin Exp Res 20:31–34, 1996

Spohr HL, Will MS, Steinhausen HS: Prenatal alcohol exposure and long-term developmental consequences. Lancet 341:907–910, 1993

Squire LR, Amaral DG, Press GA: Magnetic resonance imaging of the hippocampal formation and mammillary nuclei distinguish medial temporal lobe and diencephalic amnesia. J Neurosci 10:3106–3117, 1990

Steele TD, McCann UD, Ricaurte GA: 3,4-Methylene-dioxymethamphetamine (MDMA, "ecstasy"): pharmacology and toxicology in animals and humans. Addiction 89:539–551, 1994

Stillman R, Galanter M, Lemberger L, et al: Tetrahydrocannabinol (THC): metabolism and subjective effects. Life Sci 19:569–576, 1976

Stone DM, Stanl DC, Hanson GR, et al: The effects of 3,4-methylene dioxy-methamphetamine (MDMA) and 3,4-methylenedioxy-amphetamine (MDA) on monoaminergic systems in the rat brain. Eur J Pharmacol 128:41–48, 1986

Strang J, Gurling H: Computerised tomography and neuropsychological assessment in long-term high-dose known addicts. British Journal of Addiction 9:1011–1019, 1989

Swanson J, Holzer C, Ganju V: Violence and psychiatric disorder in the community: evidence from the Epidemiological Catchment Area Survey. Hospital and Community Psychiatry 41:761–770, 1990

Tarter RE, Schneider DU: Blackouts—relationship with memory capacity and alcoholic history. Arch Gen Psychiatry 33:1492–1496, 1976

Tarter RE, Hegedus A, Gavaler J: Hyperactivity in sons of alcoholics. J Stud Alcohol 46:259–261, 1985

Taylor P: Agents acting at the neuromuscular junction and autonomic ganglia, in Goodman and Gilman's The Pharmacological Basis of Therapeutics, 9th Edition. Edited by Hardman JG, Limbird EE. New York, McGraw-Hill, 1996, pp 177–197

Torvik A, Torp S: The prevalence of alcoholic cerebellar atrophy. A morphometric and histological study of autopsy material. J Neurol Sci 75:43–51, 1986

Tsai G, Gastfriend DR, Coyle JT: The glutamatergic basis of human alcoholism. Am J Psychiatry 152:332–340, 1995

Tsuang JW, Irwin MR, Smith TL, et al: Characteristics of men with alcoholic hallucinosis. Addiction 89:73–78, 1994

Tumeh SS, Nagel JS, English RJ, et al: Cerebral abnormalities in cocaine abusers: demonstration by SPECT perfusion brain scintigraphy. Radiology 176:821–824, 1990

Varma VK, Malhotra AK, Dang R, et al: Cannabis and cognitive functions: a prospective study. Drug Alcohol Depend 21:147–152, 1988

Victor M, Brausch C: The role of abstinence in the genesis of alcohol epilepsy. Epilepsia 8:1–20, 1967

Victor M, Adams RD, Mancall EL: A restricted form of cerebellar cortical degeneration occurring in alcoholic patients. Arch Neurol 1:579–688, 1959

Victor M, Adams RD, Collins GH: The Wernicke-Korsakoff Syndrome. A Clinical and Pathological Study of 245 Patients, 82 With Post-Mortem Examinations. Philadelphia, PA, FA Davis, 1971

Victor M, Adams RD, Collins GH: The Wernicke-Korsakoff's syndrome and other related neurologic disorders related to alcohol and malnutrition. Philadelphia, PA, FA Davis, 1989

Volkow ND, Mullani N, Gould KL, et al: Cerebral blood flow in chronic cocaine users. Br J Psychiatry 152:641–648, 1988

Volkow ND, Fowler JS, Wolf AP, et al: Changes in brain glucose metabolism in cocaine dependence and withdrawal. Am J Psychiatry 148:621–626, 1991

Walker DW, Barnes DE, Zornetzer SF, et al: Neuronal loss in hippocampus induced by prolonged ethanol consumption in rats. Science 209:711–713, 1980

Weiss SR, Raskind R, Morganstern NL, et al: Intracerebral and subarachnoid hemorrhage following use of methamphetamine ("speed"). Int Surg 53:123–127, 1970

West JR, Lind MS, Demuth RM, et al: Lesion-induced sprouting in the rat dentate gyrus is inhibited by repeated ethanol administration. Science 218:808–810, 1982

Wilkinson DA, Sanchez-Craig M: Relevance of brain dysfunction to treatment objectives: should alcohol-related cognitive deficits influence the way we think about treatment. Addictive Behaviours 6:253–260, 1981

Wolkowitz OM, Weingartner H, Thompson K, et al: Diazepam-induced amnesia: a neuropharmacological model of an "organic amnestic syndrome." Am J Psychiatry 144:25–29, 1987

Woody GE, McLellan AT, O'Brien CP, et al: Assessing psychiatric comorbidity. NIDA Res Monogr 106:152–166, 1991

World Health Organization: The ICD-10 Classification of Mental and Behavioural Disorders. Geneva, World Health Organization, 1992

Wright DG, Laureno R, Victor M: Pontine and extra-pontine myelinolysis. Brain 102:361–389, 1979

Yesavage JA, Freman AM: Acute phencyclidine (PCP) intoxication: psychopathology and prognosis. J Clin Psychiatry 39:664–666, 1978

Yu VJ, Cooper DR, Wellenstein DE, et al: Cerebral angiitis and intracerebral hemorrhage associated with methamphetamine abuse. J Neurosurg 58:109–111, 1983

CHAPTER 6

A Neuropsychiatric Approach to Aggressive Behavior

Sheldon Benjamin, M.D.

In 1991, there were 758 violent crimes for every 100,000 people in the United States, with one violent crime occurring every 17 seconds (U.S. Department of Justice 1992). This figure does not include violence that did not result in charges being filed because of mental illness, brain damage, or other reasons. No figures are available to allow calculation of the percentage of violent crimes related to psychiatric or neurological disease, but individuals with brain damage are thought to represent a minority of violent offenders (Elliott 1992).

Aggressive behavior is universal. It is essential for drive fulfillment and survival. Despite the aforementioned figures, aggressive behavior usually is not pathological. *Temperamental aggression,* related to the assertiveness that enables humans to be competitive, confers an adaptive advantage and is presumed to be part of our heredity. Only when assertiveness is inappropriate to the context does it become aggression. When temperamental aggression requires treatment, behavioral, educational, psychotherapeutic, or environmental manipulation approaches are often used. *Pathological aggression,* according to this paradigm, is more likely to be a reflection of an abnormal brain and is less likely to be genetically determined (Gualtieri 1991). It typically manifests as irritability or explosive outbursts. In contradistinction to temperamental aggression, pathological aggression often requires treatment. To attempt to eliminate aggression altogether would not be an appropriate goal for neuropsychiatric research. The investigation and treatment of pathological aggression, however, falls solidly within the purview of neuropsychiatry. Elucidating the relationship between specific brain pathologies and pathological aggression both enhances our ability to determine which individuals are at risk of becoming violent and leads to the development of specific management approaches aimed at the underlying cause of aggressive behavior in a given individual.

Pathophysiology of Aggression

Although a general link between brain damage and aggression was contained in Eugen Bleuler's description of the "organic psychosyndrome" (Bleuler 1916), the notion of a single "organic brain syndrome" producing aggression is overly simplistic and limits understanding of the complex relationships among brain areas associated with aggression. The Jacksonian concept of hierarchical control of brain function is a useful paradigm for comparing the impact of levels of central nervous system (CNS) damage on aggressive behavior. According to this model, primitive homeostatic functions are subserved by our "reptilian" brain, the hypothalamus and brainstem. The limbic system exerts control over these lower brain areas. Finally, neocortical areas allow humans higher control over limbic and brainstem areas. The frontal neocortex, for example, a critical area in the genesis of pathological aggression, modulates both limbic and hypothalamic output. In a review of the literature on aggression in animals and humans (Weiger and Bear 1988), it was demonstrated that damage at any of these levels can result in pathological aggression. Anatomic localization of these three levels is illustrated in Figure 6–1. The following discussion of levels of neural organization associated with aggression is based on this model.

Diencephalic Level

The hypothalamus monitors the internal chemical milieu, controls pituitary hormonal responses, and sends input to lower centers associated with stereotypical behaviors. Hypothalamic functions include regulation of temperature, thirst, satiety, and biological rhythms. Discrete hypothalamic lesions, relatively uncommon in humans, have been shown in animals to elicit stereotyped aggressive behavior independent of history or environmental stimuli. Bard (1928) coined the term *sham rage* for the displays of unprovoked rage behavior (hissing, autonomic excitement, arching of back, and claw extension)

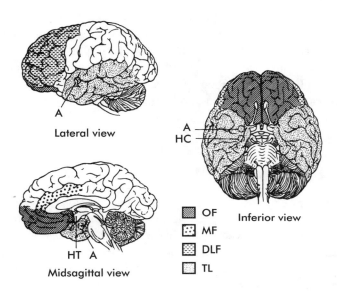

FIGURE 6-1.   CNS levels implicated in aggression. OF = orbitofrontal cortex; DLF = dorsolateral frontal cortex; MF = medial frontal cortex; A = amygdala; HT = hypothalamus; HC = hippocampus; TL = temporal lobe. Dotted circles indicate approximate locations of structures deep to the cortical surface.

evoked by section of a cat's brain just rostral to the hypothalamus. It was later shown that lateral hypothalamic stimulation in cats elicited predatory behavior toward natural prey, described as a "quiet biting attack" or "stalking attack" (Wasman and Flynn 1962).

Muricidal behavior in cats has also been induced by lateral hypothalamic injection of cholinesterase inhibitors and blocked by injection of atropine, implicating acetylcholine as a lateral hypothalamic neurotransmitter with a role in aggression (Smith et al. 1970). Bear et al. (1986) reported a fascinating case that may represent a clinical correlation of this finding in humans. Following several days of heavy application to his cat of flea powder containing an anticholinesterase agent, both man and cat developed a striking behavior change. The cat began killing large numbers of birds and mice, and the man developed "a continual rage" causing his housemate to leave for fear of attack. Within a week of discontinuing use of the offending agent, both man and cat returned to their premorbid personalities.

Stimulation of the ventromedial hypothalamus evokes a defensive posture in the animal and inhibits aggression (Roberts 1958). Bilateral destruction of the ventromedial hypothalamus induced previously friendly animals to attack their caretakers (Wheatley 1944), apparently by removing this inhibition. A famous human correlation of this observation was provided by Reeves and Plum (1969), who reported the development of bulimia, obesity, amenorrhea, diabetes insipidus, and aggressive outbursts toward approaching individuals in a 20-year-old woman who proved on postmortem examination to have a hamartoma destroying her ventromedial hypothalamus.

Limbic System Level

The limbic system, with functions subserving emotions, exerts control over the hypothalamus. The amygdala, located in the anteromedial temporal lobe, is an important link between incoming sensory and sensory association signals and outflow to the hypothalamus, a sort of bridge between externally perceived reality and basic drives. It may help assign emotional valence to perceived objects (Bear 1979). In their famous experiment, Heinrich Klüver and Paul Bucy (1939) performed bilateral anterior temporal lobectomies on sexually mature rhesus monkeys and observed a number of changes in the monkeys' behavior. These included the development of "hypermetamorphosis," or a tendency to explore their cages extensively; increased orality, or the tendency to use their mouths to examine objects; diversification of appetite and sexual practices; and what was called "tameness," or a reduction in fear toward normally fear-inducing objects (including humans). The reduced fear was believed to be a form of "psychic blindness," or loss of the emotional valence associated with perceived objects. Attempts to replicate this work, but with the animals observed in groups or in their natural habitats rather than isolated in cages, resulted in the observation that the animals were unable to assume their normal role in the social hierarchy of the group and tended toward social isolation (Kling 1972). Aggression was decreased in certain contexts but increased in others. The tameness observed in captivity may reflect not simply loss of aggressivity but a more complex loss of a sense of social appropriateness.

A Klüver-Bucy–like syndrome occurs in humans following bilateral destruction of the amygdalae resulting from herpes encephalitis, Pick's disease, or head trauma or late in the course of Alzheimer's disease. Affected individuals typically become apathetic and docile; tend to explore their environment with their hands, placing objects they encounter into their mouths; become bulimic; and become sexually preoccupied. Many develop agnosias, and nearly all show signs of aphasia and amnesia (Lilly et al. 1983).

Modulation of hypothalamic-mediated aggressive behavior by the amygdala has been demonstrated in animals. Stimulation of the dorsomedial amygdala of a cat undergoing lateral hypothalamic stimulation results in increased firing of the ventromedial hypothalamus, inhibiting cat attack behavior toward rats. Stimulation of the ventrolateral amygdala decreases firing of the ventromedial hypothalamus and facilitates the cat's attack behavior (Egger and Flynn 1967).

The opposite effect on limbic control of the hypothalamus can occur in temporolimbic epilepsy, with increased firing of the amygdala. Gastaut (1954), Geschwind (Waxman and Geschwind 1975), Bear (Bear and Fedio 1977), and others have described a constellation of personality traits in individuals with temporal lobe epilepsy (TLE) that includes a general deepening of the emotions (hyperemotionality), alterations in sexuality (typically a decrease), and a tendency to cling to each thought, idea, and action longer than dictated by the context, a trait that has been called *hypometamorphosis*. This interictal personality disturbance can thus be considered a partial inverse of the Klüver-Bucy syndrome, in which hypoemotionality, hypermetamorphosis, and hypersexuality occur (Blumer 1975; Gastaut 1954). Interictal psychosis and depression also occur at higher than predicted rates in this population (Trimble 1996).

Partial seizures are the most frequent form of acquired epilepsy, and temporolimbic foci are the most common source of partial seizures. The frequency and specificity of the aforementioned interictal personality syndrome have been the subject of debate, but the traits do seem to occur in a minority of individuals with temporolimbic seizures. Using healthy and neuromuscular disease control groups, Bear and Fedio (1977) surveyed individuals with lateralized temporolimbic seizure foci for the presence of 18 personality traits frequently described in the literature as occurring in this population. Table 6–1 lists these traits in order of decreasing ability to discriminate subjects with temporal lobe epilepsy from control subjects. A number of authors have replicated Bear and Fedio's findings of increased interictal traits in people with TLE (Hermann and Riel 1981; Mungas 1982; Nielson and Kristensen 1981; Rodin and Schmaltz 1984; Seidman 1980; Stark-Adamec and Adamec 1986). Some authors, however, failed to demonstrate the specificity of the syndrome when control groups consisted of people with generalized seizures, mixed psychiatric disorders, or neurobehavioral disorders (Hermann and Riel 1981; Rodin and Schmaltz 1984; Stark-Adamec and Adamec 1986). However, there are problems inherent in each of these control groups as well (e.g., generalized seizures involve the temporal lobes; mixed psychiatric disorders and mixed neurobehavioral disorders would be

TABLE 6–1.   Interictal traits associated with temporal lobe epilepsy

Humorlessness	Anger
Dependence	Religiosity
Circumstantiality	Hypermoralism
Sense of personal destiny	Paranoia
Obsessiveness	Sadness
Viscosity	Hypergraphia
Emotionality	Elation
Guilt	Aggression
Philosophical interest	Altered sexuality

Note.   Traits are listed in decreasing order of ability to discriminate people with temporal lobe epilepsy from control subjects.
Source.   Adapted from Bear and Fedio 1977.

expected to include many of the behavioral attributes subsumed in the temporal lobe syndrome).

Various interictal traits have been reported to occur more frequently in patients with an aura of fear (Hermann 1982) or a mediobasal focus on the electroencephalogram (EEG) (Nielson and Kristensen 1981). Further work in this direction could help determine which TLE patients are at highest risk for development of interictal personality features.

In discussing the association of aggression and epilepsy, it is important to be clear about the temporal relationship of aggression and seizures. *Ictal aggression* is rare. When it does occur, it consists of brief, unplanned outbursts toward objects or individuals in the patient's environment at the time of the seizure. Movements tend to be stereotyped, automatic, and unsustained, typically lasting about 30 seconds (Delgado-Escueta et al. 1981). Planning and carrying out a violent crime would be impossible during a complex partial seizure.

Postictal aggression is fairly common. In the postictal confusional state, an individual may be irritable and actively resist attempts at restraint, but any aggression that occurs will be unplanned, undirected, and unsustained. Epileptic prodromes of up to a few days of increased irritability terminated by a seizure can also occur.

Interictal aggression refers to aggression that occurs at a time when the individual is not having seizures. It may occur with increased frequency in individuals who manifest the interictal behavior syndrome described above. With deepened emotions, fearfulness or paranoia, and a moralistic viewpoint, aggressive behavior may be expressed as "justified rage." It may be well planned and include complex behaviors, and the individual may feel conflicted over the action taken. Aggressive behavior may occur in response to a stimulus that others, unaware of the meaning of the stimulus to the patient, perceive as trivial (Devinsky and Bear 1984). Interictal aggression has been found to occur more frequently in TLE than in primary generalized epilepsy and in left- rather than right-sided TLE foci (Devinsky et al. 1994). Compared with psychiatric inpatients with aggressive personality disorders, patients with TLE were less likely to be amnestic for aggressive acts and more likely to claim responsibility (Bear et al. 1982). Interictal aggression occasionally improves with seizure control (Walker and Blumer 1984).

The association between TLE and interictal behavior change, reported by many authors (Bear 1979; Bear and Fedio 1977; Bear and Schenk 1981; Herzog et al. 1982; Sachdev and Waxman 1981; Seidman 1980), could have numerous explanations. Apart from coincidence, which is unlikely because of the frequency of the behaviors and because their onset follows the onset of seizures, there are a number of possible explanations for this association:

- Both the seizure disorder and the behavior may be caused by the same underlying brain lesion. For example, interictal psychosis is more common among individuals with medial temporal lesions (Davison and Bagley 1969). Frontal lobe seizures can be associated with aggression in that they are sometimes accompanied by frontal lobe personality syndromes (see next section) caused by the same lesion.
- Behavioral or cognitive effects of anticonvulsants may influence the behavior. These effects include behavioral or cognitive toxicity, not only at supratherapeutic anticonvulsant levels but at standard therapeutic levels as well in some cases. Barbiturate therapy is associated with irritability, depression, and learning problems (Farwell et al. 1990; McGowan et al. 1983). Antiepileptic therapy can cause hyposexuality (Isojarvi et al. 1995). Vigabatrin (γ-vinyl-γ-aminobutyric acid [γ-vinyl GABA]) has been associated with depression, psychotic symptoms, and irritability, especially in individuals with psychiatric histories (Brodie and McKee 1990; Ring et al. 1993). Although carbamazepine or valproate is usually the best choice for individuals with seizure disorders and behavioral or psychiatric issues, these agents, like most antiepileptic drugs, can occasionally cause cognitive or behavioral problems (Trimble 1988).
- The behavior could be caused by subictal epileptic activity. Deep limbic discharges can be measured by depth electrodes in the absence of an abnormal pattern on scalp EEG in some cases.

- Though organized aggression is unlikely during a seizure, the behavior could be ictal activity mistaken for psychiatric symptoms. It is frequently difficult to detect ictal epileptic activity resulting from simple partial seizures on scalp EEG, for example. Deep frontal seizures often elude detection too.

- Behavior and seizure frequency may be related. Frequent seizures have been known, since the time of Kraepelin, to be capable of producing epileptic "twilight states," with the patient in a low-grade confusional state that may be associated with development of psychiatric symptoms and behavior or personality change (Bruens 1974). Too-tight seizure control, on the other hand, can also be associated with behavioral deterioration. The observation that seizures can sometimes result in amelioration of psychotic symptoms led von Meduna to introduce convulsive therapy in the 1930s. Some individuals with both psychosis and epilepsy have an increased propensity toward psychotic exacerbation when their seizures are well controlled and a decreased propensity toward psychosis when their seizures are poorly controlled. Landolt demonstrated the EEG correlation of this "alternating psychosis," a phenomenon called *forced normalization*, in which previously epileptiform EEG activity normalizes during psychotic symptoms and resumes when the individual is no longer psychotic (Wolf 1991). A number of explanations for this phenomenon have been suggested, including opposing effects on central monoamines, opposing γ-aminobutyric acid (GABA) and dopaminergic effects, and kindling of limbic dopaminergic neurons (Pollock 1987). It is suspected that the frequency of other behaviors, as well, may be inversely related to seizure frequency in some individuals.

- Abnormal temporolimbic discharges themselves can lead to behavior changes. The temporal lobe appears to help attribute visceral and emotional significance to perceived stimuli. Bear (1979) postulated that intermittent temporolimbic seizure discharges may result in the learning of aberrant sensorilimbic associations that would lead to unusual predilections and behavior. Because of the inverse relationship between interictal traits and the Klüver-Bucy syndrome of temporolimbic disconnection, he called his proposed mechanism *sensory-limbic hyperconnection*. Kindling theory offers a possible mechanism. *Kindling* refers to the induction of seizures or behavior changes by repetitive application to sensitive brain areas of subconvulsive electrical or chemical stimuli. The defensive rage response threshold in the cat, for example, has been permanently lowered by kindling the hypothalamus (Adamec and Stark-Adamec 1983). Although kindling observations have been confined to animal models, some researchers believe that secondary epileptogenesis or development of mirror foci in epileptic individuals may represent a human example (Morrell 1991). It is the limbic areas typically involved in temporal lobe epilepsy that are most sensitive to the kindling effect. Abnormal temporolimbic discharges may exert a more detrimental effect on personality if the seizure focus is active during crucial periods of personality development.

- Finally, it has been alleged that the experience of epilepsy alone may be sufficient to produce alterations of personality and behavior. This suggestion has not been well supported by experimental data and does not explain the apparent preferential association of interictal behavior changes with temporolimbic epilepsy.

Frontal Neocortical Level

The prefrontal cortex plays a role in social learning, anticipation of consequences of behaviors, and response selection. The orbitofrontal cortex, connected with the amygdala and hypothalamus, and via the frontal dorsolateral convexity with the rest of the brain, exerts higher control over the amygdala. Orbitofrontal damage renders an individual overly responsive to environmental changes. Trivial stimuli elicit aggression normally precluded by long-range judgment. The time, place, and strategy of the aggressive response are inappropriate to the social context. Individuals with orbitofrontal damage are impulsive, are socially disinhibited, and lack critical self-evaluation. They may be unable to anticipate the negative consequences of a given behavior. They can be silly, hyperactive, and excitable so that their behavior can resemble mania.

Damage to the dorsolateral convexity of the frontal lobe, on the other hand, typically renders the individual apathetic, with slowed psychomotor activity, lack of motivation (abulia), and, occasionally, brief aggressive outbursts. Individuals with such damage may be mistaken as depressed. Medial frontal damage involving the cingulum also causes a sluggish apathy and can result in akinetic states. Table 6–2 compares the deficits associated with lesions of the three prefrontal areas (Figure 6–1).

The division of frontal syndromes into three subtypes is not without problems. Most etiologies of frontal damage do not respect these divisions, and combination syndromes are the rule. Bilateral damage is often necessary for the emergence of frontal lobe syndromes, though milder forms may be seen with unilateral damage. In recent years, the strictly localizationist perspective has been supplanted by the concept of a distributed frontal network involving frontal lobes, caudate nuclei, and the dorsomedial nuclei of the thalamus (Mesulam 1990). Aspects of the frontal syndrome may ensue from

TABLE 6–2. Comparison of frontal syndromes

	Area of damage		
	Dorsolateral convexity	Orbitofrontal cortex	Medial FC (anterior cingulum)
Signs and symptoms	"Pseudodepressed"	"Pseudopsychopathic"	Akinetic (decreased initiation of motor behavior in milder forms)
	Abulic	May be hyperactive or look hypomanic (but affect is shallow)	Mute (decreased verbal output in milder forms)
			More pronounced with supplementary motor area involvement
	Apathetic	Irritable	Apathetic
	Unmotivated	Disinhibited	Decreased spontaneity
	Indifferent	Antisocial behavior (aggression short-lived)	Urinary incontinence
	Occasional short-lived outbursts	Inappropriate jocular affect (witzelsucht)	Gait disturbance (lower extremity weakness and sensory loss)
		Inane euphoria (moria)	
	Psychomotor retardation	Emotional lability	
	Inability to inhibit inappropriate responses	Easily influenced by environment	
		Imitation behavior	
		Utilization behavior	
		Environmental dependency	
	Motor perseveration and impersistence	Poor judgment	
	Inability to profit from mistakes	Sexual preoccupation (rare sexual aggression)	
	Decreased creativity	Lack of social tact	

Signs and symptoms (continued)	Decreased future planning	Undue familiarity	Poor organization
			Coarsening of interpersonal style
			Impulsivity
			Inability to take pleasure (especially aesthetic, social, or intellectual)
			Restricted response to pain
			Distractibility
			Impaired goal-oriented behavior
			Lack of concern for correct performance
			Lack of insight and foresight
			Inability to see ramifications of decisions
			Inability to organize daily activity or plan for future
			Decreased creativity
			Inability to pursue meaningful interpersonal relationships
Etiologies	Trauma	Trauma	Vascular
	Hydrocephalus	Tumor	Deep medial tumors
	Tumor	Anterior cerebral artery aneurysm	Hydrocephalus
	Alzheimer's disease	Pick's disease	
	Multiple sclerosis	Multiple sclerosis	

(continued)

TABLE 6–2. Comparison of frontal syndromes *(continued)*

	Area of damage		
	Dorsolateral convexity	Orbitofrontal cortex	Medial FC (anterior cingulum)
Etiologies *(continued)*	Psychosurgery	Encephalitis Psychosurgery	
Cognitive deficits	Problems shifting set[a] Pull to stimulus[b] Perseveration on multiple loops, and alternating sequences Discrepant motor and verbal behavior[c] Motor programming and sequencing deficits[d] Poor word list generation[e] Poor abstraction and categorization Segmented perception and drawing[f]	Impaired go/no-go performance[g] Pull to stimulus Intrusions on mental status tasks Performance variability Inability to preserve organization of learned material Inability to recognize social task demands in context	Impaired go/no-go performance[g] Slowness on all tasks
		Disinhibited grasp response (when supplementary motor area involved)	Disinhibited grasp response (when supplementary motor area involved)

Note. Most clinical situations involve aspects of more than one frontal syndrome. FC = frontal cortex. [a]Decreased ability to shift set refers to the inability to shift to a new task without contamination from prior tasks. The Wisconsin Card Sort task requires this skill. [b]Inability to overcome automatic pull to most salient stimulus available. For example, the patient draws hands pointing to the 10 and the 11 instead of the 11 and the 2 when asked to draw a clock with hands pointing to "10 after 11." [c]Difficulty maintaining linkage between verbal output and motor task. For example, the patient might be able to repeat "knock, cut, slap" but unable to perform the appropriate simultaneous hand movements in sequence when being taught the Luria three-step motor sequence. [d]Inability to perform a series of motor tasks in the correct order. For example, the patient may perform all three hand movements of the Luria three-step motor sequence but in the wrong order. [e]Difficulty coming up with more than a few words in a given category. The patient is given 1 minute to say all of the words he or she can think of that begin with a given letter or is asked to list as many members of a category (e.g., automobile models) as possible in 1 minute. Most high school graduates should be able to list at least 12 words. [f]When asked to copy a complex figure, the patient will proceed one segment at a time rather than noticing the overall outline of the figure. [g]The go/no-go procedure tests ability to inhibit an overlearned response. The patient is first trained to perform an alternating procedure (e.g., holding up one finger when the examiner holds up two) and then told to change the rules and refrain from responding under one condition).

Sources. Data from M. Albert, personal communication, 1986; Cummings 1985; Damasio 1985; and Mega and Cummings 1994.

damage to any of the sites in the network.

The original report, almost 150 years ago, of behavior change resulting from frontal lobe damage remains one of the better descriptions of the syndrome. Phineas P. Gage, a foreman in the blasting brigade of the Rutland and Burlington Railroad in Cavendish, Vermont, was injured September 13, 1848, when an explosion resulted in a 4-foot tamping iron being blown through his frontal lobes. Amazingly, he recovered under the care of Dr. J. M. Harlow, but his behavior was permanently changed, as captured in the following description by Dr. Harlow:

He is fitful, irreverent, indulging at times in the grossest profanity (which was not previously his custom), manifesting but little deference for his fellows, impatient of restraint or advice when it conflicts with his desires, at times pertinaciously obstinate yet capricious and vacillating, devising many plans of future operation which are no sooner arranged than they are abandoned in turn for others appearing more feasible. A child in his intellectual capacity and manifestations, he has the animal passions of a strong man. In this regard his mind was radically changed, so decidedly that his friends and acquaintances said he was "no longer Gage." (Harlow 1868, pp. 339–340)

The following case from the University of Massachusetts Neuropsychiatry Referral Center illustrates a posttraumatic mixed frontal lobe syndrome.

Bifrontal encephalomalacia and hydrocephalus following traumatic lobar hemorrhages producing mixed orbital and dorsolateral convexity frontal syndrome. A 34 year old right handed single male computer technician sustained left frontoparietal fracture, left subdural hematoma, and bifrontal parenchymal hemorrhages after falling down a flight of stairs in his home while intoxicated. His parents, also intoxicated, were unaware of the incident until discovering him the next morning. He sustained widespread bilateral frontal damage and required a ventriculoperitoneal shunt for treatment of hydrocephalus. Residual deficits included mild spastic right hemiparesis, incontinence, marked executive function difficulties, perseveration, decreased verbal fluency, stimulus-bound behavior, and a dramatic personality change. The latter included bouts of explosive laughter or shouting, impulsivity, irritability, a tendency to become overwhelmed with task complexity, concrete thinking, poor insight, denial of deficits, and markedly impaired future planning. He was apathetic about his hospitalization, though he claimed to disagree with it, and gave a different plan each week for what he wanted to do post-discharge. He would suddenly become loud and threatening, bring his face into close proximity with another individual and posture as if about to strike. His behavior was quite frightening to staff and patients. Unless intervention occurred, such interactions would end in the patient striking blows with closed fists or provoking a fight. Behavioral exacerbations were often influenced by the level of stimulation in his environment. Understanding of the behavioral changes enabled staff to implement a simple treatment plan for his aggressive outbursts. Removal from the provoking stimulus, quiet interaction, and sometimes the offer of a snack were all that was necessary to prevent escalation of his behavior.

The frontal lobes are essential for maturation of complex comportmental skills, formal operational thought, appropriate social conduct, and moral judgment (Price et al. 1990). As opposed to other childhood brain injuries—those producing aphasia, for example—from which recovery is often excellent, early life damage to the prefrontal cortex can have devastating consequences. Price et al. (1990) described an individual who developed sociopathic behavior resulting from bilateral congenital frontal subdural hematomas evacuated at 1 week of age. By age 8, he did not respond to parental discipline, could not delay gratification, tended to blame others for his problems, and was easily influenced by deviant children. He was psychiatrically hospitalized and imprisoned many times as an adult, amassing a long list of offenses, including physical and sexual assault, arson, forgery, larceny, and lewd behavior (public masturbation, bartering cigarettes for sexual favors). He often committed offenses impulsively in full view of authorities with no thought as to consequences. The social and emotional deficits of early life frontal damage may also be delayed. Eslinger et al. (1992) reported the case of a 33-year-old woman who sustained a left frontal hemorrhage at age 7. Although she exhibited cognitive slowing after the injury, social disinhibition, interpersonal conflicts, and emotional dysregulation did not appear until she was confronted with the progressively more complex social situations that develop in adolescence.

Aggression in interictal personality syndrome differs from that seen in frontal lobe syndromes. Whereas the individual with temporolimbic seizures and interictal aggression typically has a general deepening of the emotions, the individual with frontal dysfunction typically is emotionally shallow. Although the precipitant may seem trivial to an observer, interictal aggression may occur in response to a violation of the individual's rigid moral code, may be planned and long remembered, and may be seen as justified rage by that person. Frontal aggression, on the other hand, may occur in response to truly trivial provocation and be poorly planned, and the individual's anger may be short-lived.

It is not uncommon for posttraumatic seizures, personality change, and chronic vegetative symptoms to develop in a single individual with traumatic brain injury, potentially affecting all three brain levels involved in the control of aggression. In one study of 286 recurrently violent individuals evaluated in a private neurological practice, combinations of head injury and seizures were found to be common (Elliott 1982). Frontal lobe dysfunction may also be a common pathway for several etiologies of violent behavior. Raine et al. (1994) reported prefrontal hypometabolism on positron-emission tomography (PET) during a continuous performance task in a controlled study of 22 violent offenders accused of murder. Their cohort included individuals with schizophrenia, traumatic brain injury, attention-deficit disorder, substance abuse, epilepsy, and paranoid personality, so it would be difficult to conclude that violence was the only variable potentially correlating with the PET findings. However, the suggestion of prefrontal dysfunction is intriguing. The association of violent criminal offending with evidence of brain abnormality is discussed at length in Chapter 7.

Other Conditions Associated With Aggressive Behavior

Studies of episodic dyscontrol syndrome (intermittent explosive disorder) (Elliott 1992) and of marital violence (Rosenbaum and Hoge 1989) have found individuals with traumatic brain injury to be overrepresented in these conditions. Attention-deficit/hyperactivity disorder (ADHD), a frequently familial disorder presumed to reflect diffuse neurochemical or neurological dysfunction, is strongly associated with aggressive behavior. Between 10% and 50% of adolescents with ADHD develop antisocial behavior (Cantwell 1985). Twenty-three percent of children with ADHD, compared with 2% of children without ADHD, exhibited sociopathy as adults (Hechtman and Weiss 1986). ADHD frequently persists into adulthood. Though not typically hyperactive, adults with this syndrome experience instability in academic, marital, and occupational pursuits and lack the executive functions necessary to organize themselves to meet financial, personal, and occupational obligations in a timely way (Kane et al. 1990).

Certain chromosomal abnormalities have been associated with aggression. The XYY chromosomal anomaly has, in the past, been linked to violent behavior, but this association has not been proven. Klinefelter's syndrome (XXY syndrome) has been associated with EEG abnormalities and behavioral disturbances. Fragile X syndrome often includes dysmorphic features, impaired intellect, autistic symptoms, and aggressive behavior. It is the most common form of X-linked retardation and may account for 10% of retarded individuals (Rogers and Simensen 1987).

Neurochemistry and Aggression

A number of neurotransmitter systems have been implicated in aggressive behavior, but the serotonergic system has received the most attention by far. A growing literature exists on the roles of the serotonergic and arginine vasopressin systems in the control of aggressive behavior in animals. Arginine vasopressin facilitates offensive aggression among golden hamsters, whereas serotonin agonists appear to cause a reduction in aggression (Ferris et al. 1997). Coccaro (1996) noted a possible correlation between life history of aggressive behavior and cerebrospinal fluid (CSF) vasopressin levels in individuals with personality disorder. Ferris (1996) postulated that elevated brain serotonin levels may reduce aggressive behavior by means of inhibiting activity in the arginine vasopressin system.

Decreased levels of 5-hydroxyindoleacetic acid (5-HIAA), a serotonin metabolite, were found in the CSF of individuals who committed violent crimes, acts of impulsive aggression, or attempted suicide (Golden et al. 1991). Aggressive psychiatric inpatients and subjects with conduct disorder were found to have decreased numbers of serotonin transporter sites (Birmaher et al. 1990; Marazzitti et al. 1993; Stoff et al. 1987). Linnoila and colleagues (1983) found that individuals with a history of multiple crimes of violence had lower CSF 5-HIAA levels than individuals who committed only one violent crime. Low platelet serotonin uptake was associated with aggressive behavior in various populations (Golden et al. 1991). Reduced prolactin response to fenfluramine challenge correlated with impulsive aggression in men with character disorder (Coccaro et al. 1989) and violent offenders with antisocial personality (O'Keane et al. 1992). A similar correlation was demonstrated in nonhuman primates (Botchin et al. 1993). Although methodological issues complicate the interpretation of CSF metabolite, platelet-binding, and challenge studies, a number of pieces of evidence point to serotonin's role in aggression. Linnoila and Virkkunen (1992) proposed the existence of a "low serotonin syndrome" that includes early-onset impulsive aggressive behavior, early alcohol abuse, diurnal activity disturbance, decreased CSF 5-HIAA levels, increased suicide risk, family history of type II alcoholism (the strongly genetic, male-transmitted variety), and a possible tendency toward hypoglycemia. An association between the low serotonin syndrome and personality traits such as impulsivity, monotony avoidance, irritability, verbal aggressiveness, and poor socialization was also described (Virkkunen et al. 1994). Not all studies have demonstrated clear relationships between serotonin and aggression. One recent study of peripheral serotonin function in 40 patients with schizophrenia found no difference between platelet ^{3}H-paroxetine binding in aggressive and nonaggressive subjects (Maguire et al. 1997).

Norepinephrine has also been implicated in the etiology of aggressive behavior. β-Blocking agents reduce aggressive behavior in animals and in selected populations of neurologically impaired people (Greendyke et al. 1986). GABA, the major inhibitory neurotransmitter of the CNS, has some antiaggressive properties that may relate to the utility of benzodiazepines in the treatment of some aggressive individuals.

Some evidence exists of a correlation between increased CSF free testosterone levels and aggressivity as distinct from the impulsivity associated with the low serotonin syndrome (Virkkunen and Linnoila 1993; Virkkunen et al. 1994). Body builders who abuse anabolic steroids have been reported to develop aggressive behavior (Choi and Pope 1994; Parrott et al. 1994; Schulte et al. 1993; Yates et al. 1992). In sex offenders, including pedophiles, rapists, and exhibitionists, some success has been reported using medroxyprogesterone acetate (Depo-Provera) treatment (Meyer et al. 1992) and leuprolide, a gonadotropin-releasing hormone agonist (Rich and Ovsiew 1994).

Neuropsychiatric Evaluation of Aggressive Behavior

The goals of neuropsychiatric evaluation are to determine the effects of the neuropsychiatric condition on the patient; to assess the level of CNS dysfunction, the possible mechanism of the dysfunction, and the degree of reversibility of the condition; and to determine what interventions might help ameliorate the problem. Neuropsychiatric evaluation includes gathering a history; performing neurological, mental status, and cognitive examinations;

forming a hypothesis as to the cause of the patient's symptoms; suggesting further diagnostic tests, if needed, to confirm the hypothesis; and interpreting the findings to the patient, staff, and family. Neurobehavioral explanations alone are seldom sufficient for the understanding of aggressive behavior in a given individual. Integration of knowledge of an individual's development, psychodynamics, and genetics is necessary for the development of a more complete picture (Ovsiew and Yudofsky 1993).

Ninety percent of a neuropsychiatric evaluation consists of gathering the history. In the case of aggressive behavior, the history begins with obtaining as complete a description of the individual's aggression as possible. Because an individual may deny aggressive behavior for a variety of reasons, interviewing staff and family members and reviewing old records are as important as interviewing the patient. When obtaining the history of aggressive behavior, it is helpful to focus on a particular aggressive incident that is well recalled rather than talking in general terms. The history should include observations about events or changes that had been going on in the individual's life or environment before the incident, events that occurred that day, and exactly what the individual was doing immediately before the incident. Evidence of a prodrome should be sought. In the case of diencephalic aggression, the clinician might find that before the incident the individual was hypersomnic or had insatiable hunger or thirst and was prevented from satisfying those desires. The clinician should be particularly alert for signs of psychotic behavior, panic attacks, depressive mood swings, manic behavior, intoxication, or substance-withdrawal symptoms before an aggressive incident. (Pathological intoxication as a cause of aggressive behavior is discussed in Chapter 5.) In retarded or autistic individuals, an increase in motoric excitement, stereotyped behavior, or rituals may signal a coming attack. Note should be made of the response by staff or others to the patient's aggression, with particular attention given to any reactions that could be seen as reinforcing the behavior. Staff attention, for example, can be a reinforcer if it occurs or increases only after outbursts.

It is important to know whether an aggressive attack took place in clear consciousness and whether the aggression itself was well planned or directed toward a particular individual, especially if it was necessary for the patient to move or travel to target that particular individual. If consciousness is clouded, the possibility of delirium should be considered. The many causes of delirium can be found in any standard psychiatry text. Both intoxication and substance-withdrawal syndromes can produce clouding of consciousness. Aggression in the setting of impaired consciousness also raises the possibility of seizure-related phenomena, especially postictal irritability. Aggression toward people and objects in the individual's environment may be associated with impaired consciousness during partial seizures. However, aggression as a manifestation of the seizure itself is rare and would take the form of non-directed, unplanned attacks at people and objects that happen to be nearby at the time. When an aggressive incident follows a stimulus that makes the individual angry, seizure-related phenomena are unlikely. If aggression occurs after the individual has been sleeping or during what appears to be arousal from sound sleep, rapid eye movement (REM) sleep behavioral disorder (RBD) should be considered (Schenck and Mahowald 1990).

Several features of the incident itself may be of diagnostic utility. Outbursts longer than 3 minutes are unlikely to represent seizures. Time of day of episode can help identify effects of staffing patterns, hunger-related behavior, medication peak and trough effects, problems resulting from insufficient structure, neuroendocrine abnormalities, and fatigue. Amnesia for one's aggressive behavior is a surprisingly poor indicator of etiology. In one study, individuals with character disorder were more likely than patients with epilepsy to claim amnesia for their outbursts and to deny responsibility for their actions (Bear et al. 1982).

DSM-IV (American Psychiatric Association 1994) distinguishes intermittent explosive disorder from conditions that include ongoing aggression and irritability without explosive outbursts. Diagnostic criteria for intermittent explosive disorder include several discrete episodes of failure to resist aggressive impulses that result in serious assaultive acts or destruction of property; degree of aggressiveness grossly out of proportion to any precipitating psychosocial stressors; and absence of a better explanation for the aggressive episodes by another mental disorder, direct physiological effects of a substance, or a general medical condition (including head trauma). DSM-IV allows the diagnosis of intermittent explosive disorder even if generalized aggression or impulsivity is present between aggressive episodes. Note is made that individuals with narcissistic, obsessive, paranoid, or schizoid traits may be especially prone to having explosive outbursts of anger when under stress. Nonspecific EEG abnormalities, diffuse neuropsychological dysfunction, and neurological "soft" signs frequently occur. Episodic dyscontrol syndrome, described by Bach-y-Rita et al. (1971) and largely replaced in contemporary literature by intermittent explosive disorder, overlaps with but is not equivalent to the DSM-IV syndrome. The term *episodic dyscontrol* was used to describe individuals with affective aggression and no generalized irritability between attacks. The episodic dyscontrol syndrome also described individuals prone to violent outbursts with little or no provocation, the outbursts lasting minutes to hours. Included were individuals with temporal lobe epilepsy, seizurelike outbursts, pathological intoxication, and generalized violence who may have had other psychiatric and neurologic diagnoses. Further study of this population revealed that the attacks were similar to seizures in many ways, with more than half of individuals reporting auras before their outbursts and drowsiness afterward and nearly as many reporting amnesia for the episodes (Maletzky 1973). A history of childhood hyperactivity, febrile seizures, and traumatic brain injury was common. The triad of enuresis, fire setting, and cruelty to animals, held to predict adult criminal behavior (Hellman and Blackman 1966), was found in only 15%–25% of subjects (Bach-y-Rita et al. 1971; Maletzky 1973).

Irritability without explosive outbursts may have many causes, including prescription medications, traumatic brain injury, epileptic prodromes or postictal phases, and hyperthyroidism, in addition to irritability as a feature of personality, affective, psychotic, and late–luteal phase dysphoric or posttraumatic stress disorders. In individuals treated with neuroleptics, akathisia should not be overlooked as a possible etiology of aggressive behavior toward one's self or others.

In a developmentally disabled individual who has never been aggressive, new-onset aggression should trigger a medical workup to rule out dental problems, constipation, headaches or other pain, occult infection, unseen head injury, metabolic abnormality, or akathisia (if taking neuroleptics). On the other hand, if a developmentally disabled individual is chronically irritable with cyclic exacerbations, tactile defensiveness, territorial aggressiveness, or an institutionalized attitude to gratification, the clinician should rule out atypical bipolar disorder or other affective disorder, anxiety or panic disorder, and orbitofrontal syndrome (see below).

With the increased attention to neuropsychiatric factors outlined in this chapter, one must not overlook the standard psychiatric history relevant to aggression. Information should be gathered about prior suicide attempts or self-injurious behavior, aggression toward others, use of weapons, arrests, family violence, other impulsive behaviors, and substance use. Table 6–3 summarizes points to cover in taking the history of aggressive episodes.

The clinician's ability to recognize known neurobehavioral disorders that include aggression is of paramount importance. Personality changes resulting from frontal lobe syndromes and the interictal behavior syndrome of temporolimbic epilepsy have already been described. Individuals with right-hemisphere syndromes, who show impaired comprehension of pun, double entendre, sarcasm, and emotional prosody, may misperceive environmental stimuli and become delusional (Levine and Grek 1984), increasing the risk of aggressive behavior. Focal damage to right-hemisphere sites, espe-

TABLE 6–3. Items to elicit when taking history of aggressive episodes

Precipitants	Episode quality
Environmental changes	Violence directed?
Increased stimulation	Length of episode
Internal conflict	Time of day of episode
Psychosocial stressors	Clear onset and ending?
Trivial provocation	Consciousness clear or clouded?
No obvious precipitant	Amnesia for episode?
Planned attack	Remorse afterward?
Prodrome	Recognizable patterns
Sleep deprivation	New-onset aggression
Hyperphagia	Orbitofrontal syndrome
Polydipsia	Dorsolateral frontal syndrome
Psychotic symptoms	Interictal (temporal lobe epilepsy)
Anxiety/panic	behavior
Sadness/depression	Intermittent explosive disorder
Psychomotor excitement	Right-hemisphere syndrome
Euphoria	Diencephalic syndrome
Irritability	Pseudobulbar palsy
Increased rituals	Attention-deficit/hyperactivity disorder
Delirium	Self-injurious behavior (in individuals
Signs of intoxication/withdrawal	with autism or mental retardation)

cially limbic-connected and peridiencephalic areas, can be associated with manic behavior (Cummings and Mendez 1984). Schizophrenia-like psychosis has been associated with left-hemisphere damage. If the features of a given neurobehavioral syndrome appear to be present but have been stable features of the individual's personality since childhood, the possibility of a congenital neurobehavioral syndrome should be considered (Eslinger et al. 1992; Price et al. 1990; Voeller 1986; Weintraub and Mesulam 1983). Early-onset alcoholism combined with impulsive aggression should alert the clinician to the possibility of a serotonin-related aggression syndrome (Linnoila and Virkkunen 1992).

When obtaining the neuropsychiatric history, the clinician must pay particular attention to traumatic brain injury and seizures, because they commonly involve damage to the aforementioned CNS areas involved in aggression. When collecting information on past traumatic brain injuries, the clinician should inquire specifically about variables that have been related to neurological outcome, including duration of coma, of retrograde amnesia (time from last recall before impact), and of anterograde or posttraumatic amnesia (time until clear recall of new information is reestablished). Length of posttraumatic amnesia correlates best with neurobehavioral morbidity.

Specific inquiry as to how an individual's personality may have changed following injury may yield evidence of the focal neurobehavioral syndromes discussed earlier. Individuals with prior history of traumatic brain injury may be more strongly affected by further mild brain injuries.

Especially in the case of partial seizures, some patients may be unaware of their epilepsy. One must specifically inquire about common partial seizure symptoms. A history of any recurrent brief stereotypical behavioral episodes should provoke further inquiry. Simple partial seizures can occur in clear consciousness. Complex partial seizures involve a change in the level of consciousness that may range from a "spaced out" feeling to a blank stare during which the individual is completely amnestic. Automatisms typically occur during the amnestic interval. Postictal confusion and lethargy tend to be of short duration if they occur. Often a warning or aura (which, in fact, is a simple partial seizure) occurs just before a seizure in temporal lobe epilepsy. Common partial seizure symptoms are listed in Table 6–4. Review of seizure frequency data may reveal that aggression has emerged with either increased or decreased seizure activity. Awareness of the syndromes of frontal lobe epilepsy is also helpful (Broglin et al. 1992; Riggio and Harner 1992). Individuals with frontal seizures may have one of the previously mentioned frontal behavioral syndromes (which include aggression) as well as seizures that may be asymmetrical, with frenetic bimanual, postural, gestural, or bipedal automatisms. These seizures are often mistaken for psychogenic seizures and tend to have brief, if any, postictal periods.

The neurodevelopmental history may contain clues to abnormal brain development or focal learning disorders that may be associated with neurobehavioral syndromes. Table 6–5 lists points to cover in the neurodevelopmental history. Handedness is listed because of the association of anomalous dominance with brain damage. Change in handedness in childhood or left-handedness in absence of a family history of left-handedness indicates possible anomalous dominance.

A complete neurological and mental status examination, paired with knowledge of the typical syndromes associated with aggression, helps narrow the differential diagnosis. A more complete treatment of the neuropsychiatric examination can be found elsewhere (Benjamin 1997; Ovsiew 1992). Multiple cranial nerve signs point to brainstem dysfunction. Decreased arousal may also be present. Pseudobulbar palsy, which may include aggressive verbal outbursts as well as pathological laughing and crying, indicates bilateral corticobulbar tract lesions. Insatiable thirst, appetite, and sex drive, as well as lethargy, may point to diencephalic abnormalities. The neurological examination is typically normal in temporolimbic epilepsy. When present,

TABLE 6–4.   Common partial seizure symptoms

Motor
  Focal motor
  Versive
  Postural
  Phonatory
Somatosensory/special sensory
  Visual
    Spots, colored lights
    Formed hallucinations
  Auditory
  Gustatory
  Olfactory (unpleasant smells are most common)
  Vertiginous
Autonomic
Psychic
  Dysphasic
    Speech arrest
    Words
    Palilalia
  Poor or impaired memory
    Déjà vu, déjà entendu, déjà veçu
    Jamais vu, jamais entendu, jamais veçu
    Panoramic vision
    Specific memory
    Distorted time perception
  Cognitive
    Confusion
    Remoteness, depersonalization
    Forced thinking
  Affective
    Fear (negative affects are most common)
  Illusions
    Polyopsia
    Teleopsia
    Metamorphopsia
    Paracusis, echo
    Change in size or weight of limb, feels like someone else's

TABLE 6–5.   Items to elicit in the neurodevelopmental history

Gestation	Schooling
Trauma	Highest education achieved
Infection	Best and worst subjects
Maternal substance abuse	Language problems
Prematurity	Attention problems
Perinatal factors	Construction problems
Anoxia	Behavior problems
Trauma	Expulsion/suspension?
Difficult labor	Motor incoordination
Neurodevelopment	Grade point average
Cerebral palsy?	Grade repeats
Neurodevelopmental milestones	Neurological history
Onset of walking	Head injuries (with duration of loss
Onset of speech	of consciousness, posttraumatic
Toilet training	amnesia)
Handedness (including family history)	Seizures (including febrile)
Prolonged enuresis	Loss of consciousness
Fire setting	Central nervous system
Cruelty to animals	infection
Relationships	Substance use
Peer relationships	Arrests
Stability of family relationships	
Abusive relationships	

asymmetry of spontaneous smile or superior quadrantanopsia indicates contralateral temporal lobe abnormality. Decreased verbal memory is associated with left medial temporal lobe involvement, whereas nonverbal memory loss is typically associated with right temporal lobe dysfunction. Decreased confrontation naming or verbal fluency, the latter demonstrated by having the individual list as many words of a given category as possible in 1 minute, may indicate a left temporal disorder when there is normal dominance.

Olfactory deficits, motor signs (weakness, reflex asymmetry), and frontal release signs can be seen in individuals with frontal lobe damage. Forced grasping, if present, may indicate contralateral frontal damage, especially with involvement of the supplementary motor area. Motor impersistence, the inability to sustain a motor command, is more typical of right frontal deficit. With medial frontal damage, the clinician should be alert for lower extremity weakness, sensory loss, abnormal gait, and incontinence, as well as decreased spontaneous initiation of behavior progressing to akinetic mutism in more severe cases. Table 6–2 summarizes the neuropsychiatric abnormalities found in the three syndromes of frontal damage.

Once one or more hypotheses are formed on the basis of the history and neuropsychiatric examination, neurodiagnostic testing is ordered to gather supporting evidence. Focal findings on neurological examination should be investigated with structural imaging. In the setting of acute traumatic brain injury, X-ray computed tomography (CT) is typically used, as it can easily detect fractures and bleeding. Structural damage from subacute or chronic traumatic brain injury is best evaluated using CT or magnetic resonance imaging (MRI). MRI is preferred in most cases because of its superior imaging of the inferior frontal cortex, temporal lobes, and posterior fossa structures and its ability to detect small deposits of hemosiderin (for which special techniques must be used) in the case of diffuse axonal injury. However, if a patient is unable to lie still in the scanner for the approximately 30 minutes necessary for imaging, the CT scan, which can be accomplished more quickly, is preferred. Acquired partial complex seizures are highly correlated with focal brain pathology. If partial seizures have been diagnosed, MRI with coronal T2 images of the temporal lobes has the best chance of visualizing mesial temporal sclerosis, a frequent pathological finding, as well as other focal brain lesions.

When seizures are suspected clinically, a sleep EEG should be done to increase the chances of recording an epileptiform abnormality. If negative EEGs have been obtained in the sleeping and awake states, yet partial seizures are still clinically suspected, an EEG with sphenoidal leads will increase the chances of detecting a medial temporal focus.

If the aggressive behavior occurs only on arousal from sleep and the clinician suspects nocturnal seizures or RBD, a sleep EEG to rule out postictal aggression and a sleep laboratory evaluation are indicated. Polysomnography reveals electromyographic activity during REM sleep in individuals with RBD.

Functional brain imaging is now widely available in the form of single photon emission computed tomography (SPECT). Performed in many general hospital nuclear medicine departments, brain SPECT imaging measures relative cerebral perfusion. Decreased perfusion can be seen in areas of brain dysfunction that do not appear abnormal on structural brain imaging. One can often visualize abnormalities related to coup and contrecoup contusions despite normal head CT (Gray et al. 1992; Newton et al. 1992; Roper et al. 1991). SPECT perfusion deficits have been shown to correlate with neurobehavioral outcome and neuropsychological deficits (Ichise et al. 1994; Oder et al. 1992). If a given behavior is suspected of being a seizure, one can inject the SPECT tracer during the suspicious event and then transport the patient to the scanner an hour later, when behavior has come under control, to obtain the images. Focal cortical hyperperfusion is strongly correlated with active seizure foci (Van Heertum et al. 1993). Such studies have become easier with the introduction of stabilized SPECT tracers that can remain in solution up to 6 hours. When the clinician suspects a focal neurobehavioral syndrome, the SPECT scan may provide confirmatory evidence even when other studies are normal (Trzepacz et al. 1992).

Neuropsychological evaluation can be used to confirm a neurobehavioral hypothesis of focal brain dysfunction. Neuropsychological testing is most productive when the ordering clinician specifies the hypothesis being tested. Focal brain dysfunction should never be diagnosed on the basis of a single neurological, mental status, or neuropsychological finding. The most compelling evidence of focal brain abnormality is the convergence of evidence from different testing modalities. Even with a negative MRI, for instance, the combination of left inferior quadrantanopsia, difficulties with constructions, and slowing over posterior right-hemisphere leads on EEG is strongly suggestive of right parietal abnormality. Neuropsychological evaluation is also used to determine whether a decline in cognitive function has occurred (academic records may facilitate the determination), to establish a baseline against which the course of a dementia or recovery from brain damage may be charted, or to provide objective data for pharmacological trials.

Strategies for Treatment of Aggressive Behavior

Pharmacological Treatment

A number of pharmacological approaches are used in the treatment of aggression. With so many neuropsychiatric causes of aggression, it is not surprising that no single medication approach is useful for all individuals. Neuroleptics, antidepressants, antimanic agents, anxiolytics, anticonvulsants, and β-blockers all have their place. Treatment outcome may be difficult to judge, especially if the individual is removed from the setting in which the aggression occurred. Determination of treatment effect may also be complicated by disagreement among treatment team members or failure to involve the patient in monitoring treatment effect. To maximize the chances of success, a number of practices are helpful.

Before treatment is initiated, target behaviors should be identified and agreed on. In developmentally disabled individuals, only those aggressive behaviors representing a danger to the individual's own self or others should be targeted. In this group, one often sees stereotypical behaviors, including tapping, touching, striking oneself lightly, or hyperactivity, that do not actually cause damage despite staff complaints. Countable behaviors are preferred. However, in the case of individuals who are generally irritable rather than manifesting discrete outbursts, improvement measures can be agreed on in advance. Rating scales are often useful. The Overt Aggression Scale (OAS), depicted in Figure 6–2, assists in documentation of episode type, frequency, and severity (Yudofsky et al. 1986). The OAS is filled out following each aggressive episode. In developmentally disabled individuals, the OAS can be supplemented with the Aberrant Behavior Checklist (ABC), a 52-item rating scale that can be used at regular intervals to quantify agitated, loud, stereotypical, and physically aggressive behavior (Aman et al. 1985). Data collection should be carried out during a pretreatment baseline period for a duration dictated by frequency of the target behavior.

With the exception of treatment of schizophrenic exacerbations and major depression, for which it may take months to reproduce an initial therapeutic effect or to deteriorate from a prior therapeutic effect, an ABA or ABAB treatment protocol is the best way of ensuring reproducible antiaggressive effects. The letter A in this terminology refers to on-drug intervals and the letter B to off-drug intervals. If possible, one medication manipulation at a time and gradual dosage changes will help the clinician know with certainty which intervention was successful. As hospital stays have become shorter, however, this advice has become easier to implement in outpatient than inpatient populations.

Before initiating treatment with a new agent, the clinician should consider possible behavioral effects of any medications the individual is already taking. Elimination of medications known to produce depression or irritability should be undertaken first. In epileptic individuals, simplification of anticonvulsants can reduce cognitive and behavioral side effects resulting from polypharmacy, sometimes improving aggressive behavior. Certain anticonvulsants, such as barbiturates, phenytoin, and felbamate, are more prone to produce behavioral toxicity than other agents. Ideally, conversion to carbamazepine or valproate, which have both fewer neurobehavioral side effects and occasional success in the treatment of aggressive behavior, should be attempted. However, the patient's neurologist should be involved in this decision because these agents are not appropriate for all seizure types.

Because in many cases one cannot predict which agent will be most successful in a given individual, an algorithm such as the one in Figure 6–3 may be helpful. After obtaining a thorough history of the aggressive behavior, establishing the method of measuring treatment effect, following the protocol

---

Overt Aggression Scale (OAS)

Stuart Yudofsky, M.D., Jonathan Silver, M.D., Wynn Jackson M.D., and Jean Endicott, Ph.D.

Identifying Data

Name of patient	Name of rater
Sex of patient: 1 male 2 female	Date / / (mo/da/yr) Shift: 1 night 2 day 3 evening

☐ No aggressive incident(s) (verbal or physical) against self, others, or objects during the shift (check here).

Aggressive Behavior (check all that apply)

Verbal aggression	Physical aggression against self
☐ Makes loud noises, shouts angrily	☐ Picks or scratches skin, hits self, pulls hair (with no or minor injury only)
☐ Yells mild personal insults (e.g., "You're stupid!")	☐ Bangs head, hits fist into objects, throws self onto floor or into objects (hurts self without serious injury)
☐ Curses viciously, uses foul language in anger, makes moderate threats to others or self	☐ Small cuts or bruises, minor burns
☐ Makes clear threats of violence toward others or self (I'm going to kill you.) or requests to help to control self	☐ Mutilates self, makes deep cuts, bites that bleed, internal injury, fracture, loss of consciousness, loss of teeth

Physical aggression against objects	Physical aggression against other people
☐ Slams door, scatters clothing, makes a mess	☐ Makes threatening gesture, swings at people, grabs at clothes
☐ Throws objects down, kicks furniture without breaking it, marks the wall	☐ Strikes, kicks, pushes, pulls hair (without injury to them)
☐ Breaks objects, smashes windows	☐ Attacks others, causing mild to moderate physical injury (bruises, sprain, welts)
☐ Sets fires, throws objects dangerously	☐ Attacks others, causing severe physical injury (broken bones, deep lacerations, internal injury)

Time incident began: ___ ___ : ___ ___ am/pm	Duration of incident: ___ ___ : ___ ___ (hours/minutes)

Intervention (check all that apply)

☐ None	☐ Immediate medication given by mouth	☐ Use of restraints
☐ Talking to patient	☐ Immediate medication given by injection	☐ Injury requires immediate medical treatment for patient
☐ Closer observation	☐ Isolation without seclusion (time out)	☐ Injury requires immediate treatment for other person
☐ Holding patient	☐ Seclusion	

Comments

FIGURE 6–2.   The Overt Aggression Scale.

Source.   Reprinted from Yudofsky SC, Silver JM, Jackson W, et al.: "The Overt Aggression Scale for the Objective Rating of Verbal and Physical Aggression." *American Journal of Psychiatry* 143:35–39, 1986. Used with permission. Copyright 1986, American Psychiatric Association.

for new-onset aggression, and considering current medications that could themselves be causing or exacerbating the aggressive behavior, the clinician should embark on a series of careful clinical trials, the order of which is dictated by the predominant diagnostic features. Behaviors suspected of being seizure-related should be treated with anticonvulsants. Individuals with epileptiform EEGs but without clinical seizures may also respond to anticonvulsant treatment. Axis I psychiatric disorders or prodromes consistent with Axis I disorders should be treated next. Substance abuse, intermittent explosive disorder, and attentional dysfunction should be considered. Finally, a series of empirical trials of monotherapy or add-on therapy for aggression can be undertaken in an order dictated by the existing literature.

Because of the risk of tardive dyskinesia, neuroleptics should be reserved for individuals with psychosis when possible. Adequate antipsychotic treatment frequently ameliorates aggression in this population. In individuals with refractory psychosis and aggressive behavior, clozapine treatment has been shown to improve the aggression with or without improvement in the primary psychiatric disorder (Cohen and Underwood 1994; Ratey et al. 1993; Volavka et al. 1993). In animal models, the antiaggressive effect has also been observed (Dixon et al. 1994; Garmendia et al. 1992). Antipsychotic agents are also occasionally utilized in nonpsychotic individuals. Examples include individuals with Gilles de la Tourette's syndrome or dementia with "sun-downing" (nocturnal agitation related to increased confusion), or when sedative side effects are desirable for short-term treatment situations. Neuroleptics should be avoided, if possible, in patients with traumatic brain injury because of the risk of increasing cognitive slowing, decreasing motivation, or exaggerating other cognitive deficits. Animal studies have demonstrated that haloperidol inhibits amphetamine-induced acceleration in recovery from brain injury and impedes recovery when used alone (Feeney et al. 1982). Data from human stroke studies also indicate that neuroleptics impede motor recovery (Goldstein and Investigators 1995). Standard neuroleptics tend to cause akathisia, an unpleasant restless sensation that can facilitate aggression and be mistaken for increased agitation (Drake and Ehrlich 1985; Keckich 1978; Siris 1985). Neuroleptics also tend to decrease the seizure threshold. Clozapine has the greatest epileptogenic tendency among neuroleptics, but clozapine-induced seizures are easily treated, typically with valproate or phenytoin. Among standard neuroleptics, slight differences in effect on seizure threshold have been demonstrated in animal models, with molindone, pimozide, and fluphenazine having less effect than other agents (Oliver et al. 1982). Although neuroleptics should generally be avoided in nonpsychotic individuals, these agents can improve both exter-

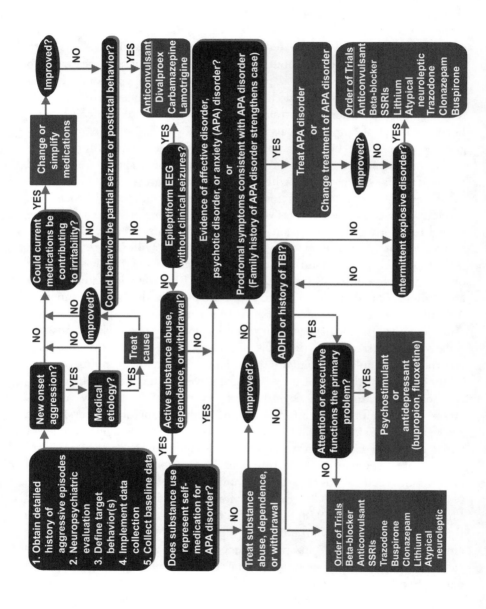

FIGURE 6–3. Algorithm for treatment of aggressive behavior. An individual may fulfill more than one set of criteria in the algorithm. Algorithm sequence is based on factors that influence medication choice, not prevalence of diagnoses or establishment of an exclusive diagnosis. Order of suggested pharmacological trials is based on the author's experience and review of the literature. Individual factors, including treatment history, sensitivity to side effects, and medical history, can alter the order of medication trials in particular individuals. ADHD = attention-deficit/hyperactivity disorder; EEG = electroencephalogram; SSRIs = selective serotonin reuptake inhibitors; TBI = traumatic brain injury.

nally directed and self-directed aggression in neurologically impaired and developmentally disabled patients and can be tried if other agents have failed. Atypical antipsychotics are preferred because of their lower rate of extrapyramidal side effects.

Aggression can occur in the context of depression or mania. When aggressive behavior occurs as part of major depression or obsessive-compulsive disorder (OCD), there may be some advantage in selecting a serotonergic antidepressant. When an individual with aggressive behavior has some elements of depression but DSM-IV criteria for the disorder are not met, a serotonergic therapy may be selected. Similarly, antimanic therapies may be tried in an aggressive individual whose condition falls short of the criteria for the bipolar disorders.

Serotonin reuptake inhibitors may be useful for aggressive behavior even when no affective component is present. Low-dose amitriptyline was reported to ameliorate aggression in patients with anoxic encephalopathy (Slabowicz and Stewart 1990). Sertraline lowered the rates of impulsive aggressive behavior of seven subjects with personality disorder in one open trial (Kavoussi et al. 1994) and ameliorated severe aggression in two subjects with Huntington's disease in another report (Ranen et al. 1996). Sertraline was found to decrease aggression and self-injurious behavior in eight of nine adult outpatients with mental retardation and autism in an open trial (Hellings et al. 1996). Trazodone has been reported to be useful in the treatment of aggression in developmentally disabled adults with dementia (Bernstein 1992; Pinner and Rich 1988; Simpson and Foster 1986) and in impulsively aggressive children (Zubietka and Alessi 1992). Clomipramine, a serotonin reuptake inhibitor, significantly decreased anger attacks and ritualized behavior in 12 autistic subjects in a placebo-controlled comparison with desipramine (Gordon et al. 1993). However, worsening of impulsivity, suicidal tendencies, and aggression has also been reported with serotonin-reuptake blockers and other antidepressants (Hawthorne and Lacey 1992; Teicher et al. 1990, 1993). The author has found the selective serotonin reuptake inhibitors (SSRIs) very useful in the treatment of irritability following traumatic brain injury.

Lithium has long been used in the treatment of aggression. Cases of lithium-responsive aggression have been reported in traumatic brain injury (Glenn et al. 1989; Haas and Cope 1985), dementia (Kunik et al. 1994), developmental disabilities (Craft et al. 1987; Langee 1990; Luchins and Dojka 1989; Pary 1991; Spreat et al. 1989), ADHD (Siassi 1982), schizophrenia (Van Putten and Sanders 1975), "organic brain syndrome" (Williams and Goldstein 1979), temporal lobe epilepsy, and antisocial personality disorder (Tupin et al. 1973). In one controlled study of 25 aggressive, developmentally disabled adults, predictors of lithium responsiveness included less than one episode per week, hyperactivity, stereotypical behavior, epilepsy, and female gender (Tyrer et al. 1984). Caution is advised in cases of brain damage, however, because lithium has been reported to decrease cognitive function in this population in concert with the antiaggression effect (Glenn et al. 1989).

When aggression occurs in the context of panic disorder or other anxiety disorders, or when there is prominent anxiety prior to an outburst, anxiolytics may be the treatment of choice. Long-acting benzodiazepines (e.g., clonazepam) are preferred over shorter acting agents (e.g., lorazepam) for chronic treatment. Short-acting benzodiazepines can be useful as premedication for tests or other anxiety-producing situations and are often useful in the treatment of acute manic behavior or agitation; however, they should be used on an ongoing basis only with great caution, because of the behavioral toxicity during peak absorption, behavioral rebound at end of dose interval, increased irritability ("paradoxical" agitation), and tolerance effects common to all benzodiazepines. Transient lowering of the seizure threshold is common during tapering of these agents following chronic use.

The serotonin$_{1A}$ agonist buspirone can have some advantages for chronic use (it is not a useful as-required [PRN] medication) because it is not sedating and does not share the aforementioned effects. It has been reported successful in the treatment of some cases of aggression in individuals with brain damage, even in the absence of prominent anxiety (Colella et al. 1992; Gedye 1991; Ratey et al. 1991, 1992; Stanislav et al. 1994), but it, too, may paradoxically increase aggression in some cases.

Anticonvulsants may be useful in the treatment of aggression even in the absence of suspected seizures, EEG abnormalities, or bipolar disorder. Phenytoin was tested as a psychoactive agent as early as 1943 (Kalinowsky and Putnam 1943). Apart from one study demonstrating some benefit

(Maletzky 1973), its utility as an antiaggression agent has not been proven (Connors et al. 1971; Gottschalk et al. 1972; Lefkowitz 1969). Carbamazepine (Hakoloa and Laulumaa 1982; Kafantaris et al. 1992; Kanjilal 1977; Keck et al. 1992; Lewin and Sumners 1992; Luchins 1983, 1984; Mattes 1984; Patterson 1987; Reid et al. 1981; Tunks and Dermer 1973; Young and Hillbrand 1994) and valproate (Giakas et al. 1990; Keck et al. 1992; Mazure et al. 1992; Mellow et al. 1993; Wilcox 1994), on the other hand, have both been used successfully for treatment of aggression. Although only a handful of controlled trials have been reported, both agents have been found useful for treating aggressive behavior in individuals with developmental disability and other organic brain syndromes (Kastner et al. 1993; Mazure et al. 1992; Mellow et al. 1993; Patterson 1987; Reid et al. 1981). In a recent open study, divalproex was shown to ameliorate chronic explosive temper outbursts and affective lability in 10 adolescents without brain damage (Donovan et al. 1997). Lamotrigine appears to behave as an anticycling agent in mood disorders and may have some antidepressant activity. Studies of lamotrigine and aggression have not yet been published.

First described by Elliott (1977) as a nonsedating treatment for belligerent behavior following acute brain damage, antinoradrenergic therapy has been shown to be successful in the treatment of aggressive behavior in adults and children with or without organic brain damage (Arnold and Aman 1991; Connor 1993; Elliott 1977; Greendyke and Kanter 1986; Greendyke et al. 1984, 1986; Lader 1988; Luchins and Dojka 1989; Mattes 1985, 1986, 1990; Polakoff et al. 1986; Ratey et al. 1983, 1986; Ruedrich et al. 1990; Sorgi et al. 1986; Yudofsky et al. 1981). β-Blockers and α-agonists (e.g., clonidine) are both used. Most studies have involved individuals with brain damage (Elliott 1977; Greendyke and Kanter 1986; Greendyke et al. 1984, 1986; Yudofsky et al. 1981), dementia (Kunik et al. 1994), or developmental disabilities (Arnold and Aman 1991; Connor 1993; Connor et al. 1997a; Luchins and Dojka 1989; Ratey et al. 1986; Ruedrich et al. 1990), but this strategy has also been reported to be useful when there is a history of ADHD (Mattes 1986) and as an add-on treatment for individuals with other primary psychiatric disorders, notably schizophrenia (Sorgi et al. 1986). Long-acting agents such as nadolol may promote compliance because they can be given on a twice-daily, and sometimes a once-daily, basis. Pindolol, with its partial sympathomimetic effect, may be better tolerated by individuals sensitive to the bradycardic effects of standard β-blockers. A comparative study of 80 patients (Mattes 1990) found carbamazepine better for patients with intermittent explosive disorder and propranolol better for aggressive patients with a history of ADHD. Some authors have advised caution in interpreting this literature pending further controlled studies (Lader 1988; Ruedrich et al. 1990).

Methylphenidate has been reported to improve aggressive behavior in patients with traumatic brain injury (Gualtieri and Evans 1988) and in those with attention-deficit disorder (Pelham et al. 1991). In a controlled study of 38 young males with traumatic brain injury, methylphenidate was found to have a statistically significant tendency to ameliorate anger (Mooney and Haas 1993). Methylphenidate appeared to worsen impulsive aggressive behavior in one case report of posttraumatic behavior change (Haas and Cope 1985). Pemoline and amantadine can also be used.

The algorithm proposed in this chapter suggests a method for determining monotherapy of aggressive behavior. In practice, however, combined pharmacotherapy commonly occurs. In a recent pharmacoepidemiological study, aggression was shown to be a significant predictor of combined pharmacotherapy in seriously emotionally disturbed youth (Connor et al. 1997b). Before adding a second agent, one should maximize treatment with the first agent. If the first agent is moderately but incompletely effective, consideration should be given toward increasing the dosage before adding another drug. If the first agent has had no effect, it should be tapered. When adding a second agent, consideration must be given to drug interactions. Adding carbamazepine, for example, may reduce the level of the initial agent, whereas adding propranolol may increase the level of other agents. Combined therapy can be advantageous in certain situations. For example, when β blockade occasionally causes dysphoria despite having produced an improvement in aggression, an SSRI can be added to control the dysphoria and further treat the aggression, rather than changing treatments.

As yet, no agents have been developed specifically for the treatment of aggression. Agents that ameliorate impulsive and predatory aggression without impairing an individual's motor and motivational behavior are needed. The quest for such agents, known as *serenics*, is well under way. Serotonin$_{1A/1B}$ receptor agonists have shown the most promise in animal models (Kravitz and Fawcett 1994). The first such agent to be tested in humans, eltoprazine, has had mixed results in the few patients treated and had to be removed from study because of untoward side effects. However, serenic agents may represent the most promising future pharmacological treatment of pathological aggression.

The literature on pharmacological management of aggression contains many more case reports than it contains controlled trials. Of the controlled trials that do exist, there are often insufficient data to rule out the presence of treatable psychiatric disorders and insufficient description to categorize the aggressive behavior. Studies comparing different psychopharmacological approaches in the treatment of aggression have been few. Every psycho-pharmacological intervention that has been used successfully for aggressive behavior has either had no effect or caused exacerbation of aggression in some cases. Therefore, it is suggested that clinicians gain experience with a variety of antiaggression agents and approach each patient's treatment as objectively as possible using a strategy such as the one described above.

Behavioral Treatment

Staff members of units specializing in psychiatric treatment, brain injury rehabilitation, and treatment of developmental disabilities must have a basic knowledge of behavioral treatment principles regardless of whether they view themselves as primarily providing behavioral therapy. Detailed reviews of behavioral management techniques in aggression can be found elsewhere (Franzen and Lovell 1987; Wong et al. 1988). A brief overview of useful behavioral principles follows.

It is difficult to undertake behavioral modification treatment outside of the inpatient or group-home setting. In general, unstructured time should be kept to a minimum on units with assaultive patients with brain damage. Staff must be educated as to what constitutes reinforcement and non-reinforcement of behavior and the importance of consistency across all shifts. If passes are part of the patient's treatment, the patient's family should be made aware of the behavioral plan. Target behaviors must be clearly defined by the treatment team. Antecedent behaviors and inadvertent reinforcing responses should be spelled out. A single behavior should be designated as the initial target for modification, and a mechanism for counting the behavior and recording the data should be put in place. Although there may be a number of maladaptive behaviors, staff must ignore behaviors other than the designated target behavior, if possible. If the designated behavior responds to treatment, a new behavior can be selected as the focus.

Once selected and defined, a given maladaptive behavior can be treated by reducing the antecedent behaviors that tend to elicit the aggressive response, rewarding the patient for performance of an alternative desirable behavior, or reducing the amount of positive reinforcement the patient receives for performing the aggressive target behavior. Reduction of antecedent behavior is tailored to the individual but may be as simple as removing the individual from overstimulating environments, presenting the individual with a few choices rather than the need to make ambiguous decisions, or attempting to involve the individual in an activity program appropriate to his or her level to reduce frustration. A common problem among individuals who resort to violence is the lack of nonviolent conflict resolution skills, especially those that are language dependent. Training in conflict resolution strategies or social skills may offer the patient an alternative to aggressive behavior. The patient can then be exposed to increasingly conflictual situations in a controlled environment and allowed to practice these techniques. Reducing positive reinforcement following target behaviors usually requires staff to withdraw attention from the individual rather than sit down and "process" the incident with him or her immediately. Obviously, certain aggressive behaviors require seclusion, restraint, or use of PRN medications, so it is often impossible to eliminate these potential reinforcers completely. However, these interventions can be carried out in a businesslike fashion with the minimum contact required.

Reward for nonperformance of the target behavior is a common approach. Most inpatient psychiatry units have a limited reinforcement system built in to the program in the form of privilege levels that must be earned. Token economies are also frequently used. Often, though, these programs are not geared to the unique problems of the individual. A program of differential reinforcement of other behaviors (DRO) is tailor-made for the individual patient. Selection of reinforcers is done according to the likes or goals of the individual. Reinforcers may be individual attention from staff, desired privileges or activities, or, if appropriate, food. The patient receives a check for each interval free of the target behavior. The decision to use a system of checks that can be accumulated toward later exchange for reinforcers or actual provision of reinforcers at the conclusion of each behavior-free interval as well as the choice of interval length must take the individual's attention span and recall ability into account. Intervals may need to be as short as 5 minutes if that is the limit of recall. After the initial period of removal of reinforcement for a target behavior, one often sees an increase in the target behavior, known as an *extinction burst*. This increase should be transient if the program is maintained. DRO programs are often successful, though they obviously require a good deal of staff consistency and can be labor intensive.

Pharmacological management of aggression is often combined with behavioral management techniques. In a well-integrated program, the two paradigms are complementary. The same behavioral data can be analyzed to assess either approach. Ideally, changes in the behavioral and pharmacological treatment plans should occur at different times so that assessment of the effect of each intervention can be made. Each treatment attempted should be summarized in the discharge summary to allow future treaters the benefit of one's experience with a given individual and to prevent loss of hard-won gains.

Conclusion

Public health facilities must develop expertise in the evaluation and management of aggression. Simply ordering neurodiagnostic tests on every individual will lead to unnecessary expense and has not been shown to improve the diagnosis and treatment of aggressive behavior. With cost-effective care a major priority, tests should be selected to confirm or narrow diagnostic hypotheses. Units treating aggressive individuals should develop standards for documentation of aggressive behavior to facilitate objective observation of pharmacological and behavioral treatments. Staff must be trained to record thorough descriptions of aggressive incidents that allow individually tailored treatment plans to be constructed. Treatment teams on units specializing in the treatment of aggressive individuals should have available to them a neuropsychiatric consultant or a neurologist sensitive to the issues reviewed in this chapter and a behavioral consultant to assist with difficult behavioral plans. Ultimately, the onus of responsibility for the neuropsychiatric evaluation and treatment of aggressive behavior falls on the public health psychiatrist, however. We must make sure that our residency training programs include sufficient neuropsychiatric background to enable general psychiatrists to meet this challenge.

An oft-forgotten approach to the reduction of aggressive behavior is prevention. Traumatic brain injury and substance abuse contribute to so many of the causes of aggression discussed in this chapter that clinicians treating this population should be at the forefront of movements to increase the use of automobile restraint devices and appropriate head protective gear for motorcycling, bicycling, and other sports and to establish and improve educational programs aimed at reducing substance abuse in school-age children.

Just as there is no unitary neurobehavioral explanation for all aggression, there are no treatments that can be applied to every case of aggressive behavior. Careful neuropsychiatric evaluation combined with consistent application of pharmacological and behavioral strategies offers the best hope of reduction of pathological aggression.

References

Adamec RE, Stark-Adamec C: Limbic kindling and animal behavior—implications for human psychopathology associated with complex partial seizures. Biol Psychiatry 18:269–293, 1983

Aman MG, Singh NN, Stewart AW, et al: The Aberrant Behavior Checklist. Psychopharmacol Bull 21:845–850, 1985

American Psychiatric Association: Diagnostic and Statistical Manual of Mental Disorders, Fourth Edition. Washington, DC, American Psychiatric Association, 1994

Arnold LE, Aman MG: Beta blockers in mental retardation and developmental disorders. J Child Adolesc Psychopharmacol 1:361–373, 1991

Bach-y-Rita G, Lion JR, Climent CE, et al: Episodic dyscontrol: a study of 130 violent patients. Am J Psychiatry 127:1473–1478, 1971

Bard P: A diencephalic mechanism for the expression of rage with special reference to the sympathetic nervous system. Am J Physiol 84:490–515, 1928

Bear DM: Temporal lobe epilepsy—a syndrome of sensory-limbic hyperconnection. Cortex 15:357–384, 1979

Bear DM, Fedio P: Quantitative analysis of interictal behavior in temporal lobe epilepsy. Arch Neurol 34:454–467, 1977

Bear D, Schenk L: Increased autonomic responses to neutral and emotional stimuli in patients with temporal lobe epilepsy. Am J Psychiatry 138:843–845, 1981

Bear DM, Levin K, Blumer D, et al: Interictal behaviour in hospitalised temporal lobe epileptics: relationship to idiopathic psychiatric syndromes. J Neurol Neurosurg Psychiatry 45:481–488, 1982

Bear DM, Rosenbaum JF, Norman R: Aggression in cat and man precipitated by a cholinesterase inhibitor. Psychosomatics 26:535–536, 1986

Benjamin S: Neuropsychiatry, in Psychiatry for Medical Students, 3rd Edition. Edited by Waldinger R. Washington, DC, American Psychiatric Press, 1997, pp 335–377

Bernstein L: Trazodone treatment of targeted aggression in a mentally retarded man (letter). J Neuropsychiatry Clin Neurosci 4:348, 1992

Birmaher B, Stanley M, Greenhill L, et al: Platelet imipramine binding in children and adolescents with impulsive behavior. J Am Acad Child Adolesc Psychiatry 29:914–918, 1990

Bleuler E: Textbook of Psychiatry. New York, Arno Press, 1916. Reprint, 1976

Blumer D: Temporal lobe epilepsy and its psychiatric significance, in Psychiatric Aspects of Neurologic Disease, Edited by Benson DF, Blumer D. New York, Grune & Stratton, 1975, pp 171–198

Botchin MB, Kaplan JR, Manuch SB, et al: Low versus high prolactin responders to fenfluramine challenge: marker of behavioral differences in adult male cynomolgus macaques. Neuropsychopharmacology 9:93–99, 1993

Brodie MJ, McKee PH: Vigabatrin and psychosis (letter). Lancet 335:1279, 1990

Broglin D, Delgado-Escueta AV, Walsh GO, et al: Clinical approach to the patient with seizures and epilepsies of frontal origin. Adv Neurol 57:59–88, 1992

Bruens JH: Psychoses in epilepsy, in Handbook of Clinical Neurology, Vol 15. Edited by Vinken PJ, Bruens JH. Amsterdam, North-Holland, 1974, pp 593–610

Cantwell DP: Hyperactive children have grown up. Arch Gen Psychiatry 42:1026–1028, 1985

Choi PY, Pope HGJ: Violence toward women and illicit androgenic-anabolic steroid use. Ann Clin Psychiatry 6:21–25, 1994

Coccaro EF: Neurotransmitter correlates of impulsive aggression in humans, in Understanding Aggressive Behavior in Children, Vol 794. Edited by Ferris CF, Grisso T. New York, New York Academy of Sciences, 1996, pp 82–89

Coccaro EF, Siever LJ, Klar HM, et al: Serotonergic studies in patients with affective and personality disorders: correlates with suicidal and impulsive aggressive behavior. Arch Gen Psychiatry 46:587–599, 1989

Cohen SA, Underwood MT: The use of clozapine in a mentally retarded and aggressive population. J Clin Psychiatry 55:440–444, 1994

Colella RF, Ratey JJ, Glaser AI: Perimenstrual aggression in mentally retarded adult ameliorated by buspirone. Int J Psychiatry Med 22:351–356, 1992

Connor DF: Beta blockers for aggression: a review of the pediatric experience. J Child Adolesc Psychopharmacol 3:99–114, 1993

Connor DF, Ozbayrak KR, Benjamin S, et al: A pilot study of nadolol for overt aggression in developmentally delayed individuals. J Am Acad Child Adolesc Psychiatry 36:826–834, 1997a

Connor DF, Ozbayrak KR, Kusiak KA, et al: Combined pharmacotherapy in children and adolescents in a residential treatment center. J Am Acad Child Adolesc Psychiatry 36:248–254, 1997b

Connors CK, Kramer R, Rothschild GH, et al: Treatment of young delinquent boys with diphenylhydantoin sodium and methylphenidate: a controlled comparison. Arch Gen Psychiatry 24:156–160, 1971

Craft M, Ismail IA, Krishnamurti D, et al: Lithium in the treatment of aggression in mentally handicapped patients: a double-blind trial. Br J Psychiatry 150:685–689, 1987

Cummings JL: Clinical Neuropsychiatry. Orlando, FL, Grune & Stratton, 1985

Cummings JL, Mendez MF: Secondary mania with focal cerebrovascular lesions. Am J Psychiatry 141:1084–1087, 1984

Damasio AR: The frontal lobes, in Clinical Neuropsychology. Edited by Heilman KM, Valenstein E. New York, Oxford University Press, 1985, pp 339–375

Davison K, Bagley CR: Schizophrenia-like psychoses associated with organic disorders of the central nervous system: a review of the literature, in Current Problems in Neuropsychiatry. British Journal of Psychiatry Special Publ No 4. Edited by Herrington RN. Ashford, Kent, UK, Headley Brothers, 1969, pp 113–184

Delgado-Escueta AV, Mattson RH, King L, et al: The nature of aggression during epileptic seizures. N Engl J Med 305:711–716, 1981

Devinsky O, Bear DM: Varieties of aggressive behavior in temporal lobe epilepsy. Am J Psychiatry 141:651–656, 1984

Devinsky O, Ronsaville D, Cox C, et al: Interictal aggression in epilepsy: the Buss-Durkee hostility inventory. Epilepsia 35:585–590, 1994

Dixon AK, Huber C, Lowe DA: Clozapine promotes approach-oriented behavior in male mice. J Clin Psychiatry 55 (suppl B):4–7, 1994

Donovan SJ, Susser ES, Nunes EV, et al: Divalproex treatment of disruptive adolescents: a report of 10 cases. J Clin Psychiatry 58:12–15, 1997

Drake RE, Ehrlich J: Suicide attempts associated with akathisia. Am J Psychiatry 142:499–501, 1985

Egger MD, Flynn JP: Further studies on the effects of amygdaloid stimulation and ablation on hypothalamically elicited attack behavior in cats, in Structure and Function of the Limbic System. Edited by Adey WR, Tokizane T. New York, Elsevier, 1967, pp 165–182

Elliott FA: Propranolol for the control of belligerent behavior following acute brain damage. Ann Neurol 1:489–491, 1977

Elliott FA: Neurologic findings in adult minimal brain dysfunction and the dyscontrol syndrome. J Nerv Ment Dis 170:680–687, 1982

Elliott FA: Violence: the neurologic contribution: an overview. Arch Neurol 49:595–603, 1992

Eslinger PJ, Grattan LM, Damasio H, et al: Developmental consequences of childhood frontal lobe damage. Arch Neurol 49:764–769, 1992

Farwell JR, Lee YJ, Hirtz DG, et al: Phenobarbital for febrile seizures—effects on intelligence and on seizure recurrence. N Engl J Med 322:364–369, 1990

Feeney DM, Gonzalez A, Law WA: Amphetamine, haloperidol, and experience interact to affect rate of recovery after motor cortex injury. Science 217:855–857, 1982

Ferris CF: Serotonin inhibits vasopressin-facilitated aggression in the Syrian hamster, in Understanding Aggressive Behavior in Children, Vol 794. Edited by Ferris CF, Grisso T. New York, New York Academy of Sciences, 1996, pp 98–103

Ferris CF, Melloni RH, Koppel G, et al: Vasopressin/serotonin interactions in the anterior hypothalamus control aggressive behavior in golden hamsters. J Neurosci 17:4331–4340, 1997

Franzen MD, Lovell MR: Behavioral treatments of aggressive sequelae of brain injury. Psychiatric Annals 17:389–396, 1987

Garmendia L, Sanchez JR, Azpiroz A, et al: Clozapine: strong antiaggressive effects with minimal motor impairment. Physiol Behav 51:51–54, 1992

Gastaut H: Interpretation of the symptoms of psychomotor epilepsy in relation to physiological data on rhinencephalic functions. Epilepsia 3:84–88, 1954

Gedye A: Buspirone alone or with serotonergic diet reduced aggression in a developmentally disabled adult. Biol Psychiatry 30:88–91, 1991

Giakas WJ, Seibyl JP, Mazure CM: Valproate in the treatment of temper outbursts (letter). J Clin Psychiatry 51:525, 1990

Glenn MB, Wroblewski B, Parziale J, et al: Lithium carbonate for aggressive behavior or affective instability in ten brain-injured patients. Am J Phys Med Rehabil 68:221–226, 1989

Golden RN, Gilmore JH, Corrigan MHN, et al: Serotonin, suicide, and aggression: clinical studies. J Clin Psychiatry 52:61–69, 1991

Goldstein LB, Sygen in Acute Stroke Investigators: Common drugs may influence motor recovery after stroke. Neurology 45:865–871, 1995

Gordon CT, State RC, Nelson JE, et al: A double-blind comparison of clomipramine, desipramine, and placebo in the treatment of autistic disorder. Arch Gen Psychiatry 50:441–447, 1993

Gottschalk LA, Couri L, Uliana R, et al: Effects of diphenylhydantoin on anxiety and hostility in institutionalized prisoners. Compr Psychiatry 14:503–511, 1972

Gray BG, Ichise M, Chung D, et al: Technetium-99m-HMPAO SPECT in the evaluation of patients with a remote history of traumatic brain injury: a comparison with x-ray computed tomography. J Nucl Med 33:52–58, 1992

Greendyke RM, Kanter DR: Therapeutic effects of pindolol on behavioral disturbances associated with organic brain disease: a double-blind study. J Clin Psychiatry 47:423–426, 1986

Greendyke RM, Schuster DB, Wooton JA: Propranolol in the treatment of assaultive patients with organic brain disease. J Clin Psychopharmacol 4:282–285, 1984

Greendyke R, Kanter D, Schuster D, et al: Propranolol treatment of assaultive patients with organic brain disease. J Nerv Ment Dis 174:290–294, 1986

Gualtieri CT: Neuropsychiatry and Behavioral Pharmacology. New York, Springer-Verlag, 1991

Gualtieri CT, Evans RW: Stimulant treatment for the neurobehavioral sequelae of traumatic brain injury. Brain Inj 2:273–290, 1988

Haas JF, Cope N: Neuropharmacologic management of behavioral sequelae in head injury: a case report. Arch Phys Med Rehabil 66:472–474, 1985

Hakoloa HP, Laulumaa VA: Carbamazepine in treatment of violent schizophrenics (letter). Lancet 1:1358, 1982

Harlow JM: Recovery from the passage of an iron bar through the head. Publications of the Massachusetts Medical Society 2:327–347, 1868

Hawthorne ME, Lacey JH: Severe disturbance occurring during treatment for depression of a bulimic patient with fluoxetine. J Affect Disord 26:205–207, 1992

Hechtman L, Weiss G: Controlled prospective fifteen year followup of hyperactives as adults. Can J Psychiatry 31:557–567, 1986

Hellings JA, Kelley LA, Gabrielli WF, et al: Sertraline response in adults with mental retardation and autistic disorder. J Clin Psychiatry 57:333–336, 1996

Hellman DS, Blackman N: Enuresis, firesetting, and cruelty to animals: a triad predictive of adult crime. Am J Psychiatry 122:1431–1435, 1966

Hermann BP: Interictal psychopathology in patients with ictal fear: a quantitative investigation. Neurology 32:7–11, 1982

Hermann B, Riel P: Interictal personality and behavioral traits in temporal lobe and generalized epilepsy. Cortex 17:125–128, 1981

Herzog AG, Russell V, Vaitukaitis JL, et al: Neuroendocrine dysfunction in temporal lobe epilepsy. Arch Neurol 39:133–135, 1982

Ichise M, Chung D, Wang P, et al: Technetium-99m-HMPAO SPECT, CT and MRI in the evaluation of patients with chronic traumatic brain injury: a correlation with neuropsychological performance. J Nucl Med 35:217–226, 1994

Isojarvi JIT, Repo M, Pakarinen AJ, et al: Carbamazepine, phenytoin, sex hormones, and sexual function in men with epilepsy. Epilepsia 36:366–370, 1995

Kafantaris V, Campbell M, Padron-Gayol MV, et al: Carbamazepine in hospitalized aggressive conduct disorder children: an open pilot study. Psychopharmacol Bull 28:193–199, 1992

Kalinowsky LB, Putnam TJ: Attempts at treatment of schizophrenia and other nonepileptic psychoses with Dilantin. Archives of Neurology and Psychiatry 49:414–420, 1943

Kane R, Mikalac C, Benjamin S, et al: Attention deficit disorder in adults, in Attention Deficit Disorder. Edited by Barkley R. Guilford, 1990, pp 613–654

Kanjilal GC: An evaluation of Tegretol in adults with epilepsy, in Tegretol in Epilepsy: Proceedings of an International Meeting. Edited by Roberts FD. Macclesfield, Cheshire, England, Geigy Pharmaceuticals, 1977, pp 55–57

Kastner R, Finesmith R, Walsh K: Long term administration of valproic acid in the treatment of affective symptoms in people with mental retardation. J Clin Psychopharmacol 13:448–451, 1993

Kavoussi RJ, Liu J, Coccaro EF: An open trial of sertraline in personality disordered patients with impulsive aggression. J Clin Psychiatry 55:137–141, 1994

Keck PE, McElroy SL, Friedman LM: Valproate and carbamazepine in the treatment of panic and posttraumatic stress disorders, withdrawal states, and behavioral dyscontrol syndromes. J Clin Psychopharmacol 12 (suppl):36S–41S, 1992

Keckich WA: Violence as a manifestation of akathisia (letter). JAMA 240:2185, 1978

Kling A: Effects of amygdalectomy on social-affective behavior in non-human primates, in The Neurobiology of the Amygdala. Edited by Eleftheriou BE. New York, Plenum, 1972, pp 511–536

Klüver H, Bucy P: Preliminary Analysis of Functions of the Temporal Lobe in Monkeys. Archives of Neurology and Psychiatry 42:979–1000, 1939

Kravitz HM, Fawcett J: Serenics for aggressive behaviors. Psychiatric Annals 24:453–459, 1994

Kunik ME, Yudofsky SC, Silver JM, et al: Pharmacologic approach to management of agitation associated with dementia. J Clin Psychiatry 55 (suppl):13–17, 1994

Lader M: Beta-adrenoreceptor antagonists in neuropsychiatry: an update. J Clin Psychiatry 49:213–223, 1988

Langee HR: Retrospective study of lithium use for institutionalized mentally retarded individuals with behavior disorders. Am J Ment Retard 94:448–452, 1990

Lefkowitz MM: Effects of diphenylhydantoin on disruptive behavior: study of male delinquents. Arch Gen Psychiatry 20:645–651, 1969

Levine DN, Grek A: The anatomic basis of delusions after right cerebral infarction. Neurology 34:577–582, 1984

Lewin J, Sumners D: Successful treatment of episodic dyscontrol with carbamazepine. Br J Psychiatry 161:261–262, 1992

Lilly R, Cummings JL, Benson DF, et al: The human Klüver-Bucy syndrome. Neurology 33:1141–1145, 1983

Linnoila M, Virkkunen M, Scheinen M, et al: Low cerebrospinal fluid 5-hydroxyindoleacetic acid concentration differentiates impulsive from non-impulsive violent behavior. Life Sci 33:2609–2614, 1983

Linnoila VM, Virkkunen M: Aggression, suicidality, and serotonin. J Clin Psychiatry 53 (suppl):46–51, 1992

Luchins DJ: Carbamazepine for the violent psychiatric patient (letter). Lancet 4:766, 1983

Luchins DJ: Carbamazepine for violent non-epileptic schizophrenics. Psychopharmacol Bull 20:569–571, 1984

Luchins DJ, Dojka D: Lithium and propranolol in aggression and self-injurious behavior in the mentally retarded. Psychopharmacol Bull 25:372–375, 1989

Maguire K, Cheung P, Crowley K, et al: Aggressive behaviour and platelet ^{3}H-paroxetine binding in schizophrenia. Schizophr Res 23:61–67, 1997

Maletzky BM: The episodic dyscontrol syndrome. Diseases of the Nervous System 34:186–189, 1973

Marazzitti D, Rotondo A, Presta S, et al: Role of serotonin in human aggressive behavior. Aggressive Behavior 19:347–353, 1993

Mattes JA: Carbamazepine for uncontrolled rage outbursts. Lancet 11:1164–1165, 1984

Mattes JA: Metoprolol for intermittent explosive disorder. Am J Psychiatry 142: 1108–1109, 1985

Mattes JA: Propranolol for adults with temper outbursts and residual attention deficit disorder. J Clin Psychopharmacol 6:299–302, 1986

Mattes JA: Comparative effectiveness of carbamazepine and propranolol for rage outbursts. J Neuropsychiatry Clin Neurosci 2:159–164, 1990

Mazure CM, Druss BG, Cellar JS: Valproate treatment of older psychotic patients with organic mental syndromes and behavioral dyscontrol. J Am Geriatr Soc 40:914–916, 1992

McGowan M, Neville B, Reynolds EH: Comparative monotherapy trial in children with epilepsy. British Journal of Clinical Practice (symposium suppl) 27: 115–118, 1983

Mega MS, Cummings JL: Frontal-subcortical circuits and neuropsychiatric disorders. J Neuropsychiatry Clin Neurosci 6:358–370, 1994

Mellow AM, Solano-Lopez C, Davis S: Sodium valproate in the treatment of behavioral disturbance in dementia. J Geriatr Psychiatry Neurol 6:205–209, 1993

Mesulam M-M: Large-scale neurocognitive networks and distributed processing for attention, language, and memory. Ann Neurol 28:597–613, 1990

Meyer WJ, Cole C, Emory E: Depo-Provera treatment for sex offending behavior: an evaluation of outcome. Bulletin of the American Academy of Psychiatry and Law 20:249–259, 1992

Mooney GF, Haas LJ: Effect of methylphenidate on brain-injury related anger. Arch Phys Med Rehabil 74:153–160, 1993

Morrell F: The role of secondary epileptogenesis in human epilepsy. Arch Neurol 48:1221–1224, 1991

Mungas D: Interictal behavior abnormality in temporal lobe epilepsy: a specific syndrome or non-specific psychopathology? Arch Gen Psychiatry 39:108–111, 1982

Newton MR, Greenwood RJ, Britton KE, et al: A study comparing SPECT with CT and MRI after closed head injury. J Neurol Neurosurg Psychiatry 55:92–94, 1992

Nielson H, Kristensen O: Personality correlates of sphenoidal EEG foci in temporal lobe epilepsy. Acta Neurol Scand 64:289–300, 1981

Oder W, Goldenberg G, Spatt J, et al: Behavioural and psychosocial sequelae of severe closed head injury and regional cerebral blood flow: a SPECT study. J Neurol Neurosurg Psychiatry 55:475–480, 1992

O'Keane V, Moloney E, O'Neill H, et al: Blunted prolactin responses to d-fenfluramine in sociopathy: evidence for subsensitivity of central serotonergic function. Br J Psychiatry 160:643–646, 1992

Oliver AP, Luchins DJ, Wyatt RJ: Neuroleptic-induced seizures: an in vitro technique for assessing relative risk. Arch Gen Psychiatry 39:206–209, 1982

Ovsiew F: Bedside neuropsychiatry: eliciting the clinical phenomena of neuropsychiatric illness, in The American Psychiatric Press Textbook of Neuropsychiatry, 2nd Edition. Edited by Yudofsky SC, Hales RE. Washington, DC, American Psychiatric Press, 1992, pp 89–125

Ovsiew F, Yudofsky S: Aggression: a neuropsychiatric perspective, in Rage, Power, and Aggression. Edited by Glick RA, Roose SP. New Haven, CT, Yale University Press, 1993, pp 213–230

Parrott AC, Choi PY, Davies M: Anabolic steroid use by amateur athletes: effects upon psychological mood states. J Sports Med Phys Fitness 34:292–298, 1994

Pary RJ: Towards defining adequate lithium trials for individuals with mental retardation and mental illness. Am J Ment Retard 95:681–691, 1991

Patterson JF: Carbamazepine for assaultive patients with organic brain disease. Psychosomatics 28:579–581, 1987

Pelham WE, Milich R, Cummings EM, et al: Effects of background anger, provocation, and methylphenidate on emotional arousal and aggressive responding in attention-deficit hyperactivity disordered boys with and without concurrent aggressiveness. J Abnorm Child Psychol 19:407–426, 1991

Pinner E, Rich CL: Effects of trazodone on aggressive behavior in seven patients with organic mental disorders. Am J Psychiatry 145:1295–1296, 1988

Polakoff SA, Sorgi PJ, Ratey JJ: The treatment of impulsive and aggressive behavior with nadolol (letter). J Clin Psychopharmacol 6:125–126, 1986

Pollock DC: Models for understanding the antagonism between seizures and psychosis. Prog Neuropsychopharmacol Biol Psychiatry 11:483–504, 1987

Price BH, Daffner KR, Stowe RM, et al: The comportmental learning disabilities of early frontal lobe damage. Brain 113:1383–1393, 1990

Raine A, Buchsbaum MS, Stanley J, et al: Selective reductions in prefrontal glucose metabolism in murderers. Biol Psychiatry 36:365–373, 1994

Ranen NG, Lipsey JR, Treisman G, et al: Sertraline in the treatment of severe aggressiveness in Huntington's disease. J Neuropsychiatry Clin Neurosci 8:338–340, 1996

Ratey JJ, Morrill R, Oxenkrug G: Use of propranolol for provoked and unprovoked episodes of rage. Am J Psychiatry 140:1356–1357, 1983

Ratey JJ, Mikkelsen EJ, Smith GB, et al: Beta-blockers in the severely and profoundly mentally retarded. J Clin Psychopharmacol 6:103–107, 1986

Ratey J, Sovner R, Parks A, et al: Buspirone treatment of aggression and anxiety in mentally retarded patients: a multiple-baseline, placebo lead-in study. J Clin Psychiatry 52:159–162, 1991

Ratey JJ, Leveroni CL, Miller AC, et al: Low-dose buspirone to treat agitation and maladaptive behavior in brain-injured patients: two case reports (letter). J Clin Psychopharmacol 12:362–364, 1992

Ratey JJ, Leveroni C, Kilmer D, et al: The effects of clozapine on severely aggressive psychiatric inpatients in a state hospital. J Clin Psychiatry 54:219–223, 1993

Reeves AG, Plum F: Hyperphagia, rage and dementia accompanying a ventromedial hypothalamic neoplasm. Arch Neurol 20:616–624, 1969

Reid AH, Naylor GJ, Kay DSG: A double-blind, placebo controlled, crossover trial of carbamazepine in overactive, severely mentally handicapped patients. Psychol Med 11:109–113, 1981

Rich SS, Ovsiew F: Leuprolide acetate for exhibitionism in Huntington's disease. Mov Disord 9:353–357, 1994

Riggio S, Harner RN: Frontal lobe epilepsy. Neuropsychiatry Neuropsychol Behav Neurol 5:283–293, 1992

Ring HA, Crellin R, Kirker S, et al: Vigabatrin and depression. J Neurol Neurosurg Psychiatry 56:925–928, 1993

Roberts WW: Escape learning without avoidance learning motivated by hypothalamic stimulation in cats. Journal of Comparative and Physiological Psychology 51:391–399, 1958

Rodin E, Schmaltz S: The Bear-Fedio personality inventory and temporal lobe epilepsy. Neurology 34:591–596, 1984

Rogers RC, Simensen RJ: Fragile X syndrome: a common etiology of mental retardation. American Journal of Mental Deficiency 91:445–449, 1987

Roper SN, Mena I, King WA, et al: An analysis of cerebral blood flow in acute closed-head injury using technetium-99m-HMPAO SPECT and computed tomography. J Nucl Med 32:1684–1687, 1991

Rosenbaum A, Hoge SK: Head injury and marital aggression. Am J Psychiatry 146:1048–1057, 1989

Ruedrich SL, Grush L, Wilson J: Beta adrenergic blocking medications for aggressive or self-injurious mentally retarded persons. Am J Ment Retard 95:110–119, 1990

Sachdev HS, Waxman SG: Frequency of hypergraphia in temporal lobe epilepsy: an index of interictal behavior syndrome. J Neurol Neurosurg Psychiatry 44:358–360, 1981

Schenck CH, Mahowald MW: Polysomnographic, neurologic, psychiatric, and clinical outcome on 70 consecutive cases with the REM sleep behavior disorder (RBD). Cleve Clin J Med 57 (suppl):10–24, 1990

Schulte HM, Hall MJ, Boyer M: Domestic violence associated with anabolic steroid abuse (letter). Am J Psychiatry 150:348, 1993

Seidman L: Lateralized cerebral dysfunction, personality and cognition in temporal lobe epilepsy. Doctoral dissertation, Boston University, 1980

Siassi I: Lithium treatment of impulsive behavior in children. J Clin Psychiatry 43:482–484, 1982

Simpson DM, Foster DL: Improvement in organically disturbed behavior with trazodone treatment. J Clin Psychiatry 47:191–193, 1986

Siris SG: Three cases of akathisia and "acting out." J Clin Psychiatry 46:395–397, 1985

Slabowicz JW, Stewart JT: Amitriptyline treatment of agitation associated with anoxic encephalopathy. Arch Phys Med Rehabil 71:612–613, 1990

Smith DE, King MD, Hoebel BG: Lateral hypothalamic control of killing: evidence for a cholinoceptive mechanism. Science 167:900–901, 1970

Sorgi PJ, Ratey JJ, Polakoff S: Beta-adrenergic blockers for the control of aggressive behaviors in patients with chronic schizophrenia. Am J Psychiatry 143:775–776, 1986

Spreat S, Behar D, Reneski B, et al: Lithium carbonate for aggression in mentally retarded persons. Compr Psychiatry 30:505–511, 1989

Stanislav SW, Fabre T, Crismon ML, et al: Buspirone's efficacy in organic-induced aggression. J Clin Psychopharmacol 14:126–130, 1994

Stark-Adamec C, Adamec R: Psychological methodology versus clinical impressions: different perspectives on psychopathology and seizures, in The Limbic System: Functional Organization and Clinical Disorders. Edited by Doane BK, Livingston KF. New York, Raven, 1986, pp 217–227

Stoff DM, Pollock L, Vitiello B, et al: Reduction of ^{3}H-imipramine binding sites on platelets of conduct disordered children. Neuropsychopharmacology 1:55–62, 1987

Teicher MH, Glod C, Cole JO: Emergence of intense suicidal preoccupation during fluoxetine treatment. Am J Psychiatry 147:207–210, 1990

Teicher MH, Glod CA, Cole JO: Antidepressant drugs and the emergence of suicidal tendencies. Drug Safety 8:186–212, 1993

Trimble MR: Anticonvulsant drugs: mood and cognitive function, in Epilepsy, Behavior, and Cognitive Function. Edited by Trimble MR, Reynolds EH. New York, Wiley, 1988, pp 135–143

Trimble MR: Biological Psychiatry, 2nd Edition. Chichester, UK, Wiley, 1996

Trzepacz PT, Hertweck PA, Starratt C, et al: The relationship of SPECT scans to behavioral dysfunction in neuropsychiatric patients. Psychosomatics 33:62–71, 1992

Tunks ER, Dermer SW: Carbamazepine in the dyscontrol syndrome associated with limbic dysfunction. J Nerv Ment Dis 14:311–317, 1973

Tupin JP, Smith DB, Clanon TL, et al: The long-term use of lithium in aggressive prisoners. Compr Psychiatry 14:311, 1973

Tyrer SP, Walsh A, Edwards DE, et al: Factors associated with a good response to lithium in aggressive mentally handicapped subjects. Prog Neuropsychopharmacol Biol Psychiatry 84:751–755, 1984

U.S. Department of Justice, Federal Bureau of Investigation: Uniform Crime Reports: Crimes in the United States 1991. Washington, DC, U.S. Government Printing Office, 1992

Van Heertum RL, Miller SH, Mosesson RE: SPECT brain imaging in neurologic disease. Radiol Clin North Am 31:881–907, 1993

Van Putten T, Sanders DG: Lithium in treatment failures. J Nerv Ment Dis 161: 255–264, 1975

Virkkunen M, Linnoila M: Brain serotonin, type II alcoholism, and impulsive violence. J Stud Alcohol Suppl 11:163–169, 1993

Virkkunen M, Rawlings R, Tokola R, et al: CSF biochemistries, glucose metabolism, and diurnal activity rhythms in alcoholic, violent offenders, fire setters, and healthy volunteers. Arch Gen Psychiatry 51:20–27, 1994

Voeller KKS: Right-hemisphere deficit syndrome in children. Am J Psychiatry 143: 1004–1009, 1986

Volavka J, Zito JM, Vitrai J, et al: Clozapine effects on hostility and aggression in schizophrenia (letter). J Clin Psychopharmacol 13:287–289, 1993

Walker AE, Blumer D: Behavioral effects of temporal lobectomy for temporal lobe epilepsy, in Psychiatric Aspects of Epilepsy. Edited by Blumer D. Washington, DC, American Psychiatric Press, 1984, pp 295–323

Wasman M, Flynn JP: Directed attack elicited from the hypothalamus. Arch Neurol 6:220–227, 1962

Waxman SG, Geschwind N: The interictal behavior syndrome of temporal lobe epilepsy. Arch Gen Psychiatry 32:1580–1586, 1975

Weiger WA, Bear DM: An approach to the neurology of aggression. J Psychiatr Res 22:85–98, 1988

Weintraub S, Mesulam M-M: Developmental learning disabilities and the right hemisphere: emotional, interpersonal, and cognitive components. Arch Neurol 40:463–468, 1983

Wheatley MD: The hypothalamus and affective behavior in cats: a study of experimental lesions with anatomic correlations. Archives of Neurology and Psychiatry 52:296–316, 1944

Wilcox J: Divalproex sodium in the treatment of aggressive behavior. Ann Clin Psychiatry 6:17–20, 1994

Williams KH, Goldstein G: Cognitive and affective responses to lithium in patients with organic brain syndrome. Am J Psychiatry 136:800–803, 1979

Wolf P: Acute behavioral symptomatology at disappearance of epileptiform EEG abnormality: paradoxical or "forced" normalization, in Advances in Neurology, Vol 55. Edited by Smith D, Treiman D, Trimble M. New York, Raven, 1991, pp 127–142

Wong SE, Woolsey JE, Innocent AJ, et al: Behavioral treatment of violent psychiatric patients. Psychiatr Clin North Am 11:569–580, 1988

Yates WR, Perry P, Murray S: Aggression and hostility in anabolic steroid users. Biol Psychiatry 31:1232–1234, 1992

Young JL, Hillbrand M: Carbamazepine lowers aggression: a review. Bulletin of the American Academy of Psychiatry and Law 22:53–61, 1994

Yudofsky S, Williams D, Gorman J: Propranolol in the treatment of rage and violent behavior in patients with chronic brain syndromes. Am J Psychiatry 138:218–220, 1981

Yudofsky SC, Silver JM, Jackson W, et al: The Overt Aggression Scale: an operationalized rating scale for verbal and physical aggression. Am J Psychiatry 143:35–39, 1986

Zubietka JK, Alessi NE: Acute and chronic administration of trazodone in the treatment of disruptive behavior disorders in children. J Clin Psychopharmacol 12:346–351, 1992

CHAPTER 7

Neuropsychiatry in the Prison

Fred Ovsiew, M.D.
Peter B. C. Fenwick, M.B., B.Chir. (Cantab.),
   D.P.M., F.R.C.Psych.

> The factors which influence the direction of human activity are so many,
> so different, and of so many orders of experience, that to consider one
> sensibly, none of the others must be forgotten.
>
> Denis Williams (1969)

In this chapter, we elaborate a clinical approach to the criminal offender. The chapter necessarily overlaps with several others in this book. Substance abusers, discussed in Chapter 5, often commit criminal acts in relation to their substance abuse, and, as reviewed below, the prevalence of substance abuse in incarcerated populations is high. This in turn implies a large population of patients infected with the human immunodeficiency virus (HIV), a neuropsychiatric problem discussed in Chapter 8 of this volume. The prevalence of acquired immunodeficiency syndrome (AIDS) in United States prisons was estimated at the end of 1990 to be 14 times the prevalence in the general population, with nearly 7,000 prisoners having AIDS; the prevalence of HIV seropositivity in New York State prisons was 17% (Morris 1995). The homeless population, discussed in Chapter 11, is frequently in contact with the criminal justice system and the police. Chapter 13 describes the alterations in sexual behavior produced by brain disease, some such deviance bringing people into the criminal justice system. Most important, violence often brings people into the criminal justice system; the physiology and management of violence are discussed in Chapter 6.

In this chapter, we show that the criminal justice system, like the public mental health system, has responsibility for a large number of patients with mental disorders, and we argue that a neuropsychiatric perspective on these disorders is valuable for the clinical practitioner and potentially for public policy. We must first, however, disclaim any intent to depreciate other perspectives. In particular, a neuropsychiatric perspective does not gainsay the legal system's concept of responsibility. Though advances in scientific understanding of offenders may ultimately alter our view of some crimes, society's concern for public safety and for punishment of offenders cannot be undercut by scientific understanding. We do not in this chapter attempt to excuse or exculpate, and our primary concern is not with psychiatric evaluation as a part of legal proceedings, but with clinical evaluation and management.

Nor does a biological perspective exclude a psychosocial perspective. To the contrary, we review evidence for relatively specific interactions between somatic factors and social factors in the pathogenesis of criminal behavior. After all, the human organism is essentially social, and its neurobiology in large part subserves the organization of its social behavior. The perspectives of sociology and criminology on social and economic factors in crime must figure into a comprehensive understanding of this societal problem.

First, we review the epidemiology of mental disorder in penal institutions, with emphasis on the few available data concerning brain disease in such settings. Then we review the studies of criminals, especially violent criminals, with respect to cerebral abnormalities. We next turn to psychopathy, a frequent correlate of criminal offending, and discuss the evidence for brain disease in this diagnostic category. On the basis of this information, we then discuss a clinical neuropsychiatric approach to the criminal offender. Finally, a brief discussion of policy implications of neuropsychiatric data is offered.

Epidemiology of Mental Disorder in Penal Systems

The United States has the world's highest incarceration rate: 2.3% of the adult population is in a jail or prison or on parole. (Jails are short-term institutions, run by cities or counties, housing those awaiting trial and misdemeanants or those sentenced to terms of less than a year. Prisons, run by the states or federal government, house felons sentenced to terms longer than a year.) The jail and prison population increased from some one-half million to more than one and a quarter million in the decade from 1983 to 1993 (Center for Mental Health Services 1995). A doubling of the jail population from 1970 to 1980 was concurrent with a substantial increase in the crime rate. However, the more-than-doubling from 1981 to 1995 occurred in the absence of an increase in crime (Morris 1995). The prevalence of psychiatric disorder in inmates is incompletely ascertained, but a few recent data should suffice to indicate the scope of the problem. In a series of methodologically sophisticated studies of inmates at intake to the Cook County (Chicago) Jail, Teplin (1990) found a point prevalence rate of more than 6% for schizophrenia, mania, and major depression ("any severe disorder"). This was two to three times higher than the rate found in a comparison sample from the Epidemiologic Catchment Area (ECA) study of community rates of mental disorders. The figure correlates remarkably well with the estimate in a survey of jailers that 7.2% of inmates are seriously mentally ill (Torrey et al. 1992).

In the Cook County study, the point prevalence of substance use disorders was 29% (Teplin 1994). The lifetime prevalence of any of these disorders—schizophrenia, mania, major depression, or substance abuse—was 61% (Teplin 1994). Perhaps most striking is the overlap of diagnoses. Of those with "any severe disorder" as defined above, more than 58% also had current diagnoses of alcohol abuse or dependence, and 33%, drug abuse or dependence (Abram and Teplin 1991). Clearly, the jails in the inner city contain hard-to-treat psychiatric patients at a fearsome rate.

Substantially similar data arise from a review of methodologically less sound studies of rates of mental disorder in United States prisons (Jemelka et al. 1993). Point prevalence of schizophrenia, for example, ranged from 1.5% to 4.4%, 2.5 to 7.3 times the rate in the general population. For major depression, rates were 3.5% to 11.4%, and for mania, 0.7% to 3.9%—each again several times the rate in a nonincarcerated sample. The authors estimated that 10%–15% of prisoners are seriously mentally ill and require treatment. By using careful methods in a Quebec prison sample, Côté and Hodgins (1990) found lifetime prevalences of major mental disorders many times higher than those in the general population, but the disorders rarely occurred alone: substance abuse or dependence or antisocial personality disorder were almost always found concurrently.

Prevalence rates of this sort are highly dependent on social conditions, police and court practices, and institutional resources. Cross-cultural and historical data must be used with care. Psychiatric factors can carry different significance in the United States, with its high crime and imprisonment rates.

These caveats notwithstanding, the statistics plainly indicate the need for appropriate psychiatric services for detainees. Indeed, such services are mandated by law (Center for Mental Health Services 1995). The need for such services may well be increasing as the availability of psychiatric inpatient services decreases (Torrey et al. 1992). Police—"streetcorner psychiatrists" (Teplin and Pruett 1992)—make quasi-clinical judgments about disposition when apprehending a person who exhibits behavior disorder (Menzies 1987). Police are "acutely aware of the reduced number of psychiatric placements available to them" (Teplin and Pruett 1992, p. 144). As Torrey and colleagues (1992) noted, "if no alternative facility is realistically available, the police may see no choice but to manufacture (or selectively apply) a criminal charge that will then permit them access to the jail." The typical encounter between a police officer and a person who is mentally ill is "not one of a crazed suspect committing a heinous crime, but . . . [one of] a person engaging in behavior harmful to himself or herself. These findings thus confirm the use of police as a major community mental health resource" (Teplin 1985, p. 597).

Data specifically addressing neuropsychiatric morbidity in arrestees are scant. The prevalence of epilepsy has been best studied. Whitman et al. (1984) found the prevalence of epilepsy to be 2.4% in the Illinois prison population. They noted that this may be an underestimate because prisoners may have been unaware of or concealed their seizure disorders and thus did not enter into the study. Nonetheless, the figure is some four times as high as a general population rate for epilepsy in young men. Similarly, though in the different social context of the United Kingdom of three decades ago, Gunn and Fenton (1969) found a rate of 0.7% for epilepsy in prisons and borstals (reformatories for youths), a rate again taken to be well above that of a comparable nonincarcerated population.

Traumatic brain injury is often mentioned as a neuropsychiatric variable in the literature; it is a plausible consequence as well as cause of disinhibited or violent criminal behavior. Unfortunately, to our knowledge no appropriate epidemiological study of the prevalence and severity of traumatic brain injury in inmate populations has been reported. An important negative study with regard to the relation between head injury and crime was undertaken in Finnish veterans of World War II. On follow-up, more than three decades after the injury, no difference in rates of imprisonment was found between veterans with head injury and a control group of uninjured veterans (Virkkunen et al. 1977). Focal lesions of the frontal lobe exerted no special influence on rates of crime (Virkkunen et al. 1976).

Teplin (1994, p. 291) found in her Chicago jail sample a point prevalence of 2% for "severe cognitive impairment" as assessed by "a brief mental status examination." The clinical characteristics of this group were not reported. In relatively early studies, the proportion of prisoners with mental retardation ranged from 8% to 30% (Santamour and West 1982). A methodologically so-phisticated prospective study in Sweden revealed that the rates of criminal behavior, especially violent crime, for intellectually handicapped men and women were markedly elevated (Hodgins 1992). Recent data, however, sug-gest that offenders with mental retardation are now more adequately identi-fied by and deflected from United States prisons, with a resulting rate of mental retardation in the prison population of about 2%, approximating that in the general population (Denkowski and Denkowski 1985).

With regard to all of the populations discussed above, elevated rates of in-carceration may not always imply elevated levels of criminality; inability to avoid arrest, to cooperate with legal defense, or to "work the system" to gain early release may lead to higher rates of imprisonment. For example, offend-ers who are mentally ill frequently are arrested at the scene of the crime or report themselves to the police (Robertson 1988). Similarly, offenders who are mentally retarded are handicapped in making use of the court and parole systems (McAfee and Gural 1988). Further, comparison with ECA data may overestimate the excess psychopathology in jails because of the socioeco-nomic skew of jail populations (see Morris 1995). Still, there can be no reasonable question but that jails and prisons house a large number of psychi-atrically and neuropsychiatrically impaired inmates.

Brain Function in Criminal Populations

Many studies have attempted to identify brain dysfunction in criminal popu-lations. Almost all, however, were strikingly deficient methodologically (Volavka et al. 1992). Often investigators study convenience samples whose relation to the entire offender population is uncertain, and control groups are frequently lacking. New technologies or idiosyncratic ones for which con-trolled data are lacking are often overly relied on. Clinical examinations are often not reported in detail; for example, "the neurological examination was negative" is hard to interpret. Violence is defined in diverse ways and often inappropriately, for example, by sole reliance on the index offense for which the offender was incarcerated. Single factors are studied, with only lip service being given to interactive variables. Nonetheless, the available data are at least suggestive. For the most part, these studies have focused on cerebral factors in either psychopathy or violence. We review the results of examination of criminal populations, with specific regard to violence, then turn to the question of the cerebral organization of individuals with psychopathy.

Genetic and Perinatal Factors

Criminal behavior, especially recidivistic violence committed disproportionately by a relatively small group of criminals, is commonly a stable characteristic with onset in early life (Moffitt et al. 1989). This makes a search for factors operating early in development a plausible strategy. Raine (1993) reviewed the evidence for a genetic contribution to criminal behavior and found strong cross-cultural support for such a contribution, with genetic factors accounting for about half the explained variance (p. 71). Nonviolent crime may be more influenced than violent crime by these unspecified genetic factors (Brennan et al. 1991), and genetic effects may be more potent in adult criminals than in juveniles (Lyons et al. 1995). In the absence of any understanding of what is inherited or how it can be recognized in individual cases, these data, however important theoretically, are of limited practical significance to the neuropsychiatric clinician.

An interesting exception is a recently described X-linked syndrome of mild mental retardation, antisocial aggressive behavior, and total absence of monoamine oxidase A (Abeling et al. 1994; Brunner et al. 1993a, 1993b). Though probably rare, the newly described entity illustrates the importance of seeking information about the family history as part of the clinical assessment.

Nongenetic congenital factors have also been studied. In a prospective study, obstetric complications, which bear a relationship to several psychiatric disorders (Ovsiew 1997), were found with significantly greater frequency in the births of people who became violent criminals than in the births of people who became property offenders or who are nonoffenders (Kandel and Mednick 1991). An elevated rate of minor physical anomalies was also found in violent offenders (Kandel et al. 1989; Moffitt et al. 1989). Such anomalies are thought to arise from a disturbance in gestation and to provide an index of brain maldevelopment easily assessed at the bedside in adults as well as children (Ovsiew 1997).

Of particular importance with regard both to perinatal complications and to minor physical anomalies is the fact that the association with violence held only for subjects reared in unstable families (Mednick and Kandel 1988). This was emphasized by Raine et al. (1994a) in a more extensive study of the same Danish birth cohort studied by Kandel et al. (1989). They found a specific association between violent crime and the interaction between birth complications and maternal rejection. The latter was defined as the mother's negative attitude toward the pregnancy plus either attempted abortion or institutionalization of the baby for at least 4 months in the first year. Poor social circumstances, such as the absence of a father, poor home conditions, and low social class, were risk factors for criminality but showed no interaction with birth complications; the correlation did not hold for nonviolent crime. Similarly, genetic factors interact with environmental ones in the genesis of criminal behavior, possibly by "genetic control of sensitivity to the environment" (Cadoret et al. 1995; Kendler 1995). These replicated findings lend specificity to the earnest eclecticism of those who speak of "multifactorial" etiologies of complex behavioral disturbances.

Head Injury

Head injury is a common cause of neuropsychiatric morbidity and can be assumed to be common in the inmate population, though systematic studies are unavailable. Many studies mention head injury as a precursor of criminal, especially violent, behavior, but clinical details are generally not provided, and the data are often unconvincing. For example, Martell (1992) found a history of "severe head injury" in 22% of 50 patients confined in a maximum security hospital for criminal offenders; however, "severe" was defined to mean that the injury caused loss of consciousness. From a neuropsychiatric point of view, many such injuries may be trivial.

An interesting set of studies examined the history of head injury in husbands who were violent toward their wives. In a pilot study of 31 consecutive men referred for marital violence, 19 (61%) had histories of "severe" head injury, defined in this study to mean only that consciousness was lost or "concussion" had been diagnosed (Rosenbaum and Hoge 1989). In only 5 of the men was the duration of unconsciousness longer than minutes. A control group was not available. In a follow-up study, 53% of batterers had suffered head injury, compared with 25% of nonviolent maritally discordant men and 16% of nonviolent men with satisfactory marriages (Rosenbaum et al. 1994). Head injury was not only a significant predictor of marital violence but a substantial one, with an odds ratio of 5.58 for the comparison with nonviolent maritally discordant men. Eleven of the 53 batterers had suffered moderate or severe injuries, as compared with 2 of the 32 men in the marital discord group. These findings have several possible explanations; effects of alcohol and socioeconomic status, for example, must be taken into account. Head injury can lead to adverse changes in personality, which could produce marital discord; further, head injury can disinhibit aggressive behavior, an alteration obviously directly relevant to marital violence (Warnken et al. 1994). The authors of these studies correctly pointed to the implications of their findings not just for clinical management of maritally violent men but also for the possibility of preventive intervention in head-injury rehabilitation programs.

In an important series of studies, Lewis and Pincus and their colleagues described neuropsychiatric findings in a variety of incarcerated populations, including death row inmates (Lewis et al. 1986, 1988). All of the 15 adults and 8 of the 14 juveniles condemned to death for murder had experienced significant head injuries. Although the descriptions of the injuries are horrifying—"beaten almost to death by father (multiple facial scars)," "beaten in head with two-by-fours by parents," etc.—for the most part medical details of these injuries were unavailable, and appropriate control groups were not studied.

Neurological Examination

Neurological "soft" signs are reliable and valid indicators of cerebral abnormality. These signs are "soft" primarily in regard to their nonlocalizing character; they are easily assessed at the bedside (Ovsiew 1997). Lewis et al. (1979) reported an excess of both focal signs and soft signs in violent delinquents compared with their nonviolent co-inmates. Subsequently, they found that soft signs distinguished violent delinquents from nondelinquent control subjects (Lewis et al. 1987). Wolff et al. (1982) also found more soft signs in delinquent youths than in a comparison group matched for socioeconomic status; that lower middle class control subjects differed significantly from upper middle class control subjects indicates the importance of careful study design. McManus et al. (1985) found that, although only 1 of 71 incarcerated adolescents had a traditional focal sign, soft signs were associated with undersocialized conduct disorders and high soft sign scores were associated with neuropsychological deficits. No control group was studied.

In his study of the inmates of a maximum-security hospital, Martell (1992) found hard signs in 65% of the 40 patients who consented to a quantitative neurological examination; soft signs were present in 50%. Blake et al. (1995) studied, at the request of the individuals' attorneys, a group of 31 individuals either charged with or convicted of murder. The examiner specifically sought putative frontal signs, such as primitive reflexes, paratonia, abnormal smooth pursuit, reduced verbal fluency, and failure on a reciprocal action task. Seven of the 31 had one frontal sign, 3 had two, and 10 had three. Diagnoses could be established in 20 of the 31 individuals. Five had fetal alcohol syndrome, 5 had mental retardation, and 4 had borderline mental retardation. One each had cerebral palsy, hypothyroidism with psychosis, cerebral palsy with mental retardation, acromegaly and borderline mental retardation, hydrocephalus, or dementia. Of these, 2 had epilepsy and 3 had a history of traumatic brain injury.

Electroencephalographic Studies

The early hope that the electroencephalogram (EEG) would provide understanding of mental processes found expression in its use to explore the basis of criminality. In these early investigations, diagnostic methods were unstated or now-outmoded EEG techniques appear primitive, and EEG interpretative practices are questionable; some "abnormalities" would now be considered normal variants. Many such early studies were reviewed by Milstein (1988). For example, Silverman (1943) found 53% of the tracings in 75 residents of the psychopathic unit at a medical center for federal prisoners definitely abnormal. A history suggestive of organic brain disease was not more or less common in those with abnormal tracings. In the EEGs of 50 delinquent boys, Jenkins and Pacella (1943) found 16% to show moderate and 6% to show severe abnormalities. A pattern suggestive of organic as opposed to social origin of criminality was inferred: "restlessness, overactivity, distractibility, short attention span, irritability, excitability, temper outbursts, and frequently impulsiveness" (Jenkins and Pacella 1943, p. 110). Levy and Kennard (1953), studying inmates of a state prison, found a 30% rate of abnormality in the EEG; violent and nonviolent offenders did not differ in rate of abnormality.

Many investigators, however, felt that the EEG abnormalities were associated with violence with relative specificity. Stafford-Clark and Taylor (1949) examined 64 prisoners charged with murder. Abnormal EEGs predominated in those who had committed apparently motiveless crimes; in the offenders whose murders arose understandably, EEGs were preponderantly normal. Hill and Pond (1952) extended these observations and noted that 14 of 18 EEGs were abnormal among those who had committed an apparently motiveless murder. Nonetheless, they believed that none of the murders was the direct result of an epileptic seizure. Driver et al. (1974) were unable to confirm this finding using similar methods at the same institution. In contrast, Howard (1984) found a correlation of bilateral paroxysmal features in the EEG with the commission of violent crimes against strangers.

Williams (1969) studied a broader sample and arrived at different conclusions. In his study of a random sample of about one-quarter of the 1,250 subjects referred to him while they were awaiting trial, about two-thirds of those rated "habitually aggressive" showed abnormal EEGs, predominantly bilateral anterior abnormalities, compared with about one-quarter of the others. When subjects with known or suspected structural brain damage were excluded, 57% of those habitually aggressive had abnormal EEGs. Williams (1969, p. 519) concluded that "a major factor in the ætiology of pathological persistent aggression is disturbance of cerebral physiology." Data from a study of patients in a maximum-security hospital (Wong et al. 1994) provided similar findings. Thirty percent of those who had undergone EEGs (21% of the total population) had abnormal study results. More specifically, 20% of the most violent had slow- or sharp-wave abnormalities in the temporal lobes, as compared with only 2.4% of the least violent.

In contrast to Williams' findings, but more consistent with the work of Stafford-Clark, the idea of episodic dyscontrol arose, with abnormal EEGs taken to indicate a paroxysmal limbic abnormality giving rise to violent behavior (Fenwick 1986). A more recent example of EEG data on episodic dyscontrol is the work of Drake et al. (1992), who studied 23 patients referred for neurophysiological studies because of episodic rage or violent behavior. Seven had abnormal EEGs, compared with only 1 of 20 age-matched patients with headache and none of 24 age-matched patients with depression. The abnormalities were diffuse slowing in 5 of the patients, 2 of whom used alcohol and 1 of whom used drugs, and focal slowing in 2 who had previously been diagnosed as epileptic. The possibility of referral bias in the selection of patients is obvious. Although the topic remains controversial, it seems likely that rare aggressive acts, even murders, occur as a consequence of limbic epileptic discharges (Fenwick 1989). The available evidence, however, does not support an important direct link between epilepsy and violence. Neither Whitman et al. (1984) nor Gunn and Bonn (1971) found a relation between epilepsy and violent offenses, despite the distinctly elevated prevalence of epilepsy in the prison. Langevin et al. (1987) found no epilepsy in 39 violent offenders, 18 of whom were murderers, and no significant difference in the prevalence of EEG abnormalities among this group compared with a control group of nonviolent criminals. However, 13% of murderers and no control subjects had temporal lobe EEG findings. In the study of murderers by Blake et al. (1995), 8 of the 20 who underwent EEG had abnormalities; 2 showed temporal slowing, 1 showed bitemporal spikes, and 1 had both slowing and sharp activity. Details of the violent acts were not provided. The investigators were impressed that only 9 of 31 had either symptoms suggestive of temporal lobe epilepsy or abnormalities on EEG or magnetic resonance imaging (MRI), and only 1 of the 9 had both symptoms and EEG findings.

Neuroimaging

Few systematic structural neuroimaging data are available in offender populations. Seventy-seven of the Broadmoor patients studied by Wong et al. (1994) underwent computed tomography (CT). Ten (13%) showed generalized abnormalities, and 17 (22%) exhibited focal abnormalities, usually temporal. Forty-one percent of the scans of the most violent patients showed focal temporal abnormalities. Nineteen of the 31 murderers studied by Blake et al. (1995) had undergone neuroimaging (MRI in 15, CT in 4). Findings were normal in all patients.

Functional imaging with positron-emission tomography (PET) was undertaken by Volkow and Tancredi (1987) in four psychiatric patients, each of whom had had at least three arrests for violent behavior. All showed left temporal abnormalities, and two additionally had frontal abnormalities. Three of the patients also had left temporal EEG abnormalities, and two showed generalized atrophy by CT. As indicated by the authors, the study must be considered preliminary. No control group was used, and little information was given about the mental state of the patients at the time of the scans. A single-case study by PET of a convicted rapist yielded inconclusive results (Garnett et al. 1988).

Subsequently, Raine et al. (1994b) used PET to examine 22 individuals accused of murder and 22 nonoffender control subjects matched for age and gender. The murderers showed reduced metabolism in superofrontal, anteromedial, and (by trend) orbitofrontal cortices. The left side was more affected than the right. Though 10 subjects had histories of head injury of unspecified severity, these subjects did not differ from the others on PET, nor could variables such as the impulsivity of the crime be correlated with the PET findings.

Neuropsychological Assessment

Neuropsychological data on juvenile criminals were comprehensively reviewed by Moffitt (1990; Moffitt and Henry 1991). Despite methodological problems, a consistent finding of verbal deficits as well as executive cognitive dysfunction was identified. Denno's (1990) important prospective study of a Philadelphia birth cohort likewise showed that abnormal language achievement at age 13–14 predicted juvenile crime. Juvenile offenders, however, may differ in important biological ways from adult offenders (Lyons et al. 1995; Raine et al. 1995b). Neuropsychological data about adult criminals are less extensive. An important negative study by Robertson et al. (1987) indicated that only a slightly lower general intelligence distinguished violent from nonviolent criminals. In certain adult populations, however, neuropsychological deficits may be highly prevalent. For example, Langevin et al. (1987) suggested that neuropsychological deficits were significant in 20%–25% of violent offenders and proposed an interaction with substance abuse. In a study of maximum-security hospital patients, at least 18% were cognitively impaired (Martell 1992). The possible neuropsychological peculiarity of psychopathic individuals is discussed below.

Serotonin

Low central serotonin levels—as indicated by low levels of its metabolite 5-hydroxyindoleacetic acid (5-HIAA) in the cerebrospinal fluid (CSF)—were initially found to be associated with suicidal behavior, especially violent attempts (Roy et al. 1990). Further studies in arsonists and violent criminals led to the suggestion that impulsivity is the common factor in a low-serotonin state. For example, in subjects who had committed homicides, serotonin was low in those who had killed a lover "during a state of intense negative affect (jealousy, frustration, or fear)" (Lidberg et al. 1985, p. 235). Roy et al. (1988) found in normal volunteers that CSF 5-HIAA correlated inversely with scores on an "urge to act out hostility" scale. In violent offenders, low CSF 5-HIAA levels predicted recidivism (Virkkunen et al. 1989). Whether impulsivity is the relevant behavioral variable remains controversial (van Praag 1991). The association of low serotonin with behavioral disturbance, including violent crime, is of considerable practical importance because of the availability of safe agents that affect central serotonin, the selective serotonin reuptake inhibitors such as fluoxetine (Prozac).

Testosterone

Testosterone bears an uncertain relationship to aggressive behavior. In animal studies, the influence of testosterone on aggression can be shown to depend on the animals' prior experience (Archer 1991). However, several types of aggressive behavior occur in animals, and human violence may parallel affective defense, which is not modulated by testosterone (Albert et al. 1993). Studies seeking an association between human male testosterone levels and aggressive behavior are complicated by the fact that levels may respond to situational variables; winning a competition itself can raise testosterone levels (Albert et al. 1993). Only a few data show a relation between testosterone and criminal behavior (Bain et al. 1987). Dabbs and his colleagues (1987) found higher-testosterone adolescent and young adult incarcerated offenders to be more violent and more commonly in trouble with prison authorities.

Virkkunen et al. (1994) found that high CSF testosterone was associated with aggressiveness in alcoholic offenders.

Psychopathy

Recognition of a personality type associated with antisocial acts and criminal behavior is of long standing. Nineteenth-century concepts such as "moral insanity" and "manie sans délire"—though not intended to have specific reference to violation of social norms—were the forerunners of the construct of psychopathy (Berrios 1993; Coid 1993; Stone 1993). The subsequent formulation of antisocial personality disorder (ASPD) in DSM-III (American Psychiatric Association 1980) shifted the focus from personality traits, such as egocentricity, arrogance, and lack of empathy, to socially unacceptable behaviors, such as stealing, truancy, and irresponsibility in work and marriage (Coid 1993; Hare et al. 1991).

The prevalence of ASPD in incarcerated populations is very high. In comparison with a community prevalence of 4.5% in males and 0.8% in females, the lifetime prevalence of ASPD in jail inmates was 49% (Teplin 1994). In prisons, rates are probably about the same (Jemelka et al. 1993). By contrast, the rate of psychopathy in prisoners was estimated by Hare et al. (1991) to be 25%–30%. The discrepancy, reflecting the bias of DSM criteria toward diagnosis by means of antisocial acts, may mean that psychopathy represents a biologically more homogeneous category. Most physiological investigations have found correlations with psychopathy but not with ASPD (Hare et al. 1991). The findings from psychophysiology are reviewed elsewhere (Raine 1993; Raine et al. 1995a) and are not described here. These paradigms and techniques arise from a tradition different from psychiatric medicine; the clinician evaluating an offender cannot order skin conductance responses or cognitive evoked potentials as clinical measures. Nonetheless, a comprehensive theory of the psychobiology of criminal behavior will ultimately need to incorporate the data suggesting underarousal, stimulus seeking, and parasympathotonia in criminals.

Whether psychopathic individuals have cognitive dysfunction has been controversial. A leading candidate for such abnormality has been executive dysfunction because of clinical observations of impulsivity, lack of empathy, poor self-monitoring, and the like in this population. In this regard, a few patients with "acquired sociopathy" have been described in whom a clinical picture and psychophysiological findings suggestive of idiopathic psychopathy were related to orbitofrontal disease (Tranel 1994). In the population of psychopathic individuals without overt cerebral disease, Gorenstein (1982) found a frontal pattern on neuropsychological tests, but he used an idiosyncratic battery. Hare (1984) was not able to replicate this result in a larger population using a more satisfactory method, nor did he and co-workers find other patterns of neuropsychological impairment (Hart et al. 1990). Newman and Wallace (1993, p. 329) concluded that there was "no convincing evidence that psychopaths display clinically significant levels of neuropsychological impairment."

However, the possibility of cerebral dysfunction not of a pattern seen in acquired brain damage must be considered, what Hare et al. (1986, p. 87) called a difference in the way psychopaths are "wired up." Studies using dichotic listening (Hare and McPherson 1984; Raine et al. 1990), event-related potentials (Jutai et al. 1987), examination of syntax-related gestures during speech ("beats") (Gillstrom and Hare 1988), and tachistoscopic presentation of verbal materials (Hare and Jutai 1988) have suggested a limitation in left-hemisphere processing resources for language. The possibility of "unusual or abnormal relations among the cortical, subcortical and limbic mechanisms responsible for the integration of verbal, emotional and social behavior" (Jutai et al. 1987, p. 175) may be inferred.

The claim that left-hemisphere dysfunction is associated with aggressive behavior irrespective of psychopathy was reviewed by Nachson (1991). Such a hypothesis is consistent with the findings summarized by Moffitt (1990; Moffitt and Henry 1991) with regard to language abnormalities in juvenile offenders, Denno's (1990) findings in children who later became adult offenders, and the PET findings described above (Raine et al. 1994b; Volkow and Tancredi 1987). It is also consistent with the findings that violence in psychiatric inpatients was associated with left-hemisphere slow-wave activity on computerized EEG (Convit et al. 1991) and that left frontal injuries were more apt than right frontal injuries to lead to hostility (Grafman et al. 1986). It is not known whether a language impairment leads to developmental social dysfunction and thus greater risk of antisocial behavior, or language disturbance is an indicator of left–hemisphere-based impairment in regulation of social behavior, or the abnormal pattern of lateralization is mediated by factors such as epilepsy and substance abuse (Hillbrand et al. 1993; Nachson 1991).

Neuropsychiatric Evaluation of the Criminal Offender

Neuropsychiatric evaluation of the criminal can take place in at least three settings. First, the neuropsychiatrist may be called on to evaluate a person charged with a crime, with regard to an insanity defense or for some other forensic purpose. Second, a psychiatrist or neurologist may work in a penal setting. Psychiatric services in jails and prisons are woefully inadequate in many instances (Center for Mental Health Services 1995; Torrey et al. 1992), and neuropsychiatric evaluation may be unavailable to incarcerated populations or be provided to an arbitrarily selected or socially and financially favored few. Third, psychiatrists in more ordinary clinical settings, especially in public health settings, frequently see patients whose history includes previous arrests or imprisonment. The complexities of the legal issues surrounding competency, insanity, and fitness to stand trial are beyond the scope of this chapter. With the foregoing data about cerebral factors in criminal behavior in mind, we offer the following ideas about neuropsychiatric evaluation.

As always in neuropsychiatry, the history is essential. In forensic cases, this may include testimony of witnesses to a criminal act as well as the more common sources of ancillary data. The family history and the developmental history, including birth complications, febrile convulsions, motor and cognitive milestones, and educational attainments, form the crucial backdrop for an understanding of a criminal career or an isolated violent act. Details of any traumatic brain injury, including the length of retrograde amnesia, coma, and posttraumatic amnesia, and of any seizures must be inquired about. In regard especially to an isolated criminal act, or one different in quality from an offender's prior crimes, a detailed account of the patient's behavior and mental state in the months and weeks before the offense should be obtained; his or her behavior, thoughts, and feelings on the day of the offense should be learned. Amnesia, confusion or altered state of consciousness, delusions, and hallucinations should be noted. Delusional misidentification is recognized as a risk factor for dangerous behavior (Silva et al. 1992) and will be particularly noted by the neuropsychiatrist, because a disturbance of face recognition may be involved in its genesis (Fleminger and Burns 1993; Silva et al. 1993). Details of alcohol and drug abuse, both remote and on the day of the crime, must be explored; information about testing for drugs of abuse should be reviewed. The patient's handedness should be learned.

A physical examination should be carried out. Soft signs, minor physical anomalies, stigmata of head injury, and characteristic findings of temporal lobe epilepsy such as asymmetry of spontaneous facial expression should be particularly noted (Ovsiew 1997). The examination of the mental state should include a particularly thorough cognitive assessment. Tasks probing verbal and figural memory to test both temporal lobes and those probing executive cognitive function should be employed. The latter tests include verbal fluency, go/no-go tasks, reciprocal action tasks, and sequential motor programs such as the ring/fist test (see Ovsiew 1997).

Paraclinical investigation of incarcerated patients may depend more on availability than indication. We regard neuroimaging—by preference with MRI, a more sensitive and precise tool for these purposes than CT—as indicated for all patients for whom there is evidence of brain dysfunction from the history and examination. Temporal lobe cuts may be indicated if a diagnosis of epilepsy is under consideration. The present role of functional neuroimaging is uncertain, and PET, single photon emission computed tomography, and functional MRI cannot be recommended for routine use. EEG is indicated if the question of epilepsy has arisen because of a disturbance of consciousness at the time of the offense or for other reasons. A second EEG with sleep deprivation and recording during sleep may be indicated if suspicion remains high for an epileptic disorder after an initial negative study. Neuropsychological assessment is of great importance if the history or examination raises a question of cognitive impairment. In view of the evidence for an association of language dysfunction with criminal behavior, special attention to this domain, along with memory and executive cognitive function, is called for.

Conclusion

The foregoing material makes some matters clear and leaves room for speculation about others. Without doubt, jails and prisons contain a large number of people with psychiatric diagnoses and a substantial number with evidence of cerebral disease. The use of jails and prisons to control mentally ill people in the absence of adequate psychiatric facilities may mean that increasingly more persons with such clinical problems will be present in the criminal justice population (Torrey et al. 1992). For neuropsychiatric purposes, it may be helpful to divide criminals into those who have careers of recidivistic offending, especially violent offending, and those whose criminal acts, especially violent acts, appear isolated from an otherwise blameless life. The latter group has been a particular topic of neuropsychiatric interest under the controversial rubric of episodic dyscontrol. For them, paroxysmal limbic abnormalities may be an important pathogenetic factor, and the neuropsychiatrist can play a helpful role in clarifying whether an organic basis exists for otherwise inexplicable behavior. However, temporal EEG abnormalities may not imply that a criminal act was committed during a seizure or the postictal period but rather serve as an index of disturbed limbic processing.

The small group of offenders who commit a disproportionate share of crimes is of intense social interest. In a probably small number of such persons, overt cerebral disease, such as the "acquired sociopathy" of orbitofrontal lesions, may be found. For an unknown fraction of recidivistic offenders, a plausible though unconfirmed formulation is that anomalies of brain organization, of genetic or perinatal origin, interact with adverse family and social factors to bring about recurrent offending. Understanding of this group is far from complete, and further research to understand the nature of both the cerebral factors and the facilitating social factors—as well as possible preventive cerebral and social factors and interventions—is clearly needed. The cerebral factors may be underappreciated in routine forensic practice, and Martell (1992, p. 889) concluded that "special attention to brain integrity would benefit forensic clinical evaluations." Neuropsychiatry seems the discipline ideally placed to clarify the relationship among cerebral dysfunction, social adversity, and personality or psychiatric disturbance.

In general, the prevalence of acquired brain disease in criminal offenders has not been ascertained. Apart from epilepsy, to our knowledge no relevant cerebral factors have been the subject of appropriate epidemiological study. Traumatic brain injury seems an excellent candidate for such examination, and the preliminary and unconfirmed reports about its role in wife battering favor the need for such data. Again, the social importance of the problem argues for better scientific understanding.

This review does not address treatment issues, which are highly complex not only scientifically but socially and politically as well. Again we state that society has a legitimate interest in protection of its members from criminal activity, and certainly neuropsychiatry cannot promise treatments effective enough to substitute for incarceration in this regard—and none at all to meet society's goals of punishment and moral censure. Still, a prerequisite for a rational approach to the problem of crime is an understanding of its nature, and neuropsychiatric understanding may change our views of some criminal acts (Fenwick 1993; Tancredi and Volkow 1988) and provide space for the "therapeutic power of the criminal law" (Wexler 1994) to operate, even if fundamental ideas regarding criminal responsibility are unaltered (Shapiro 1994). Fuller study of the issues identified above seems to us to be essential to the adoption of reasonable treatment and rehabilitative options for those accused of or imprisoned for criminal acts.

References

Abeling NGGM, van Gennip AH, Overmars H, et al: Biogenic amine metabolite patterns in the urine of monoamine oxidase A–deficient patients. A possible tool for diagnosis. J Inherit Metab Dis 17:339–341, 1994

Abram KM, Teplin LA: Co-occurring disorders among mentally ill jail detainees: implications for public policy. Am Psychol 46:1036–1045, 1991

Albert DJ, Walsh ML, Jonik RH: Aggression in humans: what is its biological foundation? Neurosci Biobehav Rev 17:405–425, 1993

American Psychiatric Association: Diagnostic and Statistical Manual of Mental Disorders, 3rd Edition. Washington, DC, American Psychiatric Association, 1980

Archer J: The influence of testosterone on human aggression. Br J Psychol 82:1–28, 1991

Bain J, Langevin R, Dickey R, et al: Sex hormones in murderers and assaulters. Behav Sci Law 5:95–101, 1987

Berrios GE: Personality disorders: a conceptual history, in Personality Disorders Reviewed. Edited by Tyrer P, Stein G. London, Gaskell, 1993, pp 17–41

Blake PY, Pincus JH, Buckner C: Neurological abnormalities in murderers. Neurology 45:1641–1647, 1995

Brennan P, Mednick S, Kandel E: Congenital determinants of violent and property offending, in The Development and Treatment of Childhood Aggression. Edited by Pepler DJ, Rubin KH. Hillsdale, NJ, Erlbaum, 1991, pp 81–92

Brunner HG, Nelen M, Breakefield XO, et al: Abnormal behavior associated with a point mutation in the structural gene for monoamine oxidase A. Science 262:578–580, 1993a

Brunner HG, Nelen MR, van Zandvoort P, et al: X-linked borderline mental retardation with prominent behavioral disturbance: phenotype, genetic localization, and evidence for disturbed monoamine metabolism. Am J Hum Genet 52:1032–1039, 1993b

Cadoret RJ, Yates WR, Troughton E, et al: Genetic-environment interaction in the genesis of aggressivity and conduct disorder. Arch Gen Psychiatry 52:916–924, 1995

Center for Mental Health Services: Double Jeopardy: Persons With Mental Illnesses in the Criminal Justice System. Rockville, MD, U.S. Department of Health and Human Services, 1995

Coid J: Current concepts and classifications of psychopathic disorder, in Personality Disorder Reviewed. Edited by Tyrer P, Stein G. London, Gaskell, 1993, pp 113–164

Convit A, Czobor P, Volavka J: Lateralized abnormality in the EEG of persistently violent psychiatric inpatients. Biol Psychiatry 30:363–370, 1991

Côté G, Hodgins S: Co-occurring mental disorders among criminal offenders. Bulletin of the American Academy of Psychiatry and Law 18:271–281, 1990

Dabbs JM, Frady RL, Carr TS, et al: Saliva testosterone and criminal violence in young adult prison inmates. Psychosom Med 49:174–182, 1987

Denkowski GC, Denkowski KM: The mentally retarded offender in the state prison system: identification, prevalence, adjustment, and rehabilitation. Criminal Justice and Behavior 12:55–70, 1985

Denno DW: Biology and Violence: From Birth to Adulthood. Cambridge, UK, Cambridge University Press, 1990

Drake ME, Hietter SA, Pakalnis A: EEG and evoked potentials in episodic-dyscontrol syndrome. Neuropsychobiology 26:125–128, 1992

Driver MV, West LR, Faulk M: Clinical and EEG studies of prisoners charged with murder. Br J Psychiatry 125:583–587, 1974

Fenwick P: Is dyscontrol epilepsy? in What Is Epilepsy?: The Clinical and Scientific Basis of Epilepsy. Edited by Trimble MR, Reynolds EH. Edinburgh, Churchill Livingstone, 1986, pp 161–182

Fenwick P: The nature and management of aggression in epilepsy. J Neuropsychiatry Clin Neurosci 1:418–425, 1989

Fenwick P: Brain, mind and behaviour. Some medico-legal aspects. Br J Psychiatry 163:565–573, 1993

Fleminger S, Burns A: The delusional misidentification syndromes in patients with and without evidence of organic cerebral disorder: a structured review of case reports. Biol Psychiatry 33:22–32, 1993

Garnett ES, Nahmias C, Wortzman G, et al: Positron emission tomography and sexual arousal in a sadist and two controls. Annals of Sex Research 1:387–399, 1988

Gillstrom BJ, Hare RD: Language-related hand gestures in psychopaths. Journal of Personality Disorders 2:21–27, 1988

Gorenstein EE: Frontal lobe functions in psychopaths. J Abnorm Psychol 91:368–379, 1982

Grafman J, Vance SC, Weingartner H, et al: The effects of lateralized frontal lesions on mood regulation. Brain 109:1127–1148, 1986

Gunn J, Bonn J: Criminality and violence in epileptic prisoners. Br J Psychiatry 118:337–343, 1971

Gunn J, Fenton G: Epilepsy in prisons: a diagnostic survey. BMJ 4:326–328, 1969

Hare RD: Performance of psychopaths on cognitive tasks related to frontal lobe function. J Abnorm Psychol 93:133–140, 1984

Hare RD, Jutai JW: Psychopathy and cerebral asymmetry in semantic processing. Personality and Individual Differences 9:329–337, 1988

Hare RD, McPherson LM: Psychopathy and perceptual asymmetry during verbal dichotic listening. J Abnorm Psychol 93:141–149, 1984

Hare RD, Williamson SE, Harpur TJ: Psychopathy and language, in Biological Contributions to Crime Causation. Edited by Moffitt TE, Mednick SA. Dordrecht, Martinus Nijhoff, 1986, pp 68–92

Hare RD, Hart SD, Harpur TJ: Psychopathy and the DSM-IV criteria for antisocial personality disorder. J Abnorm Psychol 100:391–398, 1991

Hart SD, Forth AE, Hare RD: Performance of criminal psychopaths on selected neuropsychological tests. J Abnorm Psychol 99:374–379, 1990

Hill D, Pond DA: Reflections on one hundred capital cases submitted to electroencephalography. Journal of Mental Science 98:23–43, 1952

Hillbrand M, Sokol SJ, Waite BM, et al: Abnormal lateralization in finger tapping and overt aggressive behavior. Prog Neuropsychopharmacol Biol Psychiatry 17: 393–406, 1993

Hodgins S: Mental disorder, intellectual deficiency, and crime: evidence from a birth cohort. Arch Gen Psychiatry 49:476–483, 1992

Howard RC: The clinical EEG and personality in mentally abnormal offenders. Psychol Med 14:569–580, 1984

Jemelka RP, Rahman S, Trupin EW: Prison mental health: an overview, in Mental Illness in America's Prisons. Edited by Steadman HJ, Cocozza JJ. Seattle, WA, National Coalition for the Mentally Ill in the Criminal Justice System, 1993, pp 9–23

Jenkins RL, Pacella BL: Electroencephalographic studies of delinquent boys. Am J Orthopsychiatry 13:107–120, 1943

Jutai JW, Hare RD, Connolly JF: Psychopathy and event-related brain potentials (ERPs) associated with attention to speech stimuli. Personality and Individual Differences 8:175–184, 1987

Kandel E, Mednick SA: Perinatal complications predict violent offending. Criminology 29:519–529, 1991

Kandel E, Brennan PA, Mednick SA, et al: Minor physical anomalies and recidivistic adult criminal behavior. Acta Psychiatr Scand 79:103–107, 1989

Kendler KS: Genetic epidemiology in psychiatry: taking both genes and environment seriously. Arch Gen Psychiatry 52:895–899, 1995

Langevin R, Ben-Aron M, Wortzman G, et al: Brain damage, diagnosis, and substance abuse among violent offenders. Behav Sci Law 5:77–94, 1987

Levy S, Kennard M: A study of the electroencephalogram as related to personality structure in a group of inmates of a state penitentiary. Am J Psychiatry 109:832–839, 1953

Lewis DO, Shanok SS, Pincus JH, et al: Violent juvenile delinquents: psychiatric, neurological, psychological, and abuse factors. J Am Acad Child Adolesc Psychiatry 18:307–319, 1979

Lewis DO, Pincus JH, Feldman M, et al: Psychiatric, neurological, and psychoeducational characteristics of 15 death row inmates in the United States. Am J Psychiatry 143:838–843, 1986

Lewis DO, Pincus JH, Lovely R, et al: Biopsychosocial characteristics of matched samples of delinquents and nondelinquents. J Am Acad Child Adolesc Psychiatry 26:744–752, 1987

Lewis DO, Pincus JH, Bard B, et al: Neuropsychiatric, psychoeducational, and family characteristics of 14 juveniles condemned to death in the United States. Am J Psychiatry 145:584–589, 1988

Lidberg L, Tuck JR, Åsberg M, et al: Homicide, suicide and CSF 5-HIAA. Acta Psychiatr Scand 71:230–236, 1985

Lyons MJ, True WR, Eisen SA, et al: Differential heritability of adult and juvenile antisocial traits. Arch Gen Psychiatry 52:906–915, 1995

Martell DA: Estimating the prevalence of organic brain dysfunction in maximum-security forensic psychiatric patients. J Forensic Sci 37:878–893, 1992

McAfee JK, Gural M: Individuals with mental retardation and the criminal justice system: the view from states' attorneys general. Ment Retard 26:5–12, 1988

McManus M, Brickman A, Alessi NE, et al: Neurological dysfunction in serious delinquents. Journal of the American Academy of Child Psychiatry 24:481–486, 1985

Mednick SA, Kandel E: Genetic and perinatal factors in violence, in Biological Contributions to Crime Causation. Edited by Moffitt TE, Mednick SA. Dordrecht, Martinus Nijhoff, 1988, pp 121–131

Menzies RJ: Psychiatrists in blue: police apprehension of mental disorder and dangerousness. Criminology 25:429–453, 1987

Milstein V: EEG topography in patients with aggressive violent behavior, in Biological Contributions to Crime Causation. Edited by Moffitt TE, Mednick SA. Dordrecht, Martinus Nijhoff, 1988, pp 40–52

Moffitt TE: The neuropsychology of juvenile delinquency: a critical review, in Crime and Justice: A Review of Research. Edited by Tonry M, Morris N. Chicago, IL, University of Chicago, 1990, pp 99–169

Moffitt TE, Henry B: Neuropsychological studies of juvenile delinquency and juvenile violence, in Neuropsychology of Aggression. Edited by Milner JS. Boston, MA, Kluwer Academic Publishers, 1991, pp 67–91

Moffitt TE, Mednick SA, Gabrielli WF: Predicting careers of criminal violence: descriptive data and predispositional factors, in Current Approaches to the Prediction of Violence. Edited by Brizer DA, Crowner M. Washington, DC, American Psychiatric Press, 1989, pp 15–34

Morris N: The contemporary prison: 1965–present, in The Oxford History of the Prison. Edited by Morris N, Rothman DJ. New York, Oxford University Press, 1995, pp 227–259

Nachson I: Neuropsychology of violent behavior: controversial issues and new developments in the study of hemisphere function, in Neuropsychology of Aggression. Edited by Milner JS. Boston, MA, Kluwer Academic Publishers, 1991, pp 93–116

Newman JP, Wallace JF: Psychopathy and cognition, in Psychopathology and Cognition. Edited by Dobson KS, Kendall PC. San Diego, CA, Academic Press, 1993, pp 293–349

Ovsiew F: Bedside neuropsychiatry: eliciting the clinical phenomena of neuropsychiatric illness, in American Psychiatric Press Textbook of Neuropsychiatry, 3rd Edition. Edited by Yudofsky SC, Hales RE. Washington, DC, American Psychiatric Press, 1997, pp 121–163

Raine A: The Psychopathology of Crime: Criminal Behavior as a Clinical Disorder. San Diego, CA, Academic Press, 1993

Raine A, O'Brien M, Smiley N, et al: Reduced lateralization in verbal dichotic listening in adolescent psychopaths. J Abnorm Psychol 99:272–277, 1990

Raine A, Brennan P, Mednick SA: Birth complications combined with early maternal rejection at age 1 year predispose to violent crime at age 18 years. Arch Gen Psychiatry 51:984–988, 1994a

Raine A, Buchsbaum MS, Stanley J, et al: Selective reductions in prefrontal glucose metabolism in murderers. Biol Psychiatry 36:365–373, 1994b

Raine A, Lencz T, Scerbo A: Antisocial behavior: neuroimaging, neuropsychology, neurochemistry, and psychophysiology, in Neuropsychiatry of Personality Disorders. Edited by Ratey JJ. Cambridge, MA, Blackwell Scientific, 1995a, pp 50–78

Raine A, Venable PH, Williams M: High autonomic arousal and electrodermal orienting at age 15 years as protective factors against criminal behavior at age 29 years. Am J Psychiatry 152:1595–1600, 1995b

Robertson G: Arrest patterns among mentally disordered offenders. Br J Psychiatry 153:313–316, 1988

Robertson G, Taylor PJ, Gunn JC: Does violence have cognitive correlates? Br J Psychiatry 151:63–68, 1987

Rosenbaum A, Hoge SK: Head injury and marital aggression. Am J Psychiatry 146:1048–1051, 1989

Rosenbaum A, Hoge SK, Adelman SA, et al: Head injury in partner-abusive men. J Consult Clin Psychol 62:1187–1193, 1994

Roy A, Adinoff B, Linnoila M: Acting out hostility in normal volunteers: negative correlation with levels of 5HIAA in cerebrospinal fluid. Psychiatry Res 24:187–194, 1988

Roy A, Virkkunen M, Linnoila M: Serotonin in suicide, violence, and alcoholism, in Serotonin in Major Psychiatric Disorders. Edited by Coccaro EF, Murphy DL. Washington, DC, American Psychiatric Press, 1990, pp 187–208

Santamour MB, West B: The mentally retarded offender: presentation of the facts and a discussion of the issues, in The Retarded Offender. Edited by Santamour MB, Watson PS. New York, Praeger, 1982, pp 7–36

Shapiro MH: Law, culpability, and the neural sciences, in The Neurotransmitter Revolution: Serotonin, Social Behavior, and the Law. Edited by Masters RD, McGuire MT. Carbondale, IL, Southern Illinois University Press, 1994, pp 179–202

Silva JA, Leong GB, Weinstock R: The dangerousness of persons with misidentification syndromes. Bulletin of the American Academy of Psychiatry and Law 20:77–86, 1992

Silva JA, Leong GB, Weinstock R, et al: Delusional misidentification and dangerousness: a neurobiologic hypothesis. J Forensic Sci 38:904–913, 1993

Silverman D: Clinical and electroencephalographic studies on criminal psychopaths. AMA Archives of Neurology and Psychiatry 50:18–33, 1943

Stafford-Clark D, Taylor FH: Clinical and electro-encephalographic studies of prisoners charged with murder. J Neurol Neurosurg Psychiatry 12:325–330, 1949

Stone MH: Abnormalities of Personality: Within and Beyond the Realm of Treatment. New York, WW Norton, 1993

Tancredi LR, Volkow N: Neural substrates of violent behavior: implications for law and public policy. Int J Law Psychiatry 11:13–49, 1988

Teplin LA: The criminality of the mentally ill: a dangerous misconception. Am J Psychiatry 142:593–599, 1985

Teplin LA: The prevalence of severe mental disorder among male urban jail detainees: comparison with the Epidemiologic Catchment Area Program. Am J Public Health 80:663–669, 1990

Teplin LA: Psychiatric and substance abuse disorders among male urban jail detainees. Am J Public Health 84:290–293, 1994

Teplin LA, Pruett NS: Police as streetcorner psychiatrist: managing the mentally ill. Int J Law Psychiatry 15:139–156, 1992

Torrey EF, Stieber J, Ezekiel J, et al: Criminalizing the Seriously Mentally Ill: The Abuse of Jails as Mental Hospitals. Washington, DC, Public Citizen's Health Research Group and the National Alliance for the Mentally Ill, 1992

Tranel D: "Acquired sociopathy": the development of sociopathic behavior following focal brain damage. Prog Exp Pers Psychopathol Res 1994, pp 285–311

van Praag HM: Serotonergic dysfunction and aggression control. Psychol Med 21:15–19, 1991

Virkkunen M, Nuutila A, Huusko S: Effect of brain injury on social adaptability: longitudinal study on frequency of criminality. Acta Psychiatr Scand 53:168–172, 1976

Virkkunen M, Nuutila A, Huusko S: Brain injury and criminality: a retrospective study. Diseases of the Nervous System 907–908, 1977

Virkkunen M, De Jong J, Bartko J, et al: Relationship of psychobiological variables to recidivism in violent offenders and impulsive fire setters: a follow-up study. Arch Gen Psychiatry 46:600–603, 1989

Virkkunen M, Kallio E, Rawlings R, et al: Personality profiles and state aggressiveness in Finnish alcoholic, violent offenders, fire setters, and healthy volunteers. Arch Gen Psychiatry 51:28–33, 1994

Volavka J, Martell D, Convit A: Psychobiology of the violent offender. J Forensic Sci 37:237–251, 1992

Volkow ND, Tancredi L: Neural substrates of violent behaviour: a preliminary study of positron emission tomography. Br J Psychiatry 151:668–673, 1987

Warnken WJ, Rosenbaum A, Fletcher KE, et al: Head-injured males: a population at risk for relationship aggression? Violence Vict 9:153–166, 1994

Wexler DB: Low serotonin function and the therapeutic power of the criminal law, in The Neurotransmitter Revolution: Serotonin, Social Behavior, and the Law. Edited by Masters RD, McGuire MT. Carbondale, IL, Southern Illinois University Press, 1994, pp 215–221

Whitman S, Coleman TE, Patmon C, et al: Epilepsy in prison: elevated prevalence and no relationship to violence. Neurology 34:775–782, 1984

Williams D: Neural factors related to habitual aggression: consideration of differences between those habitual aggressives and others who have committed crimes of violence. Brain 92:503–520, 1969

Wolff PH, Waber D, Bauermeister M, et al: The neuropsychological status of adolescent delinquent boys. J Child Psychol Psychiatry 23:267–279, 1982

Wong MTH, Lumsden J, Fenton GW, et al: Electroencephalography, computed tomography and violence ratings of male patients in a maximum-security mental hospital. Acta Psychiatr Scand 90:97–101, 1994

CHAPTER 8

Neuropsychiatry of Human Immunodeficiency Virus Infection

Joel K. Levy, Ph.D.
Francisco Fernandez, M.D.
Barbara L. Lachar, Ph.D.
Ann L. Friedman, Ph.D., J.D.
Zishan Samiuddin, M.D.

Human immunodeficiency virus (HIV) infection is a major health and social problem. The diseases it causes are complex, and they challenge the diagnostic and interventional skills of all who attempt to contribute to the welfare of those infected. Prevention and cure may continue to elude investigators for some time to come.

HIV infection inflicts economic havoc on infected patients. Patients may become indigent as their resources are diminished by the expense of this illness or by the loss of insurance. As they leave the workforce because of recurrent illnesses, loss of energy, or cognitive decline, patients often lose their individual health care financing and may have to rely on the public sector for this care. Also, HIV infection is a major additional economic threat to the severely and persistently mentally ill who compose a segment of the homeless in the United States and who may have to rely on provision of health care and, specifically, mental health care from public health resources. A high rate of HIV infection (as high as 20%) is reported in homeless men in New York City (Nichols et al. 1994). These homeless and chronically mentally ill patients are at risk for infection because of high rates of unprotected sexual activity and parenteral drug use (Nichols et al. 1994) and because they may be in situations in which they are physically and sexually victimized or are induced to trade sex for food, money, drugs, or shelter (Nichols et al. 1994). These chronically mentally ill patients may have, as a result of their mental illness, cognitive impairment or impaired judgment, which heightens their risk for engaging in practices that may lead to infection. This issue is further discussed in Chapter 11. The high rate of HIV infection in prisons is cited in Chapter 7.

HIV has an additional complication that directly challenges the mental health professionals. By its invasion of the central nervous system (CNS), HIV can cause a range of organic mental disorders. In this chapter, we discuss the neuropathology and neurobehavioral symptoms associated with HIV infection. One metropolitan area's response to this epidemic is detailed, and the structure of public services created in reaction to local mandates and federal resource allocations is outlined.

HIV Infection: Epidemiology and Risk Factors

The acquired immunodeficiency syndrome (AIDS) (Barre-Sinoussi et al. 1983) initially confounded public health investigators with its apparent selectivity for certain populations. However, it ultimately became known that the syndrome and related illnesses were associated with a specific virus, the human immunodeficiency virus (Barre-Sinoussi et al. 1983; Gallo et al. 1983; Levy et al. 1984). Transmission risk factors include sexual behaviors in which virus-bearing body fluids make contact with the bloodstream through breaks in mucous membranes; intravenous drug use with shared needles; and administration of blood transfusions, blood products, or blood factor concentrates infected with the virus. Infants may be infected during birth and through infected milk during lactation. Persons may be exposed in their occupational pursuits, such as in medicine, dentistry, and emergency medical intervention rendered by police, fire, and rescue personnel.

According to the Centers for Disease Control and Prevention (CDC), the current reported cumulative number of cases of fully developed AIDS is in excess of 573,000 in the United States (CDC 1997). Two to three million persons are estimated to be infected with the virus but are asymptomatic.

With regard to mental health concerns, it is projected that 7.3% of AIDS patients may develop HIV encephalopathy (Janssen et al. 1992). Young (less than 15 years old) and old (75 years or older) persons may develop encephalopathy more frequently (13% and 19%, respectively) (Janssen et al. 1992).

After the virus invades the body and incorporates itself into the host's cell nuclear material, there may be a long period of dormancy of 5–7 years before symptoms emerge (Bernad 1991; Brew et al. 1988; Hollander 1991; Koralnik et al. 1990; Mitsuyasu 1989; Rowen and Carne 1991). However, there are reported cases of cognitive and psychiatric manifestations occurring even before the onset of AIDS–case-defining criteria (opportunistic infections, characteristic malignancies, or neurological syndromes) (Beckett et al. 1987; Jones et al. 1987; Maccario and Scharre 1987; Navia and Price 1987). The risk of neurobehavioral complications is high, with up to 70%–80% of infected persons exhibiting an organic mental disorder sometime within the course of the illness (Wolcott et al. 1985). These disorders may take a number of forms, from cognitive disorders and dementia to affective disorders and psychotic disturbances. HIV-related neurological effects and dementia have been included by the CDC as an additional diagnostic criterion for the status of fully developed AIDS (CDC 1987).

What triggers the progression from dormancy to AIDS is not fully known. Although there is some dispute that lifestyle factors, including alcohol or drug use, hasten progression through the clinical stages (Kaslow et al. 1989), prudence would dictate that use of these substances could tax vulnerable organ systems, may lead patients into transmission risk situations because of impaired judgment, and may further strain possibly fragile cognitive functional capacities. Alcohol has been shown to increase HIV type 1 (HIV-1) replication in vitro (Bagasra et al. 1993) and to impair important immune functions such as natural killer cell activity (Nair et al. 1994). Conversely, reports have credited active psychological coping strategies and health-promoting behaviors, such as physical exercise, with significant improvement in hematological immune markers (Antoni et al. 1990; Goodkin et al. 1992).

Central Nervous System Pathology

Direct Effects From HIV Infection

HIV was found not only to cause immune compromise but to be neuro-degenerative as well. Electron microscopy of autopsy material revealed

(Gyorkey et al. 1987) that the virus may gain entry to the brain substance by passing through endothelial gaps in the brain capillaries. Also, it has been proposed that the virus enters the brain via infected macrophages, the so-called Trojan horse effect (Dickson et al. 1991; Schindelmeiser and Gullotta 1991; Vazeux 1991). The virus may then attach to CD4+ receptors, similar to those of the CD4+ T lymphocytes, which are present on some oligodendroglia (Pumarola-Sune et al. 1987). Pert and associates have surveyed sites for which the virus seems to have an affinity (Hill et al. 1987), which include basal ganglia and temporolimbic structures. These areas may relate to neurobehavioral symptoms associated with HIV encephalopathy.

Much of our knowledge of the central neuropathology came from the pioneering observations of Price and associates (Brew at al. 1988; Navia et al. 1986a, 1986b) and Wiley and co-workers (Masliah et al. 1992; Wiley et al. 1991). Findings included involvement of the white matter and subcortical structures, often with eventual atrophy. Cortical areas have also shown cell loss, especially in the frontal lobe (Ciardi et al. 1990; Everall et al. 1991; Ketzler et al. 1990). The result of this CNS neuropathology is often reflected in cognitive changes ranging from mild memory decline and cognitive slowing to a profound dementia (CDC 1987) (Tables 8–1 and 8–2). In search of a marker that would correlate with or predict dementia, investigators found that levels of β_2-microglobulin and neopterin are promising (Brew et al. 1992; Elovaara et al. 1989; Harrison and Skidmore 1990; Karlsen et al.

TABLE 8–1. Early signs and symptoms of HIV-related neurobehavioral impairment

Cognitive	Affective/behavioral
Memory difficulties (especially affecting verbal rote or episodic)	Apathy
Concentration/attention impairment	Depressed mood
Comprehension impairment	Anxiety
Conceptual confusion	Agitation
Visuospatial/manual constructional difficulties	Mild disinhibition
Psychomotor slowing or dyscoordination	Hallucinations
Mental tracking difficulties	
Mild frontal lobe dysfunction	
Handwriting and fine motor control difficulties	
Problem-solving difficulties	

Source. Adapted from Brew BJ, Sidtis JJ, Petito CK, et al.: "The Neurologic Complications of AIDS and Human Immunodeficiency Virus Infection," in *Advances in Contemporary Neurology.* Edited by Plum F. Philadelphia, PA, FA Davis, 1988, pp. 1–49. Used with permission.

TABLE 8–2.   Late signs and symptoms of HIV-related neurobehavioral impairment

Cognitive	Affective/behavioral
Global dementia	Severe disinhibition
Mutism	Mania
Aphasia	Delusions
Severe frontal lobe dysfunction	Severe hallucinations
Severe psychomotor retardation	Agitation
Distractibility	Paranoia
Disorientation	Severe depression
	Suicidal ideation

Source.   Adapted from Brew BJ, Sidtis JJ, Petito CK, et al.: "The Neurologic Complications of AIDS and Human Immunodeficiency Virus Infection," in *Advances in Contemporary Neurology*. Edited by Plum F. Philadelphia, PA, FA Davis, 1988, pp. 1–49. Used with permission.

1991). More recent work on the neuropathology of excitotoxins (Cotton 1990; Eriksson and Lidberg 1996; Giulian et al. 1990, 1996; Heyes et al. 1991; Kieburtz et al. 1991; Lipton 1992; Sardar et al. 1995; Schwarcz et al. 1983; Walker et al. 1989; Yoshioka et al. 1995), the role of *N*-methyl-D-aspartate (NMDA) (Kieburtz et al. 1991; Lipton 1992), receptor physiology and dysregulation (Harbison et al. 1991; Heyes et al. 1992; Kaiser et al. 1990; Lipton 1991), and the specific neurotoxicity of quinolinic acid (Cotton 1990; Giulian et al. 1990, 1996; Heyes et al. 1991, 1992; Kieburtz et al. 1991; Lipton 1992; Schwarcz et al. 1983; Sei et al. 1995) is contributing to the explanation of how neuronal tissue becomes injured indirectly by the effects of HIV infection.

Secondary Neuropathology Resulting From Opportunistic Infections and Neoplasia

When opportunistic infections or malignancies such as Kaposi's sarcoma and HIV-related lymphomas arise, or when severe neurological disease occurs, the HIV-infected patient meets one of several criteria for AIDS. This may occur at any time, though immune compromise is usually reflected by laboratory markers, namely, fewer than 200 CD4+ T lymphocytes per microliter. In fact, this low level of CD4+ T lymphocytes (or their percentage of total lymphocytes at lower than 14%) has achieved such clinical significance that the CDC has included this determination as part of their most recent revision of the AIDS surveillance case definitions (CDC 1992). Additionally, syphilis and pulmonary tuberculosis (another recent addition to the AIDS surveillance case definitions [CDC 1992]) are increasingly found as co-infections in this population and can appear as CNS infection. These opportunistic infections and malignancies may contribute to severe focal neurological disorders (Bedri et al. 1983; Beilke 1989; Belman et al. 1986; Berger et al. 1987; Bredesen et al. 1988; Budka 1989; Engstrom et al. 1989; Filley et al. 1989; Gonzales and David 1988; Gray et al. 1988; Ho et al. 1987; Jarvik et al. 1988; Lantos et al. 1989; Lenhardt and Wiley 1989; Levy 1994; Lipton et al. 1991; Masdeu et al. 1988; McArthur et al. 1987, 1990; J. K. Miller et al. 1982; Petito 1988; Portegies et al. 1991; Scaravilli et al. 1989; Snider et al. 1983; Vinters et al. 1988; Whelan et al. 1983). It thus becomes an important differential diagnostic issue to investigate and treat aggressively the cause of the neurological problem in order to postpone mortality and to seek restoration of neurobehavioral function. Bredesen and colleagues (1988) reviewed common CNS infections, as well as neoplasia and other infection- or treatment-induced complications. The range of CNS involvement in AIDS is listed in Table 8–3 (Bredesen et al. 1988).

Neuroassessment of HIV-CNS Involvement

Clinical Assessment

Cognitive history. We have found that taking a careful cognitive history can be the most helpful part of the interaction with the patient in the differential diagnosis of etiologies of cognitive dysfunction (Levy 1994). This is especially true when there is no capacity for formal neurocognitive testing in a particular clinic or other community setting. The essentials of this interview are listed in Table 8–4. Specifically, in HIV-associated minor cognitive-motor disorder and HIV-associated dementia complex, patients are often aware and complain of cognitive inefficiency, including forgetfulness and increasing cognitive disorganization. In cognitive dysfunction syndromes attributable to other intracranial opportunistic infections or cancer, there is often an obviously grossly impaired mental status or focal cognitive deficits.

The history should include questions about the patient's perception of the current problem; what type of memory function is most problematic (verbal vs. visuospatial, locations of items, names of people, remote vs. recent); and what types of problems are being experienced with attention and concentration, decision making, problem solving, planning, organization, language, perception, and motoric function. Daily functions such as sleep, appetite, hygiene, interests, motivation, and interpersonal interactions should be de-

TABLE 8–3.   AIDS-related central nervous system diseases

Primary viral (HIV) syndromes
  HIV encephalopathy
  Atypical aseptic meningitis
  Vacuolar myelopathy
Opportunistic viral illnesses
  Cytomegalovirus
  Herpes simplex virus, types I and II
  Herpes varicella zoster
  Papovavirus (progressive multifocal leukoencephalopathy)
  Adenovirus type 2
Nonviral infections
  Toxoplasma gondii
  Cryptococcus neoformans
  Candida albicans
  Aspergillus fumigatus
  Coccidioides immitis
  Mucormycosis
  Rhizopus species
  Acremonium alabamensis
  Histoplasma capsulatum
  Mycobacterium hominis tuberculosis
  Mycobacterium avium–intracellulare complex
  Listeria monocytogenes
  Nocardia asteroides
Neoplasms
  Primary CNS lymphoma
  Metastatic systemic lymphoma
  Metastatic Kaposi's sarcoma
Cerebrovascular events
  Infarction
  Hemorrhage
  Vasculitis
Complications of systemic AIDS therapy

Source.   Adapted from Bredesen DE, Levy RM, Rosenblum ML: "The Neurology of Human Immunodeficiency Virus Infection." *QJM (Oxford)* 68:665–677, 1988. Used with permission.

TABLE 8–4.   HIV neurocognitive history

Name

Age and birthday

Handedness

First language at home

Educational background

   Best subjects, grades

   Worst subjects

Occupational background

   How long?

Medical history

   Childhood diseases or injuries

   Head injuries with loss of consciousness

   Strokes

   High fevers

   Toxin exposure

   Major illness, injuries, or surgeries

   Medicines: prescription, nonprescription

Duration of diagnosis of HIV infection, AIDS

Current problem

   Change in thinking functions: how long or over what period of time?

Any change in ability to concentrate?

Any periods of confusion or mental "fuzziness," such as when talking with people in person or on the phone, watching TV or a movie, reading?

Any problem with following the train of thought?

Any difficulties with handwriting?

Any word-finding problems, difficulties with slurring or stammering?

Any slowing of thinking or understanding, trouble with mental arithmetic, such as making change or balancing checkbook?

Wear glasses?

Any blurring vision, double vision, or flashing lights in eyes?

Any change in understanding what is seen? Do things look right in their relation to each other?

Overlook things when right in front of you?

Hear any unusual sounds? See unusual things? Have any strange feelings?

Any changes in any other senses?

Decreased hearing; ringing or buzzing sounds?

Change in sense of smell or taste?

Numbness, "pins and needles," loss of feeling, tingling, or burning feelings?

Any severe pain?

TABLE 8–4.	HIV neurocognitive history *(continued)*

Memory

    Any areas of memory that are better or worse?

      Memory for recent information

      Information from way back in life

    Any difference in memory for *situations* versus rote facts and figures?

    Kinds of things most easily forgotten: names, addresses, directions, reading?

    How long can things be remembered? More notes written than used to?

    Any lapses noted?

    Any getting lost or forgetting where you are?

Any new difficulties with thinking through problems or solving them, decision making, staying organized—on job, at home?

How is sleep? Any trouble getting to sleep? Night versus daytime? Any awakenings from which you cannot immediately return to sleep?

Any inability to move any parts of the body?

Muscle weakness, twitching, spasms? Trouble walking? Coordination problems? Tremors or shakiness? Problems with dropping things? Feeling like moving more slowly? Difficulty using tools or household utensils, getting dressed, telling right from left?

Headaches or dizziness? Instances thought to be seizures (staring into space for a long time, uncontrollable movements, periods where you seemed to "lose" time, incontinence)

Changes in mood, feelings, ideas?

Mood swings, loss of patience, or change in temper? Increase in irritability? Change in amount of worry? Sense of panic?

(Continue with Hamilton Rating Scale for Depression [Hamilton 1960] and Hamilton Anxiety Scale [Hamilton 1959])

scribed. The answers to these questions can help the examiner match patient complaints to one of the criterial systems, such as the American Academy of Neurology's nomenclature (Working Group of the American Academy of Neurology 1991), for defining HIV-associated minor cognitive-motor disorder and HIV-associated dementia complex. The history must also include inquiry into any psychiatric symptoms such as the criteria for the syndromes of depression (including suicidal ideation and intent), anxiety and panic, euphoria and mania, thought disorders, substance use and abuse, and obsessional thinking and compulsive behavior. A structured interview, such as the Hamilton Scales (Hamilton 1959, 1960), inquiring into these areas can qualify and quantify these symptoms.

Mental status examination. The mental status examination is an essential part of the neurobehavioral evaluation of any patient. With a disease commonly accompanied by organic mental disorders, mental status examination is necessary to distinguish among the various diagnostic possibilities. Frequently, cognitive dysfunction is of the type associated with subcortical impairment. Standard mental status examinations, such as the Mini-Mental State Exam (Folstein et al. 1975), which are designed to assess cortical functions, such as some aspects of language, are valuable for detection of focal deficits. However, they may miss the types of memory and attention/concentration problems often associated with HIV-related cognitive impairment. More formal examinations should include extensive memory assessment of different types of retrieval, such as word list learning; timed tasks for evaluating speed of cognitive processing, such as the Trail Making Test from the Halstead-Reitan Neuropsychological Test Battery (Reitan and Wolfson 1993); and tasks for assessing organizational ability, such as a verbal fluency or set test.

Neurobehavioral evaluation. Discussion has continued over the years regarding the relationship of severity of systemic disease or level of immune compromise to cognitive function (Bornstein et al. 1991; Gibbs et al. 1990; Goethe et al. 1989; Grant et al. 1987; Handelsman et al. 1991; McAllister et al. 1992; McArthur et al. 1989; Perry et al. 1991; Redfield et al. 1986; R. A. Stern et al. 1992; Y. Stern et al. 1990; Wilkie et al. 1990a, 1990b, 1992). Originally, cognitive impairment was found in patients with invasion of the CNS by opportunistic infection or malignancy. A milder level of impairment was attributed to "subacute encephalitis," a forerunner of the current nomenclature for HIV-related cognitive-motor impairments. However, significant impairment has also been observed without opportunistic infections or neoplasia (Beckett et al. 1987), and the presence of such impairment was added to the CDC criteria for AIDS in 1987 (CDC 1987).

A large multicenter survey, the Multicenter AIDS Cohort Study (MACS), found cognitive functioning in asymptomatic patients to be similar to that in matched control subjects (McArthur et al. 1989). These negative results were comparable to results of other single studies (Gibbs et al. 1990; Goethe et al. 1989; McAllister et al. 1992; Wilkins et al. 1990). Other studies, however, involving asymptomatic seropositive patients (Grant et al. 1987; Y. Stern et al. 1990; Wilkie et al. 1990a, 1990b, 1992) versus uninfected control subjects did find differences in cognitive functioning between groups.

Although this debate over group data has continued, the clinician should keep in mind that for any individual patient, complaints at any stage of the disease with regard to memory problems, mental slowing, and difficulty with attention and concentration must be taken seriously and evaluated. Dysphoria in response to the seriousness of the illness or induced by medications or affective disturbances had been thought to cause or significantly overlay, cognitively, the difficulties attributed to the neurodestructive effects of the virus (e.g., pseudodementia of depression) (Cummings and Benson 1983). However, several studies (Kovner et al. 1989; Pace et al. 1992; Syndulko et al. 1990) have demonstrated that cognitive dysfunction in HIV patients is not correlated with mood disorder and that the level of impairment from the viral effects on neural function surpasses that expected by distraction from affective causes.

The cardinal findings of HIV cognitive impairment are similar in many reports and include problems with verbal memory, attention and concentration difficulties, slowing of information processing, slowed psychomotor speed, impaired cognitive flexibility, and, in some cases, disturbances in the nonverbal abilities of problem solving, visuospatial integration and construction, and nonverbal memory (Butters et al. 1990; Collier et al. 1992; Dunlop et al. 1992; Fernandez et al. 1989; Franzblau et al. 1991; Hart et al. 1990; Jacobs et al. 1992; Janssen et al. 1988; Kaemingk and Kaszniak 1989; Karlsen et al. 1992; Klusman et al. 1991; Krikorian and Wrobel 1991; Lunn et al. 1991; Marotta and Perry 1989; Martin et al. 1992; E. N. Miller et al. 1991; Morgan et al. 1988; Nance et al. 1990; Pajeau and Roman 1991; Perry 1990; Perry et al. 1989; Riedel et al. 1992; Rubinow et al. 1988; Ryan et al. 1992; Skoraszewski et al. 1991; Y. Stern et al. 1991; Tross et al. 1988; Van Gorp et al. 1989a, 1989b, 1991; Wilkie et al. 1990a, 1990b). Recent studies showed that psychomotor tasks, such as the Wechsler Adult Intelligence Scale Digit Symbol and Block Design (Wechsler 1981) and the Trail Making Test Part B from the Halstead-Reitan Neuropsychological Test Battery (Reitan and Wolfson 1993), and memory tasks, such as the delayed Visual Reproduction subtest from the Wechsler Memory Scale (Wechsler 1987) and delayed recall of the Rey-Osterreith Complex Figure (Meyers and Meyers 1995), were most affected in the early stages of cognitive impairment associated with HIV (Van Gorp et al. 1989a). Tasks detecting psychomotor and neuromotor disturbances of HIV-related neural dysfunction such as visuomotor reaction time (Dunlop at al. 1992; Karlsen et al. 1992; Nance et al. 1990) and fine motor dexterity as measured by pegboard activities are also sensitive measures for the early detection of impairment. A suggested test battery employing the tests listed in Table 8–5 (Fernandez and Levy 1990b) or tests that address similar functions (Butters et al. 1990) can be used to assess the critical areas of cognitive functioning in order to detect HIV involvement at an early stage.

Table 8–5.   HIV basic neuropsychological battery

General
  Mini-Mental State Exam (Folstein et al. 1975)

Memory
  Buschke-Fuld Verbal Selective Reminding Test (Buschke and Fuld 1974)
  Wechsler Memory Scale Logical Memory Passages (Wechsler 1987)
  Benton Visual Retention Test (Benton 1974)
  Rey-Osterreith Complex Figure (copy; 3- and 45-minute recall) (Meyers
    and Meyers 1995)

Language/speech
  Controlled Oral Word Association (from Benton Multilingual Aphasia
    Examination) (Benton and Hamsher 1989)
  Visual Naming Test (from Benton Multilingual Aphasia
    Examination) (Benton and Hamsher 1989)

Orientation
  Pfeiffer Short Portable Mental Status Questionnaire (Pfeiffer 1975)
  Benton Temporal Orientation Test (Benton et al. 1964)

Visuospatial
  Bender-Gestalt Test (Lacks 1984)
  Raven Progressive Matrices (Raven et al. 1984)

Intellectual/executive/psychomotor
  Similarities, Digit Span, Arithmetic, Digit Symbol from the Wechsler
    Adult Intelligence Scale or the Wechsler Adult Intelligence Scale,
    Revised (Wechsler 1981)
  Trail Making Test, Parts A and B (Reitan and Wolfson 1993)
  Wisconsin Card Sorting (Heaton et al. 1993)
  Finger Tapping Test (Reitan and Wolfson 1993)
  Grooved or Purdue Pegboard (Lezak 1995)
  Reaction Time: Simple Auditory, Simple Visual, and
    Four-Choice Visual (Pirozzolo et al. 1981)
  Shipley Institute of Living Scale (Zachary 1986)
  Stroop Color Word Test (Golden 1978)

Source.   Adapted from Fernandez F, Levy JK: "Adjuvant Treatment of HIV Dementia With Psychostimulants," in *Behavioral Aspects of AIDS and Other Sexually Transmitted Diseases.* Edited by Ostrow D. New York, Plenum, 1990a, pp. 279–286.

   The patient's everyday functional abilities can be evaluated or rated to give health care providers, family, and significant others a sense of how much impairment the individual is experiencing. One scale that has been adapted for this population is the Global Deterioration Scale (Reisberg et al. 1982). This scale has been criticized for its psychometric properties (Eisdorfer et al. 1991) but has some value for characterizing the stages of memory impairment in this disorder.

Laboratory Evaluation

HIV screening.   The Food and Drug Administration first approved testing of blood for HIV in 1985. The need for testing was accentuated by the realization that HIV-positive individuals can infect others (Fischl et al. 1987; Harris et al. 1983; Jason et al. 1986). The first HIV diagnostic test was extremely effective in detecting HIV in patients already classified as having AIDS, but developing screening tests for asymptomatic persons presented a different challenge. The number of false positive values was likely to rise if a substantial population with low prevalence rates was screened.

Currently, testing procedures rely largely on detecting antibodies to HIV core protein (p 24, which develops earliest) and envelope proteins (gp 120, gp 160, and gp 41) (Alter 1987; Leoung et al. 1990; Volberding et al. 1990). Antibodies may develop 6–8 weeks after infection and can be detected by enzyme-linked immunosorbent assay (ELISA) and confirmed by the Western blot (Chalmers et al. 1986). Diagnosis may be difficult in some infants of HIV-positive mothers because the infants can passively acquire maternal antibodies. Similarly, earlier antigen standards were often contaminated with nonviral antigens (possibly human leukocyte antigen [HLA]) from lymphocytes, with this cross-reactivity leading to a large number of false positive values. Genetic recombinant technology, as used by current ELISA testing, results in increased sensitivity and specificity (Allain et al. 1986; Backer et al. 1986; Carlson et al. 1987; Food and Drug Administration 1989; Sload et al. 1991). A sample is declared HIV-positive only after two successive ELISAs and one confirmatory Western blot because up to 70% of initially positive ELISAs are not confirmed by the second ELISA (Leoung et al. 1990; Volberding et al. 1990).

CDC standards require antibodies for any two of p 24, gp 41, gp 120/160 be present to declare a sample HIV-positive. Some specimens may not meet this standard of two bands but have one band. These samples fall into the indeterminate category and may be the result of 1) early stage of infection, 2) infection with HIV-2, or 3) truly false positive results (Busch et al. 1991; Leitman et al. 1989; Scillian et al. 1989; Van der Poel et al. 1989).

U.S. blood bank professionals are divided over whether to allow persons who persistently test indeterminate for Western blot patterns to donate blood. The period of undetectable infectivity, or *window period*, is another confounding situation. Some studies have shown detectable HIV DNA levels by polymerase chain reaction (PCR) in high-risk individuals (Hewlett et al. 1988; Jackson et al. 1990; Kleinmann et al. 1988; Leffrere et al. 1990; Lifson et al. 1989; Pezella et al. 1989; Shepard et al. 1991; Wolinsky et al. 1989).

Some investigators are skeptical about PCR because of the high false-positive rate (Hewlett et al. 1988; Leffrere et al. 1990; Pezella et al. 1989). These tests may be useful in infants in whom one cannot rely on antibody testing to confirm seroconversion. The tests for the detection of HIV antigen at their current level of development, however, have little to add to the diagnosis of HIV infection by more routine antibody testing.

The decision to have HIV antibody testing is, of course, a life-changing step because of the dysphoria that can emerge with a positive finding; the potential for loss of insurance, job, and relationships with friends and family if the finding is inadvertently publicly disclosed; and the stigma implied with associations with HIV and risk behaviors. Mental health professionals must carefully weigh the impact of such information, given their knowledge of their patient's personality, when asked if testing is recommended.

Cerebrospinal fluid.   HIV enters the CNS within 2 weeks of infection, either clinically silent and unrecognized or as acute meningoencephalitis or meningitis. Symptoms develop within 3–6 weeks of primary HIV infection. The CSF in HIV disease (Brew et al. 1992; Buffet et al. 1991; Carrieri et al. 1992; Chalmers et al. 1986; Chiodi et al. 1992; Heyes et al. 1991; Larsson et al. 1991; Lolli et al. 1990; Marshall et al. 1988, 1991; McArthur et al. 1992; Portegies et al. 1989; Reboul et al. 1989; Shaskan et al. 1992; Tartaglione et al. 1991) shows elevated protein (but <100 mg/100 mL), mononuclear pleocytosis (but <200 cells/mm^3), and normal glucose. Patients with complaints about mental functioning, with altered mental status, or with focal neurological signs should be evaluated quickly for signs of opportunistic infection such as toxoplasmosis, cryptococcal infection, herpes simplex, herpes zoster varicellosus, and cytomegalovirus (Buffet et al. 1991). This is so that appropriate anti-infective treatment can be initiated before more extensive CNS injury occurs and the possibility of a seizure disorder can be averted.

Electrophysiology.   Electrophysiological evaluation of HIV patients with cognitive and neurological complaints is helpful in establishing an organic basis for these difficulties and has demonstrated neural dysfunction before other behavior markers could (Goodin et al. 1990; Goodwin et al. 1990; Merrill et al. 1991; Ollo et al. 1990, 1991). Both electroencephalography (EEG) and specific evoked potentials have been used in this regard (Goodin et al. 1990; Goodwin et al. 1990; Merrill et al. 1991; Ollo et al. 1990, 1991; Tinuper et al. 1990). The disease may elicit an epileptic disorder (Parisi et al. 1991), and most studies have shown that the percentage of patients with abnormal EEGs increases as the systemic disease progresses, with the higher percentages of abnormalities found in more physically symptomatic patients

(Elovaara et al. 1991; Gabuzda et al. 1988; Parisi et al. 1989).

Sleep-related EEG findings have also demonstrated effects of HIV on the CNS. Polysomnography used to investigate patients' complaints of dyssomnia has uncovered gross disturbances in sleep architecture (Itil et al. 1990; Norman et al. 1990; Wiegand et al. 1991a, 1991b) secondary to HIV-CNS involvement. Evoked potential studies were able to detect abnormalities in neurologically and physically asymptomatic HIV-seropositive patients (Goodin et al. 1990; Goodwin et al. 1990; Smith et al. 1988). Brainstem auditory and somatosensory evoked potentials from tibial nerve stimulation and oculomotor activity recordings showed significant delays in latencies of response compared with those of control subjects, suggesting that evoked potentials may represent an early direct indication of neurological involvement in HIV disease, before symptoms occur.

Neuroimaging. Computed tomography (CT) and magnetic resonance imaging (MRI) (Bishburg et al. 1989; Doonief et al. 1992; Flowers et al. 1990; Freund-Levi et al. 1989; Jarvik et al. 1988; Levin et al. 1990; Post et al. 1991; Tran Dinh et al. 1990; Whelan et al. 1983) have not proved especially helpful in demonstrating direct injury by HIV. Either method is able to show atrophy, as reflected in increased ventricular size and sulcal size, and both can help to define areas of white-matter involvement. In general, imaging can be helpful to rule out certain pathological entities.

Imaging reflecting functioning of the nervous system—for example, positron-emission tomography (PET) (Brunetti et al. 1989), single photon emission computed tomography (SPECT) (Kuni et al. 1991; Masdeu et al. 1991), and regional cerebral blood flow (Schielke et al. 1990)—has shown regional metabolic abnormalities subcortically, with hypermetabolism in basal ganglia and thalamus early in the course of the disease, followed by regional and then general hypometabolism as the CNS disease progresses (Brunetti et al. 1989). PET scanning has also been used investigationally to demonstrate the therapeutic effects of antiviral treatment. PET scanning noted reversal of focal, cortical abnormalities of glucose metabolism after treatment of the AIDS dementia complex with zidovudine (Brunetti et al. 1989).

Neuropsychiatry and HIV Infection in the Public Health Setting

Overview of the Ryan White CARE Act

That HIV-positive and AIDS patients face a frightening and real risk of losing their health insurance coverage was no longer speculative by the year 1990.

Also, at that time, many localities were not prepared to care for the increasing numbers of patients who had lost their private resources and had to rely on the public sector for medical services. This, however, was the year the federal government designated the largest dollar amount for the provision of care for persons infected with HIV, by way of the Ryan White Comprehensive AIDS Resources Emergency (CARE) Act (Bowen et al. 1992; McKinney et al. 1993). This act was meant to improve the quality and availability of care for individuals living with HIV disease and for their families. Financial resources were divided into categories, or Titles I–IV. Title IV did not receive funding in 1991 and 1992.

The Health Resources and Services Administration (HRSA) of the U.S. Department of Health and Human Resources manages Titles I and II under its Bureau of Health Resources Development. HRSA also collaborates through its Bureau of Health Care Delivery Assistance with the CDC to administer Title III of the act. The titles are defined as follows:

Title I. Title I provides emergency assistance to metropolitan areas disproportionately affected by the HIV epidemic. Areas reporting more than 2,000 cases of AIDS to the CDC by March 31 of the preceding year or a per capita AIDS cumulative rate of more than 0.0025 qualify to receive these monies.

The number of eligible metropolitan areas (EMAs) has been steadily growing, with 16 qualifying to receive funds in 1991, 18 in 1992, 25 in 1993, and 34 in 1994. Grants are awarded to the chief elected official of the city or county and are to be used to deliver or enhance comprehensive HIV-related services. Services are to be provided in a cost-effective and "seamless" (with regard to continuity of care) manner. Outpatient ambulatory health and support services are to be linked with inpatient care and case management services to prevent unnecessary hospitalization and to expedite discharge from inpatient facilities.

Title II. All states are eligible to receive Title II monies to improve the quality, availability, and organization of health care and support services for individuals with HIV disease and for their families. States are required to provide continuity of care by using at least 50% of their Ryan White CARE grant funds to create and operate consortia that make this possible. Children, women, and families receive care with 15% of these funds. Additionally, HRSA may use 10% of the total appropriated Title II funds to make competitive awards under the Special Programs of National Significance (SPNS) programs. States may use grant funds either to maintain continuity of existing health coverage or to enable patients to receive medical benefits under other health insurance programs (which may include risk pools).

States reporting more than 1% of the national AIDS cases in the previous 2 years must match $1 in state funds for every $2 the federal government remits. The states' obligation has increased since 1991, when states were required to match $1 for every $5 in federal funding.

Title III. Early intervention services are supported by Title III funds. All states are eligible to receive funding.

Title IV. Title IV funds support evaluations, reports, research, and services for pediatric AIDS patients in a series of specified general provisions.

Neuropsychiatric care had only been peripherally addressed, the focus being more on the psychosocial impact of HIV/AIDS. This gap was likewise prominent among Title I recipients as well, many of whom had not allocated any funds for neurobehavioral care at all.

Houston Eligible Metropolitan Area

Spectrum of Neuropsychiatric AIDS
Care in the Houston Area

Texas, and perhaps Houston, can serve as a model of AIDS care in the country. This region might be a middle ground in the AIDS epidemic; Houston is a major urban area with the fifth largest HIV/AIDS population in the United States, and cases are spread out in other metropolitan and rural areas in the state (Fernandez and Levy 1990b). As the epidemic proceeded, it became clear that increasingly more services would be needed and a coordinated effort to provide these services would be important. A survey of the community was made to begin to tie these services together in a continuity of care.

An initial needs assessment done by the Houston HIV Biopsychosocial Services Network in 1990 revealed a lack of psychiatric services for HIV patients. From a survey of 22 existing local facilities, basic psychiatric services for all indigent patients were available from the public health Harris County Hospital District, but a complete range of services, including neurobehavioral care, was available only from widely distributed agencies. For the HIV patient, general medical care was available from a number of sources, but neuropsychiatric and neuropsychological care was absent. The initial Ryan White CARE Act, Houston area, *Requests for Proposals* incorporated these needs and made a comprehensive plan for providing multiple aspects of psychiatric care at the newly renovated Southern Pacific Railroad Hospital (originally built in 1910), which has become known as the Thomas Street Clinic. Patients were able to obtain quick referrals for their psychiatric complications, and they did not have to travel all over town to get medical services, a savings in their time, money, and ebbing stamina.

After the Thomas Street Clinic had been in operation for 2 years, a follow-up needs assessment was commissioned by the Harris County/Houston Metropolitan Area Ryan White CARE Act services governing council in 1993 (Affiliated Systems Corporation 1993). Of interest for neuropsychiatric care was the finding that 38% of respondents to the survey reported requiring psychological counseling, 60% reported substance dependency, and 12.5% reported that they had been informed they were diagnosed with dementia (the actual figure, because of sampling techniques, may be higher). Those findings led to a maintained high priority for Ryan White CARE funding of neurobehavioral services for the following year.

A third needs assessment was done in 1994 for the Ryan White CARE council (Sanderson 1994). This assessment focused more on various aspects of quality of life than strictly medical issues. Nevertheless, an average of 10%–12% of respondents reported needing "neurocognitive" services (a structured environment for promoting optimal cognitive functioning and cognitive remediation training), and 23% reported needing substance dependency (detoxification and counseling) services. These needs continued to be addressed by the Ryan White CARE Act via support of county facilities and community-based organizations until 1996, when allocation was reprioritized.

Ambulatory Neuropsychiatric-HIV Care

Fernandez and his co-workers (Levy et al. 1994) proposed a program of outpatient psychiatric services, which received Ryan White CARE support beginning in 1991. This program was designed to provide a multidisciplinary clinical effort for the delivery of ambulatory mental health services for people with HIV infection and was especially conceived to meet the needs of persons with neuropsychiatric symptoms. The services to be provided included psychiatric emergency triage to other network services, individual and group therapy (including substance dependency treatment), psychopharmacotherapy, pain management, cognitive-behavioral and physical rehabilitation, stress management, and psychophysiological services ranging from biofeedback to sleep hygiene. Pursuant to the terms of the Ryan White CARE Act, the program was also designed to link with other public sector and community-based organizations to provide a continuity of care ranging from counseling and legal services through home health care and hospice care. Part of the primary goal for this program was to offer a well-coordinated set of psychiatric and neurobehavioral services that would serve as an interface with the medical services of the public health general clinic.

The ambulatory psychiatry program developed into a component of the Thomas Street Clinic, which became an integrated medical care clinic for patients with HIV infection. The psychiatry program opened in October 1991, starting with 850 visits for the remainder of that year and building to more than 2,400 patients, with the number of follow-up visits exceeding 400 per month. This clinic accepts referrals from county hospitals, the Veterans Affairs Medical Center, community health centers, community-based organizations (e.g., AIDS Foundation Houston, Montrose Clinic, Montrose Counseling Center), physicians, nurses, chaplains, social workers, case managers, family, significant others, and the patient. An infrastructure is now in place to ensure that multiple services are provided by a coordinated, multidisciplinary team in a culturally sensitive manner, as follows:

1. Provision of basic psychiatric services that include diagnostic and emergency assessments, group and individual psychotherapy, and psychopharmacological therapy.
2. Utilization of nonpharmacological interventions to enhance functioning and quality of life for neuropsychiatrically impaired patients. These include:

   a. Memory retraining, with use of print materials, workbooks, memory notebooks, and audiocassettes.
   b. Biofeedback, which is a helpful adjunct in psychiatric treatment of anxiety and stress-distress symptomatology, pain management, and habit control disorders. This has been a successful program and is part of cognitive-behavioral rehabilitation. Biofeedback is provided for patients requiring stress reduction, as an adjunct to pain management, and for minimization of need for sedating psychotropic medication in patients with risk for or active substance dependency. Additionally, electromyelographic biofeedback is used in conjunction with occupational therapy to assist in neuromuscular reeducation, by which the muscles involved in treatment can be trained to recruit increasingly more activity, which may ultimately result in movement.

3. As part of the administration of the clinic, provision of educational and support liaison to other professional staff who are not experienced with patients with cognitive impairment. Additionally, informative in-services

and specific psychoeducational modules on cognitive loss in HIV disease are provided to enhance awareness about HIV, AIDS, and advances in research and clinical care. The psychoeducational modules summarize current issues and update knowledge about neurobehavioral complications of HIV and coordination of neurobehavioral services within the ambulatory outpatient framework for both patient and their extended care network.

4. Provision of substance abuse treatment, outpatient detoxification, and relapse prevention to comorbidly diagnosed HIV-infected patients with cognitive impairment and dementia.

When a patient presents at the Psychiatric Services Programs, he or she is briefly assessed by nursing staff and then fills out a self-report instrument—the Symptom Checklist–90 (SCL-90; Derogatis 1983). The psychiatrist then administers the Mini-Mental State Exam in the course of the interview. Several options are available to the psychiatrists on completion of the assessment:

- Emergency patients in need of admission are transferred either by ambulance or by taxicab to the psychiatric emergency room at the county hospital.
- Patients whose condition is relatively stable are followed at the clinic for nonpharmacological management and medications.
- Patients who demonstrate cognitive impairment on the mental status evaluation or who endorse complaints of cognitive dysfunction are referred for a more detailed neurocognitive evaluation. On the basis of findings from this evaluation, patients are further referred for neurocognitive remediation, either individually or in classes. Memory remediation, because of the frequency of this problem, is strongly emphasized. Both compensatory methods (e.g., notebooks) and strategies (e.g., mnemonic maneuvers) are taught. These interventions have built-in self-tests to assess the success of this training. Patients can be readmitted for refresher training, as needed.
- Patients with comorbid substance abuse or dependence are referred to the Substance Abuse Treatment Program. Many of these patients have comorbid neurocognitive impairment and/or may be self-medicating for their neurobehavioral impairment, such as patients misusing stimulants for cognition disorders or sedative/hypnotics for sleep disturbance. This group of patients usually has continued psychiatric follow-up, as well as a cognitive evaluation for placement on an appropriate psychopharmacological or neurobehavioral treatment regimen.

- Patients indicating a need or desire for psychotherapy are referred to a wide variety of community resources compatible with their issues, gender, ethnicity, sexual orientation, and geographic location. The program is unique in providing specialized medication and nonpharmacological support to ensure the comprehensive care of this patient population.

Results of an examination of predominant diagnoses of patients who have undergone referral for neurobehavioral evaluation (192 patients over the first 3 years, or 8% of all ambulatory HIV patients; 86% males, 14% females; 52% white, 38% African American, 10% Hispanic) revealed that 55% had HIV-associated dementia complex (HADC) and 24% had HIV-related minor cognitive-motor disorder (HMCMD). With regard to specific psychiatric diagnoses, 48% had a current diagnosis or history of substance dependence, 41% had a depressive mood disorder, 31% had complaints of a sleep disorder, 18% had an anxiety disorder, 7% had a psychotic disturbance, and 4% had a history of bipolar disorder. Other neurobehaviorally associated diagnoses included a history of or current seizure disorder (24%), a history of head injury (21%), a reported history of attention-deficit disorder (7%), and a stroke (4%).

Of those receiving a diagnosis of HADC or HMCMD or with specific complaints of memory problems, 53 underwent memory remediation classes at the clinic, with all eventually mastering training in a notebook method of memory compensation. Work with visual imagery for remembering and other mnemonic device training were also included in the classes. Posttests determined patients' need for retaking the course to achieve criteria mastery. Two hundred patients were referred for biofeedback, either to minimize the need for sedating psychotropic medication or for basic stress reduction. In this mastery-type learning paradigm, involving training in muscle tension reduction via electromyogram (EMG) feedback, skin warming via temperature feedback, and relaxed states via alpha/theta EEG feedback, all patients could be trained to criterion. All also reported improvement in stress-related symptoms (reduction in self-rated stress measures). Patients subjectively reported that these interventions helped them lower distress symptoms whenever necessary, and they noted that they appreciated this measure of restored self-efficacy in at least one area of their health picture.

Intermediate Care for Patients With Dementia

The Houston EMA being served by the Ryan White CARE Act faced a significant gap in services in late 1991. Although there was a dedicated hospice for AIDS patients and limited nursing home facilities for constitutionally ill indigent patients, irrespective of HIV status, there were no beds dedicated for indigent dementia care for HIV-infected patients who were constitutionally healthy. A growing number of patients met this description and needed a structured program for cognitive assistance and, perhaps, a measure of cognitive rehabilitation. The subacute care hospital, CASA—A Special Hospital, which had been established as a site for subacute care for cancer and other seriously chronically ill patients, became involved in forming the Neurocognitive Program and the Transitional Living Center residential program for HIV-positive chronically indigent, homeless, substance-dependent clients with dementia. These programs merged in 1994. Thirty-eight patients were served in 1993 and 41 participated in 1994. The funding remained incomplete for indefinite admissions to the program, but it provided for a 30- to 90-day stay to provide assessment, structured cognitive-enhancement programs, and formulation of treatment plans for postdischarge care. During these 2 years, 10% were discharged to home, 9% went to nursing homes, 19% became acutely medically ill and required admission to a general medical hospital, 10% went to another group residence, 39% were able to enter the transitional living program as a step toward independent or assisted living, and 13% went to other situations. These programs were discontinued in 1996 because of funding priority changes, and, again, this metropolitan area had no specific residential facility for the demented HIV client.

Levy and colleagues (Levy and Fernandez 1993) adapted traditionally utilized cognitive assessments and rehabilitation procedures found in brain trauma and stroke rehabilitation programs for this population of HIV-infected patients with cognitive impairment. They found that patients experiencing this program improved on assessments of activities of daily living. Treatment plans that were developed during the course of the admissions were passed on to the families and significant others, or to nursing homes, to help these patients optimize their quality of life.

Nursing Home Care

The medical complexities of HIV care, especially in later stages of the disease, have proven to be daunting to nursing home providers. Issues that appear to have impeded progress in this care provision include fear of contagion, homophobia, negative reactions to chemically dependent patients, and financial concerns on the part of providers when faced with the challenge of potential residents who have exhausted resources in their long struggle with the disease. Ultimately, the majority of patients have had to turn to the public health setting for medical care in this age of "managed care," "preexisting conditions," and health insurance that is tied to employment. In the Houston metropolitan area, there remains a dearth of nursing home beds in the public health setting. Public assistance in the form of disability payments through Medicare and Medicaid supports most HIV-infected residents in private nursing facilities. This may be an area that will get further investigation for the role the public sector will play in the future.

Conclusion

The neuropsychiatric complications of HIV infection and AIDS are a perplexing assortment of neurological, neurocognitive, and affective/behavioral effects that may arise at any time during the course of the illness. Thus, all neuropsychiatrists should maintain a high index of suspicion of even the most subtle of behavioral symptoms in previously asymptomatic persons. As the epidemic continues, these symptoms may arise in individuals other than those in the initial high-risk categories, and a careful history of possibility of exposure must be included in any workup of unusual cognitive, neurological, or neuropsychiatric symptoms. If the etiology is found to be HIV-related, prompt aggressive treatment of the conditions, perhaps using innovative measures, is warranted to maintain as high a quality of life as can be promoted for as long as possible. Many of the patients will require mental health services from publicly supported facilities because many will lose job-related benefits when they become disabled. Psychiatrists and other mental health providers working in this domain must become knowledgeable about the variety and subtlety of HIV-related cognitive, affective, and behavioral disorders in order to limit morbidity and forestall mortality. These providers must become resourceful to adapt support from various sources, such as Ryan White CARE funding, to serve the needs of these patients.

References

Affiliated Systems Corporation: Houston Area HIV Health Services Ryan White Planning Council: Needs Assessment for the Greater Houston EMA. Houston, TX, Affiliated Systems Corporation, 1993

Allain J, Laurian Y, Paul D, et al: Serological markers in early stages of human immunodeficiency virus infection in hemophiliacs. Lancet 2:1233–1236, 1986

Alter HJ: Transmission of LAV/HTLV-II by blood products. Ann Inst Pasteur Virol 138:31–38, 1987

Antoni M, August S, LaPerriere A, et al: Psychological and neuroendocrine measures related to functional immune changes in anticipation of HIV-1 serostatus notification. Psychosom Med 52:496–510, 1990

Backer U, Gathof A, Howe J, et al: A new second-generation anti-HIV-1 immunoassay using recombinant envelope and core proteins. AIDS 2:477–480, 1986

Bagasra O, Kajdacsy-Balla A, Lischner HWW, et al: Alcohol intake increases human immunodeficiency virus type 1 replication in human peripheral blood mononuclear cells. J Infect Dis 167:789–797, 1993

Barre-Sinoussi F, Chermann JC, Rey F, et al: Isolation of a T-lymphotropic retrovirus from a patient at risk for acquired immune deficiency syndrome (AIDS). Science 220:868–871, 1983

Beckett A, Summergrad P, Manschreck T, et al: Symptomatic HIV infection of the CNS in a patient without clinical evidence of immune deficiency. Am J Psychiatry 144:1342–1344, 1987

Bedri J, Weinstein W, DeGregoria P, et al: Progressive multifocal leuko-encephalopathy in acquired immunodeficiency syndrome. N Engl J Med 309:492–493, 1983

Beilke MA: Vascular endothelium in immunology and infectious disease. Review of Infectious Diseases 11:273–283, 1989

Belman AL, Lantos G, Horoupian D, et al: AIDS: calcification of the basal ganglia in infants and children. Neurology 36:1192–1199, 1986

Benton AL: Revised Visual Retention Test, 4th Edition. San Antonio, TX, Psychological Corporation, 1974

Benton AL, Hamsher KdeS: Multilingual Aphasia Examination, 2nd Edition. Manual of Instructions. Iowa City, IA, AJA Associates, 1989

Benton AL, Van Allen MW, Fogel ML: Temporal orientation in cerebral disease. J Nerv Ment Dis 139:110–119, 1964

Berger JR, Kaszovitz B, Post MJ, et al: Progressive multifocal leukoencephalopathy associated with human immunodeficiency virus infection. A review of the literature with a report of sixteen cases. Ann Intern Med 107:78–87, 1987

Bernad PG: The neurological and electroencephalographic changes in AIDS. Clin Electroencephalogr 22:65–70, 1991

Bishburg E, Eng RHK, Slim J, et al: Brain lesions in patients with acquired immunodeficiency syndrome. Arch Intern Med 149:941–943, 1989

Bornstein RA, Nasralla HA, Para MF, et al: Rate of CD4 decline and neuropsychological performance in HIV infection. Arch Neurol 48:704–707, 1991

Bowen GS, Marconi K, Kohn S, et al: First year of AIDS services delivery under Title I of the Ryan White CARE Act. Public Health Rep 107:491–499, 1992

Bredesen DE, Levy RM, Rosenblum ML: The neurology of human immunodeficiency virus infection. QJM (Oxford) 68:665–677, 1988

Brew BJ, Sidtis JJ, Petito CK, et al: The neurologic complications of AIDS and human immunodeficiency virus infection, in Advances in Contemporary Neurology. Edited by Plum F. Philadelphia, PA, FA Davis, 1988, pp 1–49

Brew BJ, Bhalla RB, Paul M, et al: Cerebrospinal fluid β_2 microglobulin in patients infected with AIDS dementia complex: an expanded series including response to zidovudine treatment. AIDS 6:461–465, 1992

Brunetti A, Berg G, DiChiro G, et al: Reversal of brain metabolic abnormalities following treatment of AIDS dementia complex with 3'-azido- 2',3'-dideoxythymidine (AZT, zidovudine): a PET-FDG study. J Nucl Med 30:581–590, 1989

Budka H: Human immunodeficiency virus (HIV)-induced disease of the central nervous system: pathology and implications for pathogenesis. Acta Neuropathol (Berl) 77:225–236, 1989

Buffet R, Agut H, Chieze F, et al: Virological markers in the cerebrospinal fluid from HIV-1 infected individuals. AIDS 5(12):1419–1424, 1991

Busch MP, Arnand ZE, McHugh TM, et al: Reliable confirmation and quantitation of human immunodeficiency virus type 1 antibody using a recombinant-antigen immunoblot assay. Transfusion 31:129–137, 1991

Buschke H, Fuld PA: Evaluation of storage, retention, and retrieval in disordered memory and learning. Neurology 11:1019–1025, 1974

Butters N, Grant I, Haxby J, et al: Assessment of AIDS-related cognitive changes: recommendations of the NIMH workshop on neuropsychological assessment approaches. J Clin Exp Neuropsychol 12:963–978, 1990

Carlson JR, Mertens SC, Yee JL, et al: Rapid, easy, and economical screening test for antibodies to human immunodeficiency virus. Lancet 1:361–362, 1987

Carrieri PB, Indaco A, Maiorino A, et al: Cerebrospinal fluid beta-2-microglobulin in multiple sclerosis and AIDS dementia complex. Neurol Res 14(3):282–283, 1992

Centers for Disease Control: Revision of the CDC surveillance case definition for acquired immunodeficiency syndrome. MMWR Morb Mortal Wkly Rep 36(suppl 1S):3S–15S, 1987

Centers for Disease Control and Prevention: 1993 revised classification system for HIV infection: expanded surveillance case definition for AIDS among adolescents and adults. MMWR Morb Mortal Wkly Rep 42:41, 1992 (No RR-17)

Centers for Disease Control and Prevention: Update: trends in AIDS incidence, deaths, prevalence—United States, 1996. MMWR Morb Mortal Wkly Rep 46(8):165–173, 1997

Chalmers TC, Aster RH, Bloom JR, et al: The impact of routine HTLV-III antibody testing of blood and plasma donors on public health. Presented at the National Institutes of Health Consensus Development Conference Statement, Bethesda, MD, July 7–9, 1986

Chiodi F, Keys B, Albert J, et al: Human immunodeficiency virus type 1 is present in the cerebrospinal fluid of a majority of infected individuals. J Clin Microbiol 30(7):1768–1771, 1992

Ciardi A, Sindair E, Scaravilli F, et al: The involvement of the cerebral cortex in human immunodeficiency virus encephalopathy: a morphological and immunohistochemical study. Acta Neuropathol 81:51–59, 1990

Collier AC, Marra C, Coombs RW, et al: Central nervous system manifestations in human immunodeficiency virus infection without AIDS. Journal of Acquired Immune Deficiency Syndromes 5:229–241, 1992

Cotton P: AIDS dementia may be linked to metabolite of tryptophan. JAMA 264: 305–306, 1990

Cummings JL, Benson DF: Dementia: A Clinical Approach. Boston, MA, Butterworths, 1983

Derogatis LR: SCL-90-R Administration, Scoring and Procedures Manual–II for the Revised Version. Towson, MD, Clinical Psychometric Research, 1983

Dickson DW, Mattiace LA, Kure K, et al: Biology of disease: microglia in human disease, with an emphasis on acquired immune deficiency syndrome. Lab Invest 64:135–156, 1991

Doonief G, Bello J, Todak G, et al: A prospective controlled study of magnetic resonance imaging of the brain in gay men and parenteral drug users with human immunodeficiency virus infection. Arch Neurol 49:38–43, 1992

Dunlop O, Bjørklund RA, Abedelnoor M, et al: Five different tests of reaction time evaluated in HIV seropositive men. Acta Neurol Scand 8:260–266, 1992

Eisdorfer C, Cohen D, Paveza GJ, et al: An empirical evaluation of the Global Deterioration Scale for staging Alzheimer's disease. Am J Psychiatry 149:190–194, 1991

Elovaara I, Iivanianen M, Portiainer E, et al: CSF and serum β-2-microglobulin in HIV infection related to neurological dysfunction. Acta Neurol Scand 79:81–87, 1989

Elovaara I, Saar P, Valle S-L, et al: EEG in early HIV-1 infection is characterized by anterior dysrhythmicity of low maximal amplitude. Clin Electroencephalogr 22:131–140, 1991

Engstrom JW, Lowenstein DH, Bredesen DE: Cerebral infarctions and transient neurologic deficits associated with acquired immunodeficiency syndrome. Am J Med 86:528–532, 1989

Eriksson T, Lidberg L: Decreased plasma ratio of tryptophan to competing large neutral amino acids in human immunodeficiency virus type 1 infected subjects: possible implications for development of neuro-psychiatric disorders. J Neural Transm 103:157–164, 1996

Everall I, Luthert PJ, Lantos PL: Neuronal loss in the frontal cortex in HIV infection. Lancet 337:1119–1121, 1991

Fernandez F, Levy JK: Adjuvant treatment of HIV dementia with psychostimulants, in Behavioral Aspects of AIDS and Other Sexually Transmitted Diseases. Edited by Ostrow D. New York, Plenum, 1990a, pp 279–286

Fernandez F, Levy JK: Mental health implications of AIDS, in Mental Health Research in Texas: Retrospect and Prospect. Proceedings of the Seventh Robert Lee Sutherland Seminar in Mental Health. Edited by Bonjean C, Foss D. Austin, TX, The Hogg Foundation for Mental Health, 1990b, pp 229–251

Fernandez F, Holmes VF, Levy JK, et al: Consultation-liaison psychiatry and HIV-related disorders. Hospital and Community Psychiatry 40:146–153, 1989

Filley CM, Franklin GM, Heaton RK, et al: White matter dementia. Clinical disorders and implications. Neuropsychiatry Neuropsychol Behav Neurol 1:239–254, 1989

Fischl MA, Richman DD, Grieco MH, et al: The efficacy of AZT in the treatment of patients with AIDS and ARC. N Engl J Med 317:185–187, 1987

Flowers CH, Mafee MF, Crowell R, et al: Encephalopathy in AIDS patients: evaluation with MR imaging. Am J Neuroradiol 11:1235–1245, 1990

Folstein MF, Folstein SE, McHugh PR: Mini-Mental State: a practical method for grading the cognitive state of patients for the clinician. J Psychiatr Res 12: 189–198, 1975

Food and Drug Administration: Guideline for the Prevention of Human Immunodeficiency Virus (HIV) Transmission by Blood Products. Rockville, MD, Food and Drug Administration, 1989

Franzblau A, Letz R, Hershman D, et al: Quantitative neurologic and neurobehavioral testing of persons infected with human immunodeficiency virus type 1. Arch Neurol 48:263–268, 1991

Freund-Levi Y, Saaf J, Wahlund L-O, et al: Ultra low field brain MRI in HIV transfusion infected patients. Magn Reson Imaging 7:225–230, 1989

Gabuzda DA, Levy SR, Chiappa KH: Electroencephalography in AIDS and AIDS-related complex. Clin Electroencephalogr 19:1–6, 1988

Gallo RC, Sarin PS, Gelmann EP, et al: Isolation of human T-cell leukemia virus in acquired immune deficiency syndrome. Science 220:865–867, 1983

Gibbs A, Andrewes DG, Szmukler G, et al: Early HIV-related neuropsychological impairment: relationship to stage of viral infection. J Clin Exp Neuropsychol 12:766–780, 1990

Giulian D, Vaca K, Noonan CA: Secretion of neurotoxins by mononuclear phagocytes infected with HIV-1. Science 250:1593–1595, 1990

Giulian D, Yu J, Li X, et al: Study of receptor-mediated neurotoxins released by HIV-1-infected mononuclear phagocytes found in human brain. J Neurosci 16: 3139–3153, 1996

Goethe KE, Mitchell JE, Marshall DW, et al: Neuropsychological and neurological function of human immunodeficiency virus seropositive asymptomatic individuals. Arch Neurol 46:129–133, 1989

Golden CJ: Stroop Color and Word Test. A Manual for Clinical and Experimental Uses. Wood Dale, IL, Stoelting Company, 1978

Gonzales MF, David RL: Neuropathology of acquired immunodeficiency syndrome. Neuropathol Appl Neurobiol 14:345–363, 1988

Goodin DS, Aminoff MJ, Chernoff DN, et al: Long latency event-related potentials in patients infected with human immunodeficiency virus. Ann Neurol 27: 414–419, 1990

248   NEUROPSYCHIATRY AND MENTAL HEALTH SERVICES

Goodkin K, Blaney NT, Feaster D, et al: Active coping style is associated with natural killer cell cytotoxicity in asymptomatic HIV-1 seropositive homosexual men. J Psychosom Res 36:635–650, 1992

Goodwin GM, Chiswick A, Egan V, et al: The Edinburgh cohort of HIV-positive drug users: auditory event-related potentials show progressive slowing in patients with Centers for Disease Control stage IV disease. AIDS 4:1243–1250, 1990

Grant I, Atkinson JH, Hesselink JR, et al: Evidence for early central nervous system involvement in the immunodeficiency syndrome (AIDS) and other human immunodeficiency virus (HIV) infections: studied with neuropsychological testing and magnetic resonance imaging. Ann Intern Med 107:828–836, 1987

Gray F, Gherard R, Keohane C, et al: Pathology of the central nervous system in 40 cases of acquired immune deficiency syndrome (AIDS). Neuropathol Appl Neurobiol 14:365–380, 1988

Gyorkey F, Melnick JL, Gyorkey P: Human immunodeficiency virus in brain biopsies of patients with AIDS and progressive encephalopathy. J Infect Dis 155:870–876, 1987

Hamilton M: The assessment of anxiety states by rating. Br J Med Psychol 32:50–55, 1959

Hamilton M: A rating scale for depression. J Neurol Neurosurg Psychiatry 23:56–62, 1960

Handelsman L, Aronson M, Maurer G, et al: Neuropsychological and neurological manifestations of HIV-1 dementia in drug users. J Neuropsychiatry Clin Neurosci 4:21–28, 1991

Harbison MA, Kim S, Gillis JM, et al: Effect of the calcium channel blocker verapamil on human immunodeficiency virus type 1 replication in lymphoid cells. J Infect Dis 164:43–60, 1991

Harris C, Small CB, Klein RS, et al: Immunodeficiency in female sexual partners of men with the AIDS. N Engl J Med 308:1181–1184, 1983

Harrison NA, Skidmore SJ: Neopterin and beta-2 microglobulin levels in asymptomatic HIV infection: the predictive value of combining markers. J Med Virol 32:128–133, 1990

Hart RP, Ward JB, Klinger RL, et al: Slowed information processing as an early cognitive change associated with AIDS and ARC. J Clin Exp Neuropsychol 12:72, 1990

Heaton RK, Chalume GJ, Talley JL, et al: Wisconsin Card Sorting Test. Manual. Odessa, FL, Psychological Assessment Resources, 1993

Hewlett IK, Gregg RA, Ou C-Y, et al: Detection in plasma of HIV-specific DNA and RNA by polymerase chain reaction before and after seroconversion. Journal of Clinical Immunoassay 11:161–164, 1988

Heyes MP, Brew BJ, Martin A, et al: Quinolinic acid in cerebrospinal fluid and serum in HIV-1 infection: relationship to clinical neurological status. Ann Neurol 29:202–209, 1991

Heyes MP, Brew BJ, Saito K, et al: Inter-relationships between quinolinic acid, neuroactive kynurenines, neopterin and β_2-microglublin in cerebrospinal fluid and HIV-1-infected patients. J Neuroimmunol 40:71–80, 1992

Hill JM, Farrar WL, Pert CB: Autoradiographic localization of T4 antigen, the HIV receptor, in human brain. Int J Neurosci 32:687–693, 1987

Ho DD, Pomerantz RJ, Kaplan JC: Pathogenesis of infection with human immunodeficiency virus. N Engl J Med 317:278–286, 1987

Hollander H: Neurologic and psychiatric manifestations of HIV disease. J Gen Intern Med 6(Jan/Feb suppl):S24–S31, 1991

Itil TM, Ferracuti S, Freedman AM, et al: Computer-analyzed EEG (CEEG) and dynamic brain mapping in AIDS and HIV related syndrome: a pilot study. Clin Electroencephalogr 21:140–144, 1990

Jackson JB, Mac Donald KL, Caldwell J, et al: Absence of HIV infection in blood donors with indeterminate Western blot tests for antibody to HIV-1. N Engl J Med 322:217–222, 1990

Jacobs D, Peavy G, Velin R, et al: Verbal memory in asymptomatic HIV-infection: evidence of subcortical dysfunction in a subgroup of patients. J Clin Exp Neuropsychol 14:101, 1992

Janssen RS, Saykin AJ, Kaplan JE, et al: Neurological complications of human immunodeficiency virus infection in patients with lymphadenopathy syndrome. Ann Neurol 23:49–55, 1988

Janssen RS, Nwanyanwu OC, Selik PM, et al: Epidemiology of human immunodeficiency virus encephalopathy in the United States. Neurology 42:1472–1476, 1992

Jarvik JG, Hesselink JR, Kennedy C, et al: Acquired immunodeficiency syndrome. Magnetic resonance patterns of brain involvement with pathologic correlation. Arch Neurol 45:731–736, 1988

Jason JM, McDougal JS, Dixon G, et al: HTLV III antibody and immune status of household contacts and sexual partners of persons with hemophilia. JAMA 255:212–215, 1986

Jones GH, Kelly CL, Davies JA: HIV and onset of schizophrenia. Lancet 1:982, 1987

Kaemingk KL, Kaszniak AW: Neuropsychological aspects of human immunodeficiency virus infection. The Clinical Neuropsychologist 3:309–326, 1989

Kaiser PK, Offerman JT, Lipton SA: Neuronal injury due to HIV-1 envelope protein is blocked by anti-gp120 antibodies but not by anti-CD4 antibodies. Neurology 40:1757–1761, 1990

Karlsen NR, Reinvang I, Frøland SS: Serum level of neopterin, CD8+ cell count, and neuropsychological function in HIV-infected patients. J Clin Exp Neuropsychol 14:101, 1991

Karlsen NR, Reinvang I, Frøland SS: Slowed reaction time in asymptomatic HIV-positive patients. Acta Neurol Scand 86:242–246, 1992

Kaslow RA, Blackwelder WC, Ostrow DG, et al: No evidence for a role of alcohol or other psychoactive drugs in accelerating immunodeficiency in HIV-1-positive individuals. JAMA 261:3424–3429, 1989

Ketzler S, Weis S, Haug H, et al: Loss of neurons in the frontal cortex in AIDS patients. Acta Neuropathol (Berl) 80:92–94, 1990

Kieburtz KD, Epstein LG, Gelbard HA, et al: Excitotoxicity and dopaminergic dysfunction in the acquired immunodeficiency syndrome dementia complex: therapeutic implications. Arch Neurol 48:1281–1284, 1991

Kleinmann S, Fitzpatrick I, Secord K, et al: Follow-up testing and notification of anti-HIV Western blot atypical (indeterminate) donors. Transfusion 28:280–282, 1988

Klusman LE, Moulton JM, Hornbostel LK, et al: Neuropsychological abnormalities in asymptomatic HIV seropositive military personnel. J Neuropsychiatry Clin Neurosci 3:422–428, 1991

Koralnik IJ, Beaumanoir A, Häusler R, et al: A controlled study of early neurologic abnormalities in men with asymptomatic human immunodeficiency virus infection. N Engl J Med 323:864–870, 1990

Kovner R, Perecman E, Lazar W, et al: Relation of personality and attentional factors to cognitive deficits in human immunodeficiency virus-infected subjects. Arch Neurol 46:274–277, 1989

Krikorian R, Wrobel AJ: Cognitive impairment in HIV infection. AIDS 5:1501–1507, 1991

Kuni CC, Phame FS, Meier MJ, et al: Quantitative I-123-IMP brain SPECT and neuropsychological testing in AIDS dementia. Clin Nucl Med 16:174–177, 1991

Lacks P: Bender Gestalt Screening for Brain Dysfunction. New York, Wiley, 1984

Lantos PL, McLaughlin JE, Scholtz CL, et al: Neuropathology of the brain in HIV infection. Lancet 1:309–311, 1989

Larsson M, Hagberg L, Forsman A, et al: Cerebrospinal fluid catecholamine metabolites in HIV-infected patients. J Neurosci Res 28:406–409, 1991

Leffrere JJ, Mariotti M, Ferre-Le-Ceour F, et al: PCR testing in HIV-1 seronegative haemophilia (letter). Lancet 336:1386, 1990

Leitman SF, Klein HG, Melpoder JJ, et al: Clinical implications of positive tests for antibodies to human immunodeficiency virus type 1 in asymptomatic blood donors. N Engl J Med 32:197–924, 1989

Lenhardt TM, Wiley CA: Absence of humorally mediated damage within the central nervous system of AIDS patients. Neurology 39:278–280, 1989

Leoung GS, Feigel DW, Montgomery AB, et al: Aerosolized pentamidine for prophylaxis against PCP. N Engl J Med 323:769–775, 1990

Levin HS, Williams DH, Borucki MJ, et al: Magnetic resonance imaging and neuropsychological findings in human immunodeficiency virus infection. Journal of Acquired Immune Deficiency Syndromes 3:757–762, 1990

Levy JA, Hoffman AD, Kramer SM, et al: Isolation of lymphocytopathic retroviruses from San Francisco patients with AIDS. Science 225:840–842, 1984

Levy JK: Neuropsychiatric complications of HIV. Continuing Medical Education Course presented at the American Psychiatric Association Sesquicentennial Annual Meeting, Philadelphia, PA, May 21, 1994

Levy JK, Fernandez F: Memory rehabilitation in HIV encephalopathy (abstract). Clin Neuropathol 12 (suppl 1):S27–S28, 1993

Levy JK, Fernandez F, Samiuddin Z: Psychiatric factors of patients in an HIV outpatient clinic. Paper presented at the American Psychiatric Association Forty-Sixth Institute on Hospital and Community Psychiatry, San Diego, CA, October 3, 1994

Lezak MD: Neuropsychological Assessment, 3rd Edition. New York, Oxford University Press, 1995

Lifson AR, Stanley M, O'Malley P, et al: Evaluation of the polymerase chain reaction in a well-characterized cohort of homosexual and bisexual men. Presented at the Fifth International Conference on AIDS, Montreal, Canada, June 8, 1989

Lipton RB, Ferairu ER, Weiss G, et al: Headache in HIV-1-related disorders. Headache 31:518–522, 1991

Lipton SA: Calcium channel antagonists and human immunodeficiency virus coat protein-mediated neuronal injury. Ann Neurol 30:110–114, 1991

Lipton SA: Models of neuronal injury in AIDS: another role for the NMDA receptor. Trends Neurosci 15:75–79, 1992

Lolli F, Colao MG, De Maio E, et al: Intrathecal synthesis of anti-HIV antibodies in AIDS patients. J Neurol Sci 99:281–289, 1990

Lunn S, Skydzbjerg M, Schulsinger H, et al: A preliminary report on the neuropsychologic sequelae of human immunodeficiency virus. Arch Gen Psychiatry 48:139–142, 1991

Maccario M, Scharre DW: HIV and acute onset of psychosis. Lancet 2:342, 1987

Marotta R, Perry S: Early neuropsychological dysfunction caused by human immunodeficiency virus. J Neuropsychiatry Clin Neurosci 1:225–235, 1989

Marshall DW, Brey RL, Cahill WT, et al: Spectrum of cerebrospinal fluid findings in various stages of human immunodeficiency virus infection. Arch Neurol 45:954–958, 1988

Marshall DW, Brey RL, Butzin CA, et al: CSF changes in a longitudinal study of 124 neurologically normal HIV-1-infected U.S. Air Force personnel. Journal of Acquired Immune Deficiency Syndromes 4:777–781, 1991

Martin EM, Robertson LC, Sorensen DJ, et al: Speed of memory scanning is not affected in early HIV-1 infection (abstract). J Clin Exp Neuropsychol 14:102, 1992

Masdeu JC, Small CB, Weiss L, et al: Multifocal cytomegalovirus encephalitis in AIDS. Ann Neurol 23:97–99, 1988

Masdeu JC, Yudd A, Van Herrtum RL, et al: Single-photon-emission computed tomography in human immunodeficiency virus encephalopathy: a preliminary report. J Nucl Med 32:1471–1475, 1991

Masliah E, Achim CL, Nianfeng GE, et al: Spectrum of human immunodeficiency virus-associated neocortical damage. Ann Neurol 32(5):321–329, 1992

McAllister RH, Herns MV, Harrison MJG, et al: Neurologic and neuropsychological performance in HIV seropositive men without symptoms. J Neurol Neurosurg Psychiatry 55:143–148, 1992

McArthur JC, Sipos E, Chupp M, et al: Immunocytochemical staining of blood and cerebrospinal fluid mononuclear cells in AIDS-spectrum disorders (abstract). Neurology 37(1):319, 1987

McArthur JC, Cohen BA, Selnes OA, et al: Low prevalence of neurological and neuropsychological abnormalities in otherwise healthy HIV-1-infected individuals: results from Multicenter AIDS Cohort Study. Ann Neurol 26:601–611, 1989

McArthur JC, Ashe J, Jabs D: Diagnosis and treatment of neurologic disorders in AIDS and other sexually transmitted diseases, in Behavioral Aspects of AIDS and Other Sexually Transmitted Diseases. Edited by Ostrow D. New York, Plenum, 1990, pp 207–234

McArthur JC, Nance-Sproson TE, Griffin DE, et al: The diagnostic utility of elevation in cerebral spinal fluid β_2-microglobulin in HIV-1 dementia. Neurology 42:1707–1712, 1992

McKinney MM, Wieland MK, Bowen GS, et al: States' responses to Title II of the Ryan White CARE Act. Public Health Rep 108:4–11, 1993

Merrill PT, Paige GD, Abrams RA, et al: Ocular motor abnormalities in human immunodeficiency virus infection. Ann Neurol 30:130–138, 1991

Meyers JE, Meyers KR: Rey Complex Figure Test and Recognition Trial Professional Manual. Odessa, FL, Psychological Assessment Resources, 1995

Miller EN, Satz P, Visscher B: Computerized and conventional neuropsychological assessment of HIV-1-infected homosexual men. Neurology 41:1608–1616, 1991

Miller JK, Barrett RE, Britton CB, et al: Progressive multifocal leukoencephalopathy in a male homosexual with T-cell immune deficiency. N Engl J Med 307:1436–1438, 1982

Mitsuyasu RT: Medical aspects of HIV spectrum disease. Psychiatr Medicine 7:5–22, 1989

Morgan MK, Clark ME, Hartman WL: AIDS-related dementias: a case report of rapid cognitive decline. J Clin Psychol 44:1024–1028, 1988

Nair MP, Kumar NM, Kronfol ZA, et al: Selective effect of alcohol on cellular immune responses of lymphocytes from AIDS patients. Alcohol 11:85–90, 1994

Nance M, Pirozzolo FJ, Levy JK, et al: Simple and choice reaction time in HIV-seronegative, HIV-seropositive and AIDS patients. VIth International Conference on AIDS, Abstracts, Vol 2. San Francisco, CA, June 22, 1990, p 173

Navia BA, Price RW: The acquired immunodeficiency syndrome dementia complex as the presenting or sole manifestation of human immunodeficiency virus infection. Arch Neurol 44:65–69, 1987

Navia BA, Jordan BD, Price RW: The AIDS dementia complex, I: clinical features. Ann Neurol 19:517–524, 1986a

Navia BA, Cho E-S, Petito CK, et al: The AIDS dementia complex, II: neuropathology. Ann Neurol 19:525–535, 1986b

Nichols S, Akman J, Beckett A, et al: AIDS training curriculum. Module 8: AIDS and the severely and persistently mentally ill (SPMI). Washington, DC, American Psychiatric Association, 1994, pp 155–177

Norman SE, Chediak AD, Kiel M, et al: Sleep disturbances in HIV-infected homosexual men. AIDS 4:775–781, 1990

Ollo C, Litman R, Rubinow D, et al: Neuropsychological correlates of smooth pursuit eye movements in HIV disease. J Clin Exp Neuropsychol 12:73, 1990

Ollo C, Johnson R Jr, Grafman J: Signs of cognitive change in HIV disease: an event-related brain potential study. Neurology 41:209–215, 1991

Pace PL, Fama R, Bornstein RA: Depression and neuropsychological performance in asymptomatic HIV infection. J Clin Exp Neuropsychol 14:101, 1992

Pajeau AK, Roman GC: HIV encephalopathy and dementia. Psychiatr Clin North Am 15:455–466, 1991

Parisi A, Strosselli M, DiPerri G, et al: Electroencephalography in the early diagnosis of HIV-related subacute encephalitis: analysis of 185 patients. Clin Electroencephalogr 20:1–5, 1989

Parisi A, Strosselli M, Pan A, et al: HIV-related encephalitis presenting as convulsant disease. Clin Electroencephalogr 22:1–4, 1991

Perry SN: Organic mental disorders caused by HIV: update on early diagnosis and treatment. Am J Psychiatry 147:696–710, 1990

Perry S, Belsky-Barr D, Barr WB, et al: Neuropsychological function in physically asymptomatic, HIV-seropositive men. J Neuropsychiatry Clin Neurosci 3:296–302, 1989

Perry S, Fishman B, Jacobsberg L, et al: Relationships over 1 year between lymphocyte subsets and psychosocial variables among adults with infection by human immunodeficiency virus. Arch Gen Psychiatry 49:396–401, 1991

Petito CK: Review of central nervous system pathology in human immunodeficiency virus infection. Ann Neurol 23(suppl):S54–S57, 1988

Pezella M, Rossi P, Lombardi V, et al: HIV viral sequences in seronegative people at risk detected by in situ hybridisation and polymerase chain reaction. BMJ 298:713–716, 1989

Pfeiffer E: SPMSQ: Short Portable Mental Status Questionnaire. J Am Geriatr Soc 23:40–44, 1975

Pirozzolo FI, Christensen KJ, Ogle KM, et al: Simple and choice reaction time in dementia: clinical implications. Neurobiol Aging 2:113–117, 1981

Portegies P, Epstein LG, Hung STA, et al: Human immunodeficiency virus type 1 antigen in cerebrospinal fluid. Correlation with clinical neurologic status. Arch Neurol 46:261–264, 1989

Portegies P, Algra PR, Hollak CEM, et al: Response to cytarabine in progressive multifocal leucoencephalopathy in AIDS (letter). Lancet 337:680–681, 1991

Post MJD, Berger JR, Quencer RM: Asymptomatic and neurologically symptomatic HIV-seropositive individuals: prospective evaluation with cranial MR imaging. Radiology 178:131–139, 1991

Pumarola-Sune T, Navia BA, Cordon-Cardo C, et al: HIV antigen in the brains of patients with the AIDS dementia complex. Ann Neurol 21:490–496, 1987

Raven JC, Court JH, Raven J: Manual for Raven's Progressive Matrices and Vocabulary Scales. London, HK Lewis, 1984

Reboul J, Schuller E, Pialoux G, et al: Immunoglobulins and complement components in 37 patients infected by HIV-1 virus: comparison of general (systemic) and intrathecal immunity. J Neurol Sci 89:243–252, 1989

Redfield RR, Wright DC, Tramont EC: The Walter Reed staging classification of HTLV-III/LAV infection. N Engl J Med 314:131–132, 1986

Reisberg B, Ferris SH, de Leon MJ, et al: The Global Deterioration Scale (GDS): an instrument for the assessment of primary degenerative dementia (PDD). Am J Psychiatry 139:1136–1139, 1982

Reitan RM, Wolfson D: The Halstead-Reitan Neuropsychological Test Battery: Theory and Clinical Interpretation. Tucson, AZ, Neuropsychology Press, 1993

Riedel R-R, Helmsteadter C, Bülau P, et al: Early signs of cognitive deficits among human immunodeficiency virus-positive hemophiliacs. Acta Psychiatr Scand 85:321–326, 1992

Rowen D, Carne CA: Neurological manifestation of HIV infection. Int J STD AIDS 2:79–90, 1991

Rubinow DR, Berrettini CH, Brouwers P, et al: Neuropsychiatric consequences of AIDS. Ann Neurol 23(suppl):S24–S26, 1988

Ryan JJ, Paolo AM, Skrade M: Rey auditory verbal learning test performance of a federal corrections sample with acquired immunodeficiency syndrome. Int J Neurosci 64:177–181, 1992

Sanderson MR: Greater Houston EMA HIV+ community needs assessment. Houston, TX, Office of Community Projects, Graduate School of Social Work, University of Houston, September 1994

Sardar AM, Bell JE, Reynolds GP: Increased concentrations of the neurotoxin 3-hydroxykynurenine in the frontal cortex of HIV-1-positive patients. J Neurochem 64:932–935, 1995

Scaravilli F, Daniel SE, Harcourt-Webster N, et al: Chronic basal meningitis and vasculitis in acquired immunodeficiency syndrome. A possible role for human immunodeficiency virus. Arch Pathol Lab Med 113:192–195, 1989

Schielke E, Tatsch K, Pfister HW, et al: Reduced cerebral blood flow in early stages of human immunodeficiency virus infection. Arch Neurol 47:1342–1345, 1990

Schindelmeiser J, Gullotta F: HIV-p24-antigen-bearing macrophages are only present in brains of HIV-seropositive patients with AIDS-encephalopathy. Clin Neuropathol 10:109–111, 1991

Schwarcz R, Whetsell WO, Mangano RM: Quinolinic acid: an endogenous metabolite that produces axon-sparing lesions in the rat brain. Science 219:316–318, 1983

Scillian JJ, McHugh TM, Busch MP, et al: Early detection of antibodies against DNA-produced HIV proteins with a flow cytometric assay. Blood 73:2041–2048, 1989

Sei S, Saito K, Stewart SK, et al: Increased human immunodeficiency virus (HIV) type 1 DNA content and quinolinic acid concentration in brain tissue from patients with HIV encephalopathy. J Infect Dis 172:638–647, 1995

Shaskan EG, Brew BJ, Rosenblum M, et al: Increased neopterin levels in brains of patients with human immunodeficiency virus type 1 infection. J Neurochem 59(4):1541–1546, 1992

Shepard HW, Ascher MS, Busch MP, et al: A multicenter proficiency trial of gene amplification (PCR) for the detection of HIV-1. Journal of Acquired Immune Deficiency Syndromes 4:277–283, 1991

Skoraszewski MJ, Ball JD, Mikulka P: Neuropsychological functioning in HIV-infected males. J Clin Exp Neuropsychol 13:278–290, 1991

Sload EM, Pitt E, Chiarello RJ, et al: HIV testing, state of the art. JAMA 266: 2861–2865, 1991

Smith T, Jakobsen J, Gaub J, et al: Clinical and electrophysiological studies of human immunodeficiency virus–seropositive men without AIDS. Ann Neurol 23: 295–297, 1988

Snider ND, Simpson DM, Nielsen S, et al: Neurological complications of acquired immune deficiency syndrome: analysis of 50 patients. Ann Neurol 14:403–418, 1983

Stern RA, Singer NG, Silva SG, et al: Neurobehavioral functioning in a non-confounded group of asymptomatic HIV-seropositive homosexual men. Am J Psychiatry 149:1099–1102, 1992

Stern Y, Sano M, Marder K, et al: Subtle neuropsychological changes in HIV+ gay men. J Clin Exp Neuropsychol 12:48, 1990

Stern Y, Marder K, Bell K, et al: Multidisciplinary baseline assessment of homosexual men with and without human immunodeficiency virus infection, III: neurologic and neuropsychologic findings. Arch Gen Psychiatry 48:131–138, 1991

Syndulko K, Singer E, Fahychandon B, et al: Relationship of self-rated depression and neuropsychological changes in HIV-1 neurological dysfunction (abstract). J Clin Exp Neuropsychol 12:72, 1990

Tartaglione TA, Collier AC, Coombs RW, et al: Acquired immunodeficiency syndrome: cerebrospinal fluid findings in patients before and during long-term oral zidovudine therapy. Arch Neurol 48:695–699, 1991

Tinuper P, de Carolis P, Galeotti M, et al: Electroencephalogram and HIV infection: a prospective study in 100 patients. Clin Electroencephalogr 21:145–150, 1990

Tran Dinh YR, Mamo H, Cervorni J, et al: Disturbances in the cerebral perfusion of human immune deficiency virus-1 seropositive asymptomatic subjects: a quantitative tomography study of 18 cases. J Nucl Med 31:1601–1607, 1990

Tross S, Price RW, Navia B, et al: Neuropsychological characterization of the AIDS dementia complex: a preliminary report. AIDS 2:81–88, 1988

Van der Poel CL, Lelie PN, Reesink HW, et al: Blood donors with indeterminate anti p24 reactivity in HIV-1 Western blot: absence of infectivity to transfused patients and in virus cultures. Vox Sang 56:162–167, 1989

Van Gorp WG, Miller E, Satz P, et al: Neuropsychological performance in HIV-1 immunocompromised patients (abstract). J Clin Exp Neuropsychol 11:35, 1989a

Van Gorp WG, Mitrushina M, Cummings JL, et al: Normal aging and the subcortical encephalopathy of AIDS: a neuropsychological comparison. Neuropsychiatry Neuropsychol Behav Neurol 2:5–20, 1989b

Van Gorp WG, Satz P, Hinkin C, et al: Metacognition in HIV-1 seropositive asymptomatic individuals: self-ratings versus objective neuropsychological performance. J Clin Exp Neuropsychol 13:812–819, 1991

Vazeux R: AIDS encephalopathy and tropism of HIV for brain monocytes/macrophages and microglial cells. Pathobiology 59:214–218, 1991

Vinters HV, Guerra WG, Eppolito L, et al: Necrotizing vasculitis of the nervous system in a patient with AIDS-related complex. Neuropathol Appl Neurobiol 14: 417–424, 1988

Volberding PA, Latgakos SW, Koch MA, et al: AZT in asymptomatic HIV infection: a controlled trial in persons with fewer than 500 CD4 positive cells per cubic millimeter. N Engl J Med 322:941–949, 1990

Walker DG, Itagaki J, Berry K, et al: Examination of brains of AIDS cases for human immunodeficiency virus and human cytomegalovirus nucleic acids. J Neurol Neurosurg Psychiatry 52:583–590, 1989

Wechsler D: Wechsler Adult Intelligence Scale—Revised. San Antonio, TX, Psychological Corporation, 1981

Wechsler D: Wechsler Memory Scale—Revised. San Antonio, TX, Psychological Corporation, 1987

Whelan MA, Kricheff II, Handler M, et al: Acquired immunodeficiency syndrome: cerebral computed tomographic manifestations. Radiology 149:477–484, 1983

Wiegand M, Möller AA, Schreiber W, et al: Alterations of nocturnal sleep in patients with HIV infection. Acta Neurol Scand 83:141–142, 1991a

Wiegand M, Möller AA, Schreiber W, et al: Nocturnal sleep EEG in patients with HIV infection. Eur Arch Psychiatry Clin Neurosci 240:153–158, 1991b

Wiley CA, Masliah E, Morey M, et al: Neocortical damage during HIV infection. Ann Neurol 29:651–657, 1991

Wilkie FL, Eisdorfer C, Morgan R, et al: Cognition in early human immunodeficiency virus infection. Arch Neurol 47:433–440, 1990a

Wilkie F, Guterman A, Morgan R, et al: Cognition and electro-physiologic measures in early HIV infection (abstract). J Clin Exp Neuropsychol 12:48, 1990b

Wilkie FL, Morgan R, Fletcher MA, et al: Cognition and immune function in HIV-1 infection. AIDS 6:977–981, 1992

Wilkins JW, Robertson KR, Vander Horst C, et al: The importance of confounding factors in the evaluation of neuropsychological changes in patients infected with human immunodeficiency virus. Journal of Acquired Immune Deficiency Syndrome 3:938–942, 1990

Wolcott DL, Fawzy FI, Pasnau RO: Acquired immunodeficiency syndrome and consultation-liaison psychiatry. Gen Hosp Psychiatry 7:280–292, 1985

Wolinsky SM, Rinaldo CR, Kwok S, et al: Human immunodeficiency virus type 1 (HIV-1) infection a median of 18 months before a diagnostic Western blot: evidence from a cohort of homosexual men. Ann Intern Med 111:961–972, 1989

Working Group of the American Academy of Neurology AIDS Task Force: Nomenclature and research case definitions for neurologic manifestations of human immunodeficiency virus-type 1 (HIV-1) infection. Neurology 41:778–785, 1991

Yoshioka M, Bradley WG, Shapshak P, et al: Role of immune activation and cytokine expression in HIV-1-associated neurologic diseases. Advances in Neuroimmunology 5:335–358, 1995

Zachary RA: Shipley Institute of Living Scale. Revised Manual. Los Angeles, Western Psychological Services, 1986

CHAPTER 9

Neuropsychiatry and Persons With Developmental Disabilities

Ruth M. Ryan, M.D.

$\mathbf{D}$evelopmental disabilities are usually defined as impairments in physical, emotional, or cognitive maturity that interfere with the person's ability to function in activities of daily living and have their onset during the developmental period (usually before age 21 years). Mental retardation usually refers to IQ less than 70 (greater than 2 standard deviations below the mean for the given population). The incidence of mental retardation is 3%, and the prevalence is 1%, though there is some controversy about these figures (Munro 1986). The difference between incidence and prevalence is related to reduced life-span of persons with mental retardation. Gender differences (more males than females) are attributed to cultural differences in expectations that influence reporting, increased vulnerability to sex-linked disorders, and alleged increased aggressiveness of males in Western cultures (Koranyi 1986; Munro 1986).

Years ago, the IQ test was incorrectly thought to predict emotional maturity and eventual functional ability. Intelligence testing, per se, predicts only the person's ability to function in school; it does not predict functioning in any other context (Munro 1986). Functional inventories, such as the American Association on Mental Retardation Adaptive Behavior Scales, were developed to provide a more complete catalog of skills and needs. The American

Association on Mental Retardation has also recently revised the definition of mental retardation to reflect a comprehensive list of physical, emotional, cognitive, and other needs, rather than a list of deficits (American Association on Mental Retardation 1992; Macmillan et al. 1993).

Dysmorphology, the study of physical anomalies, has often been linked with studies of disability. However, 1 in 50 children is born with a congenital physical anomaly, and only a small minority suffer a disability related to this abnormality (Wilson 1987). The cause of mental retardation is unknown in the majority of individuals. The identifiable causes include multisystem abnormalities resulting from chromosome abnormalities; multisystem damage from infections, exogenous teratogens (toxins), or accumulated toxins in metabolic abnormalities; mechanical pressure on the brain (developmental skull abnormalities); and hypoxemic or mechanical trauma (Koranyi 1986). Mild mental retardation (IQ greater than 55) is 7–10 times more frequent than moderate (IQ 40–55), severe (IQ 25–40), and profound (IQ less than 25) mental retardation. The cause of mental retardation is known in 30%–40% of persons with IQs greater than 55 and 60%–70% of persons with IQs less than 55 (Schaefer et al. 1994)

Specific learning disabilities involve difficulties with perception and concept formation that may be observed in childhood and persist into adulthood. Overt symptoms may include attention difficulties, poor motor skills, inadequate perceptual development, immature emotional and social development, and faulty language and cognitive development. If these symptoms are not recognized as part of learning disorders, the individual may collect other diagnostic labels, many of which imply psychiatric disorders or character flaws (Newill et al. 1984). Persons with learning disabilities can be distinguished from persons with poor educational preparation (Gregg and Hoy 1989). Isolated difficulty with language acquisition is almost never attributable to social deprivation or conflicts and is more likely the result of a combination of mechanical and neurological abnormalities (Resnick and Rapin 1991).

Dyslexia, also called reading disability, is regarded as the most common learning disability. Prevalence is estimated at 4%–5%. Symptoms include an unusual manner of holding the writing instrument, delayed first word, word and letter reversals, and difficulty comprehending and producing written communication. The problem with written communication is typically inconsistent with the rest of the person's functioning. This condition is commonly familial and may be associated with dominant temporal and parietal lobe dysfunction (Duane 1991).

Various neuroanatomical abnormalities occur in persons with dyslexia. Neuroanatomical abnormalities in the left perisylvian area were described in

1985 (Galaburda et al. 1985). Corresponding abnormalities on the electroencephalogram (EEG) occur in both the expected left mediotemporal and anterotemporal regions, as well as the less expected anterofrontal regions (Duffy and McAnulty 1990). Increasing refinement of anatomical study has revealed that structural abnormalities include asymmetry characterized by delayed growth of the left posterior hemisphere sites (Bigler 1992; Galaburda 1992, 1993a, 1993b). A theory that linked immune abnormalities, left-handedness, and neurodevelopmental disorder with talent has received mixed data reviews (Flannery and Liederman 1995; Hellige 1994; Previc 1994; Tinnessen et al. 1993). Musical talent may also be associated with this abnormality (McNamara et al. 1994). Abnormal auditory anatomy may be present in dyslexia (Galaburda et al. 1994). Consistent leftward asymmetry of the parietal operculum may be of significance with regard to consistent right-handedness; non–right-handedness and lack of asymmetry are associated with various learning disabilities.

Abnormalities occur in the magnocellular pathway (also called the transient visual pathway), which mediates processing of rapid visual transitions at low contrasts involved in motion perception, stereopsis, and saccade suppression (Galaburda 1993b; Galaburda and Livingstone 1993; Habib et al. 1995). Functional magnetic resonance imaging (fMRI) reveals failure of moving stimuli stimulation of the related task functioning in the magnocellular visual subsystem, and linguistic stimuli may be treated as nonlinguistic stimuli (increased negativity on the right, rather than on the left, hemisphere) (Eden et al. 1996; Galaburda 1993a, 1993b). Structural neuroimaging findings regarding brain size, surface area, and structures must be viewed with caution in that factors such as age and gender influence brain size. Studies that control for these factors have not found any significant differences between brains of people with dyslexia and those without dyslexia (Njiokiktjien et al. 1994; Rademacher et al. 1993; Schultz et al. 1994). More sophisticated MRI studies may be necessary to reveal any significant differences (Leonard et al. 1993). Anomalous cerebral morphology in the bilateral frontal and the left temporoparietal areas is strongly associated with developmental dyslexia. The anterior portion corpus callosum may be abnormal (small) as well (Hynd et al. 1995). Another study found the posterior corpus callosum to be enlarged and the anterior portion normal (Rumsey et al. 1996). Along with the inconsistent reports of structure, increasing evidence points to plasticity of the structures that remain. Indeed, children with larger insults to the brain seem to have even greater plasticity and subsequent acquisition of skills that otherwise seem anatomically improbable (Bigler 1992).

Social-emotional learning disabilities (Voeller 1991) are specific difficulties with understanding and producing nonverbal communication with other people. Deficits in intuition are associated with other interpersonal difficulties as well. Some have suggested that this condition is similar to Asperger's syndrome (Wing 1981). Persons with social-emotional learning disabilities may be regarded as odd or eccentric and may be incorrectly labeled as schizoid (Ryan 1992). Children with right-hemisphere lesions perform more poorly on tests of affect recognition than do children with left-hemisphere lesions (Voeller and Hanson 1988).

Nonverbal learning disabilities, also called learning disorders of the right hemisphere, are seen in no more than 10% of people with learning disabilities. The term *right-hemisphere learning disability* may be too inclusive. Specific deficits include defects in mathematical and simultaneous or visuospatial reasoning. This can lead to getting lost easily, inability to respond quickly in athletics, inability to read a page of music (likened to a topographical map), inability to be on time, inaccurately imitating required dressing patterns, and an extreme tendency to focus on detail. Though not hampered by the deficits in intuition and nonverbal communication of persons with social-emotional learning disabilities, individuals with nonverbal learning disabilities who are not recognized as having these disabilities and not assisted may experience intense ridicule and damage to self-esteem. The specific neuroanatomical findings are uncertain; however, the apparently higher frequency of this condition in people with Turner's syndrome and females with fragile X syndrome has suggested further study of the X chromosome in these conditions (Denckla 1991).

Developmental disability resulting from frontal lobe injury early in life is reviewed in Chapter 6.

Numerous additional psychiatric problems are seen in adults with unrecognized learning disabilities. These problems include anxiety, poor attention, immature behavior, prolonged dependence on families, depression, substance abuse, self-doubt, and marital problems. Persons with these presentations should receive developmental assessment regarding unusual learning styles in childhood and their adult residua (Denckla 1993). Understanding and assistance with the learning disabilities can assist with these problems (Gajar 1992; Polloway et al. 1992; Spreen 1989). The diagnostic guidelines require that the clinician make certain that cognitive errors are not caused by mental retardation, a primary emotional disorder, or a specific area of brain damage. The assessment procedure involves review of all school records, medical records, and vocational records, along with behavioral observations, and multiaxial IQ testing with special attention to discrepancies, by a qualified specialist in this area (Newill et al. 1984).

Psychiatric Epidemiology and Risk Factors

At least one-third of persons with developmental disabilities (mental retardation or primary infantile autism) have a psychiatric condition (Eaton and Menolascino 1982; S. Reiss et al. 1982b; Stark et al. 1988). Persons with developmental disabilities are more frequently exposed to stresses, such as medical illnesses, abuse, trauma, and an "affectionless control" type of programming, that provoke psychiatric illnesses in predisposed persons. Persons with developmental disabilities are vulnerable to the full range of psychiatric illnesses (Sovner and Hurley 1989), and these can be diagnosed and treated using standard procedures adapted to the person's communication style (Szymanski et al. 1991). Updated epidemiological studies suggest that the most commonly seen conditions are anxiety disorders and mood disorders (Ancill and Juralowicz 1995; King et al. 1994; Ryan 1993). The evaluation of aggressive behavior in persons with developmental disabilities is discussed in Chapter 6. Dysmorphic features, per se, do not increase the risk of serious psychiatric disorders (McNeil et al. 1992).

Comorbidity

Neuropsychiatric Effects of Past Treatments

Persons with developmental disabilities are sexually, physically, and emotionally abused more frequently than other people (Sobsey 1994). Historically, persons with developmental disabilities who were subjected to abuse were not provided preventive therapy because of a myth that these treatments could not be effective (Sobsey 1994). Institutions for persons with mental retardation were often understaffed (one staff member per 100 patients) and lacking in basics such as clothing, nutrition, basic medical care, and physical safety (Blatt 1970; Blatt and Kaplan 1966). Well-staffed and well-supplied agencies were often rewarded for keeping people "controlled," "compliant," and "obedient," a type of affectionless control (Donnellan et al. 1988). Families were told to institutionalize (often with threats that their male offspring with mental retardation would become rapists) and forget about their family member with mental retardation ("pretend they have died"). Families were described in the psychiatric literature as "pathological" if they insisted on keeping contact with their sibling or child with a developmental disability. Even in the present day, there have been calls for active or passive killing ("euthanasia") of persons with developmental disabilities (U.S. Commission on

Civil Rights 1989). Chronic abuse and neglect may be associated with distorted development of limbic, serotonergic, β-adrenergic, endorphin, and dopaminergic systems, thus increasing risks for mood and anxiety disorders (Charney et al. 1993; Goldfeld et al. 1988; Ito et al. 1993; Jorge et al. 1993; Reiss and Benson 1984; Teicher et al. 1993).

General Medical Comorbidity

It has been demonstrated (King et al. 1994; Ryan and Sunada 1997) that 70%–72% of individuals with developmental disabilities who present for mental health treatment have comorbid medical conditions. This is approximately twice the rate in persons with developmental disabilities who do not present for mental health care and is twice that seen in persons who present for mental health care who do not have developmental disabilities. The most common conditions seen were undertreated or unrecognized epilepsy and undertreated or unrecognized endocrine conditions (especially hypothyroidism). Other conditions included undiagnosed movement disorders, severe head injuries, and metabolic illness. Malignancies were more common in younger people and were usually found at later stages. The general principles drawn from these data are that common conditions present in unusual ways (e.g., hypothyroidism presenting with agitation), that uncommon conditions present more often (e.g., well-nourished people presenting with beriberi, adults presenting with Wilson's disease), and that the physical examination may be unrevealing. Also, some data suggest that at least half the time more than one problem is present (Ryan and Sunada 1997). Psychiatrists in the community setting are already painfully familiar with the reluctance of some colleagues to complete thorough evaluations of persons with mental health needs. This reluctance is magnified with regard to persons who also have developmental disabilities. The skill of the community psychiatrist in making certain that appropriate evaluation occurs is essential.

Psychoactive Nonpsychiatric Medications

Increased medical comorbidity is also associated with increased use of nonpsychiatric medications with negative psychoactive effects. Persons with developmental disabilities are especially vulnerable to psychiatric side effects because of the combination of the need to perform at their peak to cope with community challenges (an impairment of 10 IQ points is more meaningful when a person has an IQ of 40 at the outset), increased medical fragility, and frequent use of multiple medications. Medications that are especially commonly used and toxic include phenytoin (deactivation of many antidepressants, depression, rage attacks) and barbiturate anticonvulsants (hyperactivity, rage, depression), histamine$_2$ blockers (irritability, psychosis, problems with concentration, magnification of toxicities of other medications), β-blockers (problems with physical and cognitive performance, depression, sleep disturbance, psychosis), and diuretics (depression). Whenever an individual is receiving a medication, the psychiatric effects should be considered ("Drugs Which Cause Psychiatric Symptoms" 1989).

Treatment Goals

Treatment goals are similar to those for persons without developmental disabilities: reduction in painful or disabling symptoms; participation in satisfying work, social, and relationship activities; and the best possible physical health. Federal guidelines specify that persons with developmental disabilities are entitled to the same health services as other citizens. This information, coupled with the reality that persons with developmental disabilities are usually served in public systems, suggests that persons with developmental disabilities will present to the community psychiatrist for diagnosis and treatment.

Psychiatric Diagnosis

Positive outcomes are associated with comprehensive treatment by a team using ongoing specific diagnostic assessments. The actual habilitative treatments can be provided by nonprofessionals, with educational support from consulting specialists (Ellenor 1977; Lew et al. 1990; Ryan et al. 1991; Sprague et al. 1992). Nonspecific diagnoses (such as "atypical psychosis" or "behavior disorder") or diagnoses that attribute behavior to the developmental disability are no longer felt to be useful (Szymanski et al. 1991). In the past, clinicians declined to make specific diagnoses when individuals referred for assessment did not use spoken communication. Numerous inventories are now available to assist the clinician in developing a comprehensive diagnostic assessment (Aman 1991; Gedye 1992; Sovner and Hurley 1990; Sovner and Lowry 1990; Szymanski 1977). In addition, many centers find it useful to develop in-house instruments for use with nonverbal individuals. Another critical piece of information is the behavior specialist's functional assessment and motivational assessment (O'Neill et al. 1990; Repp et al. 1990). This is different from the occupational therapist's functional assessment of what the person can do; the behavior specialist's functional analysis focuses on why the person emits a particular behavior of concern (communication of discomfort? attention seeking? escape demands?) and what factors in the person's life reinforce the continuing use of the behavior.

This information can be useful in a variety of ways. For example, if the person's environment does nothing to perpetuate the behavior of concern yet the person emits behavior that appears designed to elicit punishment from others, this can be a presentation of depression. A careful diagnostic assessment can be useful in confirming this impression. Further, if the person is provided excellent consistent behavior programming and the behavior persists, or symptom substitution (emergence of another symptom of equal or greater intensity that serves the same "function") is observed, this is a clear indication of some other, unaddressed factor (such as a psychiatric or other medical illness) influencing the person's health. In addition, if the environmental factors thought to be driving a particular behavior have been alleviated and there is little or no improvement, an additional undiagnosed factor may be present. The same behavior in the same person can mean something different every time it occurs. Just as a person may be tearful when happy, again when sad, and again when in pain, a person who bangs his or her head to indicate distress may do so to express depression, anxiety, the pain of a headache, or boredom. Thus, each time a behavior occurs, the complete assessment must be done, unless some obvious stress is immediately identified, and alleviation of the stress attenuates the behavior.

Treatment

Psychotropic medication use for people with developmental disabilities follows similar guidelines as for people who do not have developmental disabilities. Special attention should be paid to side effects and medication interaction effects. The most common errors are overuse of sedation and undertreatment of depression. Use of psychotropic medication, particularly antipsychotic medication, for suppression of behavior or convenience of staff is unacceptable (American Psychiatric Association 1993; American Psychiatric Association, Practice Guideline for Mental Health Care of Persons With Developmental Disabilities, in development). The medications most commonly prescribed for persons with developmental disabilities are low-potency antipsychotic medications. Thioridazine and mesoridazine were specifically marketed to institutions for people with developmental disabilities and were described as completely safe without long- or short-term side effects (Gadow and Kalachnik 1981; Hill et al. 1985; Intaglia and Rinck 1985; Tu 1979). The extensive use of these medications has resulted in an epidemic of tardive dyskinesia and tardive akathisia (Crabbe 1989; Smith and Davis 1976). The term *tardive akathisia* has been overapplied to describe any agitation any person with a developmental disability experienced while withdrawing from neuroleptics. The more specific and rare syndrome description refers to intractable motor restlessness and drivenness; at the extreme, affected individuals may be unable to stay seated while asleep (Gualtieri and Sovner 1989). When an assessment shows that a neuroleptic is not indicated, the drug should be tapered gradually. The recommended rate to avoid disabling rebound withdrawal phenomena is 10% every 4–8 weeks (Crabbe 1993). This gradual rate can also help avoid frequent changes of dose, which are associated with increased risk of tardive akathisia and tardive dyskinesia (Crabbe 1989; Gualtieri et al. 1984). The most frequent outcome of the gradual medication reduction is the unmasking of whatever illness, if any, the person has, usually an anxiety or a mood disorder (Ancill and Juralowicz 1995; King et al. 1994; Ryan 1997). The unmasking allows implementation of more specific treatment and ultimately more favorable clinical outcome. It is rare that the person actually has schizophrenia or a schizophrenia-spectrum condition. These appear to be as rare in this population as in any other (approximately 1%–2%), when proper diagnostic criteria are used, and many symptoms suggestive of psychosis turn out to be dissociative phenomena (Ancill and Juralowicz 1995; Ancill et al. 1994; King et al. 1994; Ryan 1993).

Modern behaviorism applied to persons with developmental disabilities, sometimes called *habilitation,* is individualized and person-centered (rather than symptom-centered). It is desirable to tailor approaches to the person's specific interests, goals, and psychiatric needs. Numerous procedures for eliciting this information from persons who do not use spoken communication are available (Aman 1991). Approaches that focused on extinguishing inconvenient behaviors without regard to cause are no longer believed to be useful (Carr et al. 1990). For example, rewarding a person for staying quiet and still all day is contraindicated if the person is found to have Tourette syndrome (Ryan 1993). Ignoring and redirecting crying behavior in a person with major depression is contraindicated. People with posttraumatic stress disorder should not be encouraged or pushed to develop relationships with people who remind them of abusers and should be provided supportive assistance during dissociative episodes (Ryan 1994b). Punishment techniques (defined as procedures that cause pain, fear, or embarrassment) have been explored extensively and are never indicated. Nonnaturalistic punishment techniques (electric shock, hot pepper sauce to the mouth, striking, cold water splashed in the face) may force the person into temporary compliance, but the rebound of behaviors after the removal of the punishment can be extreme.

Typically, punishment techniques control behavior only if increasing intensity or threat of increasing intensity of punishment is continued indefinitely (LaVigna and Donnellan 1986; Rodden 1996; Singer and Irvin 1987). This method of control has led to a number of deaths (State of Massachusetts v BRI 1994). The psychological effects of the use of punishment techniques, particularly when applied to control behaviors that the person was thought to be able to control but were actually involuntary, can be devastating. Some more egregious examples are striking, shocking, and restraining people for "stereotypical movements" later diagnosed as tics of Tourette syndrome (Ryan 1993); applying restraints to persons experiencing dissociative phenomena, such as flashbacks of sexual abuse that occurred while restrained (Ryan 1994b); and in various ways punishing persons experiencing temporal lobe seizure peri-ictal phenomena (Carr et al. 1990).

Psychotherapy can be useful for persons with developmental disabilities in the same situations where it is indicated for persons without developmental disabilities. Specific needs include grief work, work in processing trauma, work on poor self-esteem, cognitive-behavioral approaches to anxiety and depression, and psychosocial work in schizophrenia (Ancill et al. 1994; Bialer 1964; Stavrakaki and Klein 1986; Szymanski et al. 1991). The most common errors are failure of the therapist to develop a mutual "language" (verbal or nonverbal) and failure to develop a respectful therapeutic alliance. This is analogous to the situation of any person brought to a therapist who has a different agenda from that of the individual. Therapy that focuses on a cosmetic change to please someone other than the individual may be associated with temporary, superficial results, but long-term improvement is not seen. Long-term positive outcomes are possible and may actually require less time than might be required for treatment of a similar problem in a person without a developmental disability (Stavrakaki and Klein 1986). Similarly, therapy that is designed to make someone comply with a reversible intolerable situation is ineffective. (When it is effective, it is called *brainwashing* and is unethical.) Publications that regularly report on the newer psychotherapy techniques include *The Habilitative Mental Healthcare Newsletter* and *The NADD Newsletter*. Most standard techniques can be successfully adapted to persons with developmental disabilities; language style may need to be adjusted (Bialer 1964; Stavrakaki and Klein 1986; Szymanski et al. 1991).

Other nonmedication therapies with varying levels of research support include sensory integration therapy (occupational therapy), therapeutic touch (Krieger 1986), massage, and various culture-specific healing techniques (Kleinman et al. 1978). The community psychiatrist working in successful collaboration with the community is well served by continuing familiarity with these arts. Various nutritional therapies are being tested; the serotonin diet holds some promise as part of the treatment of mood and obsessive-compulsive disorders (Gedye 1993). Exercise and physical therapies can be useful as well.

Treatment Settings

After extensive experimentation with various types of institutionalization, most workers conclude that communities and the people living in them are healthiest with fullest possible inclusion of all members, including people with developmental disabilities. The current preferred placements are individualized and avoid the obsolete "readiness" model, a now thoroughly disproven approach that suggests that people can be prepared ("made ready") for a preferred situation, such as paid employment, in some other, nonsimilar setting. Programming persons in setting A prepares them for setting A and does not help them toward preparing for setting B. The concept of the institutional setting as a center of excellence has been expanded. Common practice had been to send the challenging individual to the institutional center of excellence to be fixed and sent back to his or her community. Workers in Colorado (Ryan et al. 1991), New Mexico (Ludwig 1994), British Columbia (British Columbia Mental Health Society 1992), and other areas have focused on the concept of the traveling team, moving the expertise typically confined to centers of excellence into the person's community, collaborating with the community team, and providing on-site consultation and ongoing teaching and follow-up. The center of excellence may be a useful setting for completion of thorough physical, neurological, and laboratory evaluations, as well as numerous medical consultations. Persons who are a danger to self or others and do not voluntarily accept supports in the community may benefit from temporary placement in institutional settings. The primary emphasis is on facilitation of independence through linkage with the person's family and home community and avoidance of permanent institutionalization (Menolascino 1991).

Myths

Myths about mental retardation have interfered with the achievement of best possible clinical outcomes. One of the more pernicious is the myth that certain behaviors, such as self-injury or assaultiveness, are "normal" for people with mental retardation or are attributable directly to mental retardation.

These behaviors are not "normal" for anyone and, when they occur, are an indication of some disorder (American Psychiatric Association 1993). The disorder may be environmental stress or part of problematic training (by which the person has been conditioned to emit these behaviors) or may be a sign of a psychiatric or other medical problem. Failure by the treating clinician to assess the individual thoroughly and to collaborate with the individual's team leads to ineffective or damaging treatments, which lead to a worsening of symptoms and a perpetuation of myths (Griffiths 1989). Other disproven myths that persist and interfere with optimal treatment are that people who do not use spoken communication cannot benefit from psychotherapy (Stavrakaki and Klein 1986), that IQ predicts emotional maturity (Balla and Zigler 1979), and that people with extensive emotional or physical needs require or do better with institutionalization (Szymanski et al. 1991). The neuropsychiatrist in the community setting must often rely on information from collaborators who may distort information based on such myths.

Neuropsychiatry and Developmental Syndromes

Developmental syndromes that affect cognitive ability may also affect emotional health as well as other body systems that influence mental health. It can be helpful to identify developmental syndromes, in that rapidly increasing numbers of specific medication and nonmedication treatments are available, and the increased understanding of the physiological risks of the condition may assist the clinician in anticipating and treating complications before they cause extreme distress. The risks of identifying these conditions relate to a tendency to overattribute emotional/behavioral characteristics to the developmental syndrome, a version of the diagnostic overshadowing (S. Reiss et al. 1982b) that has been a factor in the tendency to attribute behavioral symptoms to mental retardation. This is an especially important risk when conditions are newly recognized and only a few people with the condition have been studied (Rosen 1993). In addition, information regarding the functional prognosis of persons with developmental syndromes must be viewed with extreme caution. For example, extensive literature regarding persons with Down's syndrome stated that their life-span was limited to less than 30 years and that there was no hope of toilet training or learning to talk. Some people with Down's syndrome have attended college, lived into their 70s, married, and reared children ("Declining Mortality From Down Syndrome" 1990).

The clinician should also exercise extreme caution when proposing that people obtain developmental assessment to evaluate their own or their siblings' risk of transmission of the condition; asking people to undergo an extensive workup for the purpose of helping to avoid creating more people like themselves sends a message that can be damaging to the treatment alliance.

The following characteristics in an adult or child should prompt developmental medical evaluation: unexplained mental retardation; unusual or "dysmorphic" physical characteristics; very unusual food preferences; a family or personal history of multiple miscarriages; and a family history of mental retardation, congenital physical anomalies, or deaths from unexplained metabolic diseases. A developmental evaluation includes thorough physical examination, family examination/tree diagram, and numerous laboratory tests. A thorough physical examination is followed by a comparison of the person's physical features with standard descriptions of people without developmental disabilities and variations (Jones 1988).

Laboratory screening tests include chromosome karyotype (with high resolution of areas of interest, identified from the physical examination or history, or special probes, such as in suspected cases of fragile X syndrome); serum and urine amino acids, organic acids, and mucopolysaccharides; serum very long chain fatty acids; serum liver function studies; ammonia, lactate, pyruvate, electrolytes, and thyroid function studies; complete blood count; and other tests based on clinical history. Close consultation with a developmental evaluation center may be useful. University-affiliated programs, also called "JFK Centers," or developmental pediatricians are recommended. These centers are generally set up both to conduct evaluations directly and to instruct clinicians in local areas how to proceed with their own evaluation. Chromosome studies are more useful when there has been enough preliminary work to provide guidance to the laboratory providing the study. For example, a standard karyotype, which shows the number and general shapes of the chromosomes, would be adequate to look for a condition such as Down's syndrome but would be inadequate to look for Prader-Willi syndrome (which would require high-resolution studies of chromosome 15). Down's syndrome and Prader-Willi syndrome might appear somewhat similar in an infant. Minimum imaging studies typically include magnetic resonance imaging (MRI) of the brain and plain films of the rest of the skeleton. (MRI is superior to computed tomography [CT] with regard to sensitivity, the exception being that CT is superior with regard to detecting small calcifications, which might be of interest in inherited parathyroid abnormalities or complications of tuberous sclerosis. The risks of anesthesia to permit MRI scanning are generally minimal compared with the risks of unmonitored sedation and nontreatment of conditions missed on the less sensitive CT scan.) Bone density films may be indicated in certain suspected cases of dwarfism. Electrophysiological studies such as electromyography and electroencephalography would be suggested by history of varying levels of consciousness, ataxia, or muscle weakness. Viral studies of spinal fluid and serum titers would be suggested by history of exposure and suggestive clinical symptoms; the usual screen includes toxoplasmosis, rubella, Coxsackievirus, herpes, and human immunodeficiency virus (Jones 1988, Chapters 2 and 3; Koranyi 1986).

Beyond the usual indications described above, when should the neuropsychiatrist consider pursuing a detailed developmental evaluation? A simple guiding principle is that emotional and physical health is a reasonable goal for people with developmental disabilities. If all of the available information about a person is being used and the subsequent comprehensive intervention plan is implemented without success, then it is likely that the database is incomplete. Because the influence of developmental syndromes can change over time, a developmental medical evaluation can be indicated even in situations in which the issues of concern have not been lifelong. Descriptions of the longer-term course of most developmental syndromes are only rarely available and do not account for variations in types. For this reason, it is not useful to try to limit the screening diagnostic testing on the basis of clinical history; there is not enough comparison descriptive material available to exclude most conditions. Mortality rates, morbidity, and costs are improved by meticulous medical management (Carter and Jancar 1983; Ryan and Sunada 1994, 1997).

Neuropsychiatric Issues in Selected Conditions

Down's Syndrome

Down's syndrome, seen in 1 in 660 live births, is the most common genetic condition associated with mental retardation (Jones 1988). Physical features may include small head with shortened A-P diameter, relatively enlarged tongue, lateral epicanthal folds, midfacial hypoplasia, hypotelorism, small ears, high arched palate, short incurved fifth finger, hyperflexibility, muscular hypotonia, gap between first and second toes, and short broad hands. Not all characteristics are seen in all individuals. Karyotyping is essential for diagnosis, in that several other conditions may look superficially similar, particularly in childhood, yet have different physiologic implications. Down's syndrome is most commonly produced by trisomy 21; however, D-G translocations, mosaics, and partial aneuploidy can be seen as well (Pueschel and Pueschel 1992). Down's syndrome is a prominent example of a condition in which individuals have been stereotyped as "cute" or especially carefree and pleasant. However, people with Down's syndrome have a number of painful physical conditions and are vulnerable to the full range of psychiatric conditions. Years ago, it was speculated that the physiology of persons with Down's syndrome might preclude mania (Sovner et al. 1985). Subsequent reports of mania in persons with Down's syndrome disconfirm this (McLaughlin 1987; Ryan 1993). Specific conditions to which persons with Down's syndrome are vulnerable and that frequently are associated with psychiatric symptoms include endocrine conditions (especially hypothyroidism), autoimmune disorders (such as systemic lupus erythematosus), adult-onset seizures, sleep apnea, blood dyscrasias, and infections (upper respiratory and pulmonary especially). Other common conditions do not influence mental health as directly but may be associated with altered behavior unaccompanied by explicit complaints. Atlantoaxial dislocation can produce progressive ataxia, incontinence, paresthesias, and reduced proprioception. The person may become hesitant about activities or may rub the fingertips, behaviors that may be inappropriately dismissed. Gastroesophageal reflux can be associated with a choking sensation to which the person may respond by jamming a fist or large objects in the mouth. The dental anomalies frequently seen in this condition can be associated with abscesses not easily seen on surface examination. Abrupt squatting may be seen in persons with worsening cardiac conditions (Pueschel and Pueschel 1992).

Histologic changes of Alzheimer's disease are seen in the brains of older people with Down's syndrome; however, development of clinical Alzheimer's disease is not ubiquitous. Indeed, a number of persons who appear to manifest this progressive dementia actually have reversible conditions, such as depression (Warren et al. 1989) and sensory impairments (Hewitt et al. 1985). Early studies that examined the frequency of Alzheimer's disease in persons with Down's syndrome do not mention screening for the dozens of other biomedical conditions that can cause pseudodementia. Neurological signs of cortical changes, such as gait changes and frontal release signs, may occur unaccompanied by changes in personality or cognition (Owens et al. 1971; Thase et al. 1988).

Factors associated with a favorable outcome in persons with Down's syndrome are implementation of stimulation activities as soon as the diagnosis is suspected and meticulous ongoing evaluation and management of these complicating medical conditions (Pueschel and Pueschel 1992). Misinformed professionals who expect little developmentally have a negative effect on the parent-child interaction and thus may slow the child's progress (Miller 1988).

Fragile X Syndrome

Fragile X syndrome is the second most common chromosomal condition associated with mental retardation (Webb et al. 1987). Physical features in affected males and penetrant females include macroorchidism, prominent jaw, prominent forehead, thickened nasal bridge, large low-set ears, large hands, hyperextensible joints, and pale blue irides. Occasional abnormalities include mitral valve prolapse, torticollis, kyphoscoliosis, cleft palate, and cutis laxa. Diagnosis is traditionally made through specialized chromosomal analysis; cells are grown on folate-deficient media, which will provoke a fracture of the arm of the X chromosome in 10%–40% of cells. One hundred cells are counted, and demonstration of the marker in 10% or more of the cells is considered a positive study. Eighty percent of males and 30% of females with this marker are affected (Jones 1988, pp. 126–127). A recently developed DNA probe technique appears to be a more sensitive test (Rousseas et al. 1991). The recent discoveries of the genetics in fragile X syndrome have taught the new genetic paradigm of *genetic anticipation*, that is, the severity of the disorder increases in successive generations (Ross et al. 1993).

The phenotypic expression of the fragile X syndrome involves two steps: the expansion of DNA within the gene (Yu et al. 1991) and the methylation (deactivation and stabilization) of the DNA. The methylation deactivates the protein encoded at the fragile X site. The absence of the protein is correlated with the intensity of the expression of the disorder (Pieretti et al. 1991; Yu et al. 1991). Fragile X syndrome is an example of a condition in which investigators have labored to describe a behavioral phenotype, only to discover that with study of increasing numbers of subjects the behavioral generalizations are not substantiated (Freund et al. 1992; A. L. Reiss et al. 1988; Wolff et al. 1988). What appears to be consistent is an indirect style of verbal expression, sometimes called *cluttering*, and a higher incidence of psychopathologies of various types (Freund and Reiss 1991; A. L. Reiss et al. 1989). If a person is asked, "How do you feel about going for a ride?" the cluttering response might be "Cars run on gas, you need oil too." There are also physical discomforts and sensory integration deficits, stressors that may unmask any psychiatric conditions to which the person may be vulnerable and that the person may try to manage through a variety of physical movements that may appear autistic-like. These may remit with appropriate sensory integration treatment (Hagerman and Sobesky 1989), which can be designed by an occupational therapist specializing in this area. Persons with fragile X syndrome are also more vulnerable to cardiac abnormalities, vasculitides, and endocrine conditions such as hypothyroidism (Jones 1988, pp. 126–127). Consideration of these possibilities is indicated when there are behavioral changes.

Phenylketonuria

Phenylketonuria is a relatively common metabolic disorder in which affected individuals are unable to convert phenylalanine to tyrosine. Untreated persons develop mental retardation and may have an increased incidence of seizures. Persons treated from infancy with a specialized diet (restricted phenylalanine, supplementation of tyrosine) may have normal intelligence, behavior, and performance. Years ago, it was assumed that if the person did not receive dietary treatment early, use of the diet in adulthood would be of little utility (because IQ would not be substantially affected). However, dietary treatment, even late in life, is associated with improvements in behavior.

Phenylketonuria provides an example of the profound effects of physical discomfort on behavior. Persons with untreated phenylketonuria have often been described as "internally preoccupied," "hyperkinetic," or even "autistic-like" (Chen and Hsiao 1989) An understanding of the physiological processes involved can be illuminating and contribute to more effective treatment. In untreated phenylketonuria, the person builds up toxic levels of phenylalanine and is deficient in tyrosine. In addition to the disruptions in neurotransmitter systems, production of skin pigments is disrupted, with drying, discoloration, texture changes, and intense pruritus. This constant discomfort is a stress that can provoke a variety of psychological reactions and is alleviated with dietary treatment. Though late treatment may not substantially affect IQ, the mood and comfort improvements warrant a careful trial (Brunner et al. 1987; Danks and Cotton 1987; Fishler et al. 1987; Harper and Reid 1987; Kawashima et al. 1988). An adequate trial of diet is one that lowers serum phenylalanine into the normal range, with supplementation of tyrosine adequate to produce a normal level, both for a minimum of 6 months. The literature on increasing the appeal of the phenylketonuria diets is expanding to address concerns in this area (Fehrenbach and Peterson 1989; Hayes et al. 1987). When the diet is not successful or not possible, the neuropsychiatrist may see optimal treatment outcome when focusing on addressing the intense discomforts of this condition (itching, gastroesophageal reflux, temperature dysregulation) rather than suppressing the behaviors that are emitted in response to these discomforts.

Prader-Willi Syndrome

Prader-Willi syndrome is a condition of gonadal agenesis associated with hypotonia and muscle weakness/early fatigue, poor feeding early in life, small stature, tiny hands and feet, facial abnormalities (epicanthal folds, very small midline structures), persistent high-pitched voice, and subsequent development of central obesity. IQ is usually 40–60, though affected individuals with normal intelligence have been described (Jones 1988, pp. 170–173). Full diagnostic criteria emerged in 1983, and the most recent consensus criteria include behavioral as well as physical features that change as the person ages (Holm et al. 1993). In untreated individuals, morbid obesity with associated complications and early death are common. Behaviors frequently seen include strict adherence to rituals, persistent picking at sores, sleep disturbances, and hyperphagia. The diagnosis is made through recognition of the clinical features, though most patients also carry a characteristic deletion on paternally derived chromosome 15. In Prader-Willi syndrome, a specific understanding of the neuroanatomical abnormalities and associated physiological changes can be of use in the mental health assessment. The specific anatomical abnormality is proposed to be hypoplasia of the hypothalamus (Ledbetter et al. 1987; Manchester 1994), possibly leading to reduced or absent gonadotropin production. In addition, hypothalamic signals regarding satiety are minimal or absent. Oxytocin neurons in the hypothalamic paraventricular nucleus are thought to inhibit food intake and are sometimes termed *satiety cells*. Persons with Prader-Willi syndrome have a 28% reduction in the total activity of these cells and a 38% reduction in total cell number. Oxytocin activity was reduced by an average of 54%, with wide variation among individuals. Delayed or absent satiety was observed, though persons with Prader-Willi syndrome ate three times as much food as did control subjects. This may be the neuroanatomical basis for the absence of satiety in persons with Prader-Willi syndrome (Swaab et al. 1995). In addition, γ-aminobutyric acid (GABA) function in the brains of persons with Prader-Willi syndrome is abnormal; the increased circulating GABA probably compensates for a reduction in GABAergic receptors. This is found in persons with Prader-Willi syndrome and in persons with Angelman syndrome; both of these conditions involve abnormalities of the 15q10–13 site (Ebert et al. 1997; Lalande et al. 1994; Wagstaff et al. 1991). There is also a generalized lack of autonomic reactivity and parasympathetic tone, which may account for the generally low body temperature, unusual patterns of self-stimulation, and lack of vomiting (DiMario et al. 1994; Holm et al. 1993). Persons with mosaicism may have partial capacities in these areas, including partial fertility in rare individuals. Precocious puberty has been reported in a few individuals.

IQ is normal in 12%, borderline in 29%, and in the mildly retarded range in 41%. One study suggested that people who had never been obese had a mean IQ 20 points higher than those who were or had been obese (Cassidy and Ledbetter 1989). Most people with Prader-Willi syndrome were expected to die in the third or fourth decade, but much older survivors are reported (Goldman 1988). Hypothyroidism is rarely found (Bhate et al. 1989). People with Prader-Willi syndrome do not produce adequate testosterone to support full muscle strength and never or only rarely feel they have had enough to eat. In addition, hormones that help with metabolism of fats are not produced in usual quantities, and metabolism of fatty stores is delayed. The person may eat excessively and accumulate fat, which the muscles are increasingly less able to support and maneuver. As muscles are stressed, there are increasing complications of pickwickian syndrome and sleep apnea (Clarke et al. 1989), an overreliance on rituals to conserve energy, reduced skin sensations, and mounting complications of obesity such as diabetes, heart disease, and skeletal discomfort (Greenswag 1987; Holm et al. 1993). A combination of careful and sensitive management of diet (with appropriate nonpunitive alternative activities) and an exercise program that focuses on walking appears to be useful from the general health standpoint (Silverthorn and Hornak 1995). Aggressive management of sleep apnea and problems that interfere with ambulation is indicated. Serotonergic antidepressants, which may assist with obsessiveness and appetite suppression and do not contribute to weight gain, may be useful in treating depression and anxiety disorders (including obsessive-compulsive disorder), which are commonly seen (Stein et al. 1994).

Williams Syndrome

Williams syndrome is a rare condition that combines unusual physical features, cognitive deficits, and the rare phenomenon of verbal abilities in excess of other cognitive abilities. Physical features include medial eyebrow flare, hoarse voice, short palpebral fissures, depressed nasal bridge, epicanthal folds, small and low-set ears, prominent mouth, and anteverted nares (Jones 1988, pp. 106–107). Internal complications may include bladder diverticula, supravalvular aortic stenosis, and renal artery stenosis, which can all be progressive. Persons with Williams syndrome are described as having a loquacious personality, special skills with regard to remembering song melodies and lyrics, and copious verbal fluency. They may speak at length, yet have little or no understanding of the content of the speech. The significance to the neuropsychiatrist is that reliance on the person's verbal productions may lead to misdiagnosis; the clinician should use nonverbal diagnostic methods for person who demonstrate this or any other condition in which verbal fluency exceeds cognitive understanding (Bradley and Udwin 1989; Sunada 1993).

Asperger's Syndrome

Asperger's syndrome was originally included in the differential diagnosis of autism. There is no specific radiologic or biochemical test; the diagnosis is based on clinical findings. The core deficits are absence of intuition and inability to understand or competently produce nonverbal communication. Symptoms include a singsong speech pattern, with neologisms, unusual grammatical structure, pronoun substitutions, and pedantic content. The person may understand and use complex words but make errors with simple words. Facial expressions may be absent, inconsistent with speech content, or abruptly exaggerated. Gestures may be limited, eccentric, or clumsy. Social interactions are seriously impaired, though the person does not necessarily want to withdraw from contact with others. Errors occur frequently regarding how close to stand to people, how to initiate a conversation, eye contact, movements, physical contact, and speech content. Hygiene may be marked by simultaneous extremes; the person may take three showers per day but never brush his or her teeth. Clothing tends to be extremely repetitive (the same color, texture, and brand all the time) and often oddly conservative. Increased comfort with objects as opposed to people may be observed.

Affected individuals may have exceptional technical skills in some areas (such as repairing machinery without instructions) but be unable to perform other apparently simpler activities of daily living (such as making long-distance telephone calls). Repetitive acts such as cleaning and checking may occur. However, in contrast to persons with primary obsessive-compulsive disorder, the person with Asperger's syndrome sees the acts as reasonable and can say when the acts are "finished." Sleep patterns may be erratic in that the person may stay awake for extended periods of time while finishing a project. Under stress, the person with Asperger's syndrome may exhibit extreme anxiety, with magnification of all of the eccentric personality characteristics, but without psychosis, clear mood cycling, or delirium. DSM-IV specifies that the symptoms of concern cannot be directly attributable to mental retardation (American Psychiatric Association 1994).

Single photon emission computed tomography of persons with Asperger's syndrome reveals right-hemispheric abnormalities, including right temporal hypoperfusion with a central area of increased perfusion with frontal polar hyperperfusion, generalized right-hemispheric hypoperfusion, and reduced right frontal and occipital perfusion. A smaller right cerebellar hemisphere is seen as well (McKelvey et al. 1995). Dysfunction of frontosubcortical systems is more pronounced in persons with Asperger's syndrome and Tourette syndrome than in persons with Tourette syndrome alone (Berthier et al. 1993). Abnormalities of the corpus callosum have also been found, but this may be a coincidental finding (David et al. 1993).

The point of interest for the neuropsychiatrist is that although the person with Asperger's syndrome may appear to have one or two symptoms of a host of Axis I conditions (obsessive-compulsive disorder, bipolar disorder, schizophrenia spectrum conditions, Tourette syndrome, or panic disorder), treatment based on these diagnoses will not be particularly helpful. Treatment of Asperger's syndrome is primarily educational (though some people also elect to use some medication for intractable anxiety), focused on teaching the person didactically what other people learn intuitively. Explicit descriptions of behavior are likely to be useful for the person; examination and review of videotapes of others' interactions and videotaping of the person's own interactions can be more helpful than attempting to medicate the eccentricities. For example, one man with Asperger's syndrome was romantically attracted to women who wore certain types of eyeglasses. He was thwarted in his efforts to obtain companionship when he would walk up to women who were unknown to him, stating, "You are wearing exactly the right type of eyeglasses. I would like to have sexual intercourse with you." Numerous attempts to treat his "obsessions" and "psychotic beliefs" with medications were not useful, and the side effects were uncomfortable. To achieve his therapeutic goal (romantic companionship), it was necessary to instruct him that people might not necessarily understand the honor that his invitation bestowed and that observing and emulating a different ritual might be more helpful for him (Ryan 1992, 1994a; Wing 1981).

For the Community Psychiatrist

The psychiatrist working in the community setting may face obstacles of ongoing hostility between mental health and developmental disabilities service agencies, tendencies to oversimplify the person with developmental disability and mental health needs, high turnover of relatively untrained direct care staff, and limited availability of specialized consultants. A process of deciding whether the mental health need or the developmental disability is "primary" is artificial, when every indication is that the person requires assistance with all needs, no matter how the paperwork ranks them. Another issue is that of various nonprofessional or professional members of the service team declaring ownership of various areas of information and need and not tolerating discussion by others of parts of that issue. Thus, behavior specialists may not accept ideas from direct care staff or psychiatrists, or direct care staff may feel reluctant to make psychiatric diagnostic speculations. The people who work with the person every day have the most detailed and important information about the individual, yet in some settings are not included in meetings.

Finally, some consultation structures exclude the individual being evaluated from almost all of the process, thus allowing the person pronouncing diagnosis minimal actual time with the individual. Several adjustments to standard procedures may alleviate these difficulties, provide a more useful treatment plan, and ultimately save money. Some community psychiatrists find it useful to require written input from a large selection of direct-care providers well in advance of the consultation. An in-house instrument or one of the standardized instruments (Aman 1991) can be a useful format. The Behavior Pharmacology Clinics of Colorado require completion of a plain-language questionnaire that includes a medical review of systems, psychiatric review of systems, environmental analysis, and functional analysis (Ryan et al. 1991). The community psychiatrist makes a useful investment of time when making consultation visits with the person's entire team in the person's living and work settings. When the psychiatrist insists on team participation in diagnostic assessment and speculation, information flows more freely and outcomes are more favorable (Griffiths 1989; Hurley and Sovner 1989; Szymanski et al. 1991).

Successful community psychiatrists are already well aware that there is nothing particularly mysterious about psychiatric or other medical concepts, other than perhaps the terminology used. The time spent teaching direct-care staff about relevant psychiatric or other medical concepts is quickly repaid when the well-informed staff improve their work on the basis of an improved understanding of the person's situation. The psychiatrist can videotape lectures so that the information can be part of the new staff orientation package. Frequently, direct-care staff can combine medical technology and modern behavioral technology to create innovative approaches. The amount of training and pay is unrelated to success; the amount of support and respect accorded staff is highly correlated to success. In addition, the time the psychiatrist spends listening to in-service training on newer behavioral techniques or other relevant issues is doubly repaid; the didactic information is useful, and the explicit demonstration of respect for other areas of expertise contributes to team cohesion.

Most clinicians discover that the information learned from the developmental disabilities field is useful in all areas of neuropsychiatry (Szymanski et al. 1991). Regular collaborative contact is also important to team cohesion; if there is contact only in association with crises, then the person must always be in crisis to obtain care, and the care becomes much more of an emotional and financial drain to the system. Just as the psychiatrist may need to "humanize" the technical medical information for staff, there may also be a need to "humanize" the individual requiring evaluation to medical consultants in other specialties who may resist working with people with developmental disabilities. When the team is functioning optimally, the care tends to be most effective. The only exceptions are situations in which the team is oriented toward subjugation and control, rather than health and growth. Signs of a well-functioning team are increasing health, growth, and assertiveness of the client being served; positive regard for and inclusion of the person being served; regular meetings that are almost never avoided by any team members; an appreciation of transdisciplinary discussion (the direct-care staffer can speculate on psychiatric issues, the psychologist can propose sensory integration assessment, and so on); and intense curiosity among the team regarding ways to continually go forward. When the team is communicating well, the process of accurate, specific, and comprehensive diagnosis flows easily, as does the process of continuing assessment and refinement of treatment. The community psychiatrist, used to working in respectful collaboration with teams, can often be a leader in facilitating this successful type of process.

Conclusion

Persons with developmental disabilities and mental health needs can be treated successfully in the community. Successful treatments are comprehensive and are developed from ongoing individualized team assessment. Neuropsychiatric issues of particular concern are those related to specific developmental syndromes and point up the importance of understanding neuroanatomical correlates, physical discomfort, and medical comorbidity. Specific diagnoses may also reduce overattribution of symptoms to untreatable causes. Skills common to successful community psychiatrists, such as team collaboration and willingness to work on-site, are important in optimizing success.

References

Aman MG: Assessing psychopathology and behavior problems in persons with mental retardation: a review of available instruments. Report prepared for the National Institute of Mental Health (No ADM 91–1712), Bethesda, MD, 1991

American Association on Mental Retardation: Mental retardation: the new definition. American Association on Mental Retardation Training Institute, 1992

American Psychiatric Association: Diagnostic and Statistical Manual of Mental Disorders, 4th Edition. Washington, DC, American Psychiatric Association, 1994

American Psychiatric Association, Committee on Psychiatric Services for Persons With Mental Retardation and Developmental Disabilities: Psychiatry and Mental Retardation: A Curriculum Guide. Washington, DC, American Psychiatric Press, 1993

Ancill RJ, Juralowicz P: Epidemiology of psychiatric disorders in persons with developmental disabilities referred for evaluation. Psychiatric Services Conference Proceedings. Washington DC, American Psychiatric Association, 1995

Ancill RJ, Holliday S, Higgenbottam J: Schizophrenia: Exploring the Spectrum of Psychosis. Toronto, Wiley, 1994

Balla D, Zigler E: Personality development in retarded persons, in Handbook of Mental Deficiency, Psychological Theory and Research. Edited by Ellis NR. Hillsdale, NJ, Erlbaum, 1979, pp 143–168

Berthier ML, Bayes A, Tolosa ES: Magnetic resonance imaging in patients with concurrent Tourette's disorder and Asperger's syndrome. J Am Acad Child Adolesc Psychiatry 32:633–639, 1993

Bhate MS, Robertson PE, Davison EV, et al: Prader-Willi syndrome with hypothyroidism. Journal of Mental Deficiency Research 33:235–244, 1989

Bialer I: Psychotherapies and other adjustment techniques with the mentally retarded, in Mental Retardation: Appraisal, Education, and Rehabilitation. Edited by Baumeister AA. Chicago, IL, Aldine, 1964, pp 138–180

Bigler E: The neurobiology and neuropsychology of adult learning disorders. Journal of Learning Disabilities 25:488–506, 1992

Blatt B: Exodus From Pandemonium. Boston, MA, Allyn & Bacon, 1970

Blatt B, Kaplan F: Christmas in Purgatory. Boston, MA, Allyn & Bacon, 1966

Bradley EA, Udwin O: Williams' syndrome in adulthood: a case study focusing on psychological and psychiatric aspects. Journal of Mental Deficiency Research 33:175–184, 1989

British Columbia Mental Health Society: Summary of Outreach Services to Persons With Mental Handicap and Mental Illness. Vancouver, British Columbia Mental Health Society, 1992

Brunner RL, Brown EH, Berry HK: Phenylketonuria revisited: treatment of adults with behavioral manifestations. J Inherit Metab Dis 10:171–173, 1987

Carr EG, Robinson S, Palumbo LW: The wrong issue: aversive vs. nonaversive treatment. The right issue: functional vs. nonfunctional treatment, in Perspectives on the Use of Nonaversive and Aversive Interventions for Persons With Developmental Disabilities. Edited by Repp C, Singh NN. New York, Plenum, 1990, pp 361–379

Carter G, Jancar J: Mortality in the mentally handicapped: a 50 year survey in the Stoke Park group of hospitals (1930–1980). Journal of Mental Deficiency Research 27:143–156, 1983

Cassidy SB, Ledbetter DH: Prader-Willi syndrome. Neurol Clin 7:37–53,1989

Charney DS, Deutsch AY, Krystal JH, et al: Psychobiological mechanisms of posttraumatic stress disorder. Arch Gen Psychiatry 50:294–305, 1993

Chen CH, Hsiao KJ: A Chinese classic phenylketonuric manifested as autism. Br J Psychiatry 155:251–253, 1989

Clarke DJ, Waters J, Corbett JA: Adults with Prader-Willi syndrome: abnormalities of sleep and behaviour. J R Soc Med 82:21–24, 1989

Crabbe H: A Guidebook for the Use of Psychotropic Medication in Persons With Mental Illness and Mental Retardation. Report for the State of Connecticut Department of Mental Retardation, Hartford, 1989

Crabbe H: Tardive akathisia in persons with developmental disabilities, in National Association for the Dually Diagnosed Annual Meeting Synopsis. Kingston, NY, National Association for the Dually Diagnosed, 1993

Danks DM, Cotton RGH: Future developments in phenylketonuria. Enzyme 38:296–301, 1987

David AS, Wacharasindhu A, Lishman WA: Severe psychiatric disturbance and abnormalities of the corpus callosum: review and case series. J Neurol Neurosurg Psychiatry 56:85–93, 1993

Declining mortality from Down syndrome—no cause for complacency (editorial). Lancet i:888–889, 1990

Denckla MB: Academic and extracurricular aspects of nonverbal learning disabilities. Psychiatric Annals 21:717–724, 1991

Denckla MB: The child with developmental disabilities grown up: adult residua of childhood disorders. Neurol Clin 11:105–125, 1993

DiMario FJ, Dunham B, Burleson JA, et al: An evaluation of autonomic nervous system function in patients with Prader-Willi syndrome. Pediatrics 93:76–81, 1994

Donnellan AM, LaVigna GW, Negri-Schultz N, et al: Progress Without Punishment. New York, Teachers College Press, 1988

Drugs which cause psychiatric symptoms. Med Lett Drugs Ther 31:113–118, 1989

Duane DD: Dyslexia: neurobiological and behavioral correlates. Psychiatric Annals 21:703–708, 1991

Duffy F, McAnulty G: Neuropsychological heterogeneity and the definition of dyslexia: preliminary evidence for plasticity. Neuropsychologia 28:555–571, 1990

Eaton E, Menolascino F: Psychiatric disorders in the mentally retarded: types, problems, and challenges. Am J Psychiatry 139:1297–1303, 1982

Ebert MH, Schmidt DE, Thompson T, et al: Elevated plasma GABA levels in individuals with either Prader-Willi or Angelman's syndrome. J Neuropsychiatry Clin Neurosci 9:75–80, 1997

Eden GF, VanMeter JW, Rumsey JM, et al: Abnormal processing of visual motion in dyslexia revealed by functional brain imaging. Nature 382:66–69, 1996

Ellenor GL: Reducing irrational antipsychotic polypharmacy prescribing. Hospital Pharmacology 12:369–376, 1977

Fehrenbach AMB, Peterson L: Parental problem-solving skills, stress, and dietary compliance in phenylketonuria. J Consult Clin Psychol 57:237–241, 1989

Fishler K, Azen CG, Henderson R, et al: Psychoeducational findings among children treated for phenylketonuria. American Journal of Mental Deficiency 92:65–73, 1987

Flannery KA, Liederman J: Is there really a syndrome involving the co-occurrence of neurodevelopmental disorder, talent, non-right handedness and immune disorder among children? Cortex 31:503–515, 1995

Freund LS, Reiss AL: Cognitive profiles associated with the fra(X) syndrome in males and females. Am J Med Genet 38:542–547, 1991

Freund LS, Reiss AL, Hagerman R, et al: Chromosome fragility in obligate female carriers of the fragile X chromosome. Arch Gen Psychiatry 49:54–60, 1992

Gadow KD, Kalachnik J: Prevalence and pattern of drug treatment for behavior and seizure disorders of TMR students. American Journal of Mental Deficiency 85:588–595, 1981

Gajar A: Adults with learning disabilities: current and future research priorities. Journal of Learning Disabilities 25:507–519, 1992

Galaburda A: Neurology of developmental dyslexia. Current Opinion in Neurology and Neurosurgery 5:71–76, 1992

Galaburda A: Developmental dyslexia (editorial). Rev Neurol (Paris) 149:1–3, 1993a

Galaburda A: Neuroanatomic basis of developmental dyslexia. Neurol Clin 11: 161–173, 1993b

Galaburda A, Livingstone M: Evidence for a magnocellular defect in developmental dyslexia. Ann N Y Acad Sci 682:70–82, 1993

Galaburda A, Sherman G, Rosen G, et al: Developmental dyslexia: four consecutive patients with cortical anomalies. Ann Neurol 18:222–233, 1985

Galaburda A, Menard M, Rosen G: Evidence for aberrant auditory anatomy in developmental dyslexia. Proc Natl Acad Sci U S A 91:8010–8013, 1994

Gedye A: Recognizing obsessive-compulsive disorder in clients with developmental disabilities. The Habilitative Mental Healthcare Newsletter 11:74–77, 1992

Gedye A: Evidence of serotonergic reduction of self-injurious movements. The Habilitative Mental Healthcare Newsletter 12:53–56, 1993

Goldfeld AE, Mollica RF, Pesavento BH, et al: The physical and psychological sequelae of torture. JAMA 259:2725–2729, 1988

Goldman JJ: Prader-Willi syndrome in two institutionalized older adults. Ment Retard 26:97–102, 1988

Greenswag LR: Adults with Prader-Willi syndrome: a survey of 232 cases. Dev Med Child Neurol 29:145–152, 1987

Gregg N, Hoy C: Coherence: the comprehension and production abilities of college writers who are normally achieving, learning disabled, and underprepared. Journal of Learning Disabilities 22:370–372, 390, 1989

Griffiths D: Quality assurance for behavior interventions. Psychiatric Aspects of Mental Retardation Reviews 8:74–80, 1989

Gualtieri CT, Sovner R: Akathisia and tardive akathisia. Psychiatric Aspects of Mental Retardation Reviews 8:83–88, 1989

Gualtieri CT, Quade D, Hicks RE, et al: Tardive dyskinesia and other clinical consequences of neuroleptic treatment of children and adolescents. Am J Psychiatry 141:20–23, 1984

Habib M, Robichon F, Levrier O, et al: Diverging asymmetries of temporo-parietal cortical areas: a reappraisal of Geschwind/Galaburda theory. Brain Lang 48: 238–258, 1995

Hagerman RJ, Sobesky WE: Psychopathology in fragile X syndrome. Am J Orthopsychiatry 59:142–152, 1989

Harper M, Reid H: Use of restricted diet in the treatment of behaviour disorder in a severely mentally retarded adult female phenylketonuric patient. Journal of Mental Deficiency Research 31:209–212, 1987

Hayes JS, Rarback S, Berry B, et al: Managing PKU: an update. American Journal of Maternal and Child Nursing 12:119–123, 1987

Hellige JB: Babies, bath water, and the chicken's way out. Brain Cogn 26:228–235, 1994

Hewitt KE, Carter G, Jancar J: Ageing in Down's syndrome. Br J Psychiatry 147: 58–62, 1985

Hill BK, Balow EA, Bruininks RH: A national study of prescribed drugs in institutions and community residential facilities for mentally retarded people. Psychopharmacol Bull 21:279–284, 1985

Holm VA, Cassidy SB, Butler MG, et al: Prader-Willi syndrome: consensus diagnostic criteria. Pediatrics 91:398–402, 1993

Hurley AD, Sovner R: Creating behavioral programs: nine principles. Psychiatric Aspects of Mental Retardation Reviews 8:18–22, 1989

Hynd GW, Hall J, Novey ES, et al: Dyslexia and corpus callosum morphology. Arch Neurol 52:32–38, 1995

Intaglia J, Rinck C: Psychoactive drug use in public and community residential facilities for mentally retarded persons. Psychopharmacol Bull 21:268–278, 1985

Ito Y, Teicher MH, Glod CA, et al: Increased prevalence of electrophysiologic abnormalities in children with physiological, physical, and sexual abuse. J Neuropsychiatry Clin Neurosci 5:401–408, 1993

Jones KL: Smith's Recognizable Patterns of Human Malformations, 4th Edition. Philadelphia, PA, WB Saunders, 1988

Jorge RE, Robinson RG, Starkstein SE, et al: Depression and anxiety following traumatic brain injury. J Neuropsychiatry Clin Neurosci 5:369–374, 1993

Kawashima H, Kawano M, Masaki A, et al: Three cases of untreated classical PKU: a report on cataracts and brain calcification. Am J Med Genet 29:89–93, 1988

King BH, DeAntonio C, McCracken JT, et al: Psychiatric consultation in severe and profound mental retardation. Am J Psychiatry 151:1802–1808, 1994

Kleinman A, Eisenberg L, Good B: Culture, illness, and care: clinical lessons from anthropological and cross-cultural research. Ann Intern Med 88:251–258, 1978

Koranyi EK: Mental retardation: medical aspects. Psychiatr Clin North Am 9:635–645, 1986

Krieger D: The Therapeutic Touch: How to Use Your Hands to Help or Heal. New York, Prentice-Hall, 1986

Lalande M, Sinnett D, Glatt K, et al: Fine mapping of the GABA-A subunit gene cluster in chromosome 15q11q13 and assignment of GABRG3 to this region: report of the Second International Workshop of Human Chromosome 15 MAPPING (abstract). Cytogenet Cell Genet 67:17, 1994

LaVigna G, Donnellan A: Alternatives to Punishment: Solving Behavior Problems With Nonaversive Strategies. New York, Irvington, 1986

Ledbetter DH, Greenberg F, Holm VA, et al: Conference report: Second Annual Prader-Willi Syndrome Scientific Conference. Am J Med Genet 28:779–790, 1987

Leonard CM, Voeller KK, Lombardino LJ, et al: Anomalous cerebral structure in dyslexia revealed with magnetic resonance imaging. Arch Neurol 50:461–469, 1993

Lew M, Zaslow-Creme B, Lepler S: Effective consultation with community programs. The Habilitative Mental Healthcare Newsletter 9:65–69, 1990

Ludwig B: The Transdisciplinary Support and Assessment Clinic (TEASC). Summary of a New Outreach Program. University of New Mexico, Albuquerque, NM, 1994

MacMillan DL, Siperstein GN: Conceptual and psychometric concerns about the 1992 AAMR definition of mental retardation. Am J Ment Retard 98:325–335, 1993

Manchester D: Update on Genetics. Presented at the Roundhouse Conference for Children With Disabilities, References From The Children's Hospital, Denver, CO, October 1994

McKelvey JR, Lambert R, Mottron L, et al: Right-hemisphere dysfunction in Asperger's syndrome. J Child Neurol 10:310–314, 1995

McLaughlin M: Bipolar affective disorder in Down's syndrome. Br J Psychiatry 151:116–117, 1987

McNamara P, Flannery KA, Obler LK, et al: Special talents in Geschwind's and Galaburda's theory of cerebral lateralization: an examination in a female population. Int J Neurosci 78:167–176, 1994

McNeil TF, Blennow G, Lundberg L: Congenital malformations and structural developmental anomalies in groups at high risk for psychosis. Am J Psychiatry 149: 57–61, 1992

Menolascino FJ: Mental illness in persons with mental retardation: training and treatment for the 1990s and beyond. The NADD Newsletter 8:1–5, 1991

Miller JF: The developmental asynchrony of language development in children with Down syndrome, in The Psychobiology of Down Syndrome. Edited by Nadel L. Cambridge, MA, MIT Press, 1988, pp 12–46

Munro JD: Epidemiology and extent of mental retardation. Psychiatr Clin North Am 9:591–624, 1986

Newill BH, Goyette CH, Fogarty TW: Diagnosis and assessment of the adult with specific learning disabilities. Journal of Rehabilitation 34–39, 1984

Njiokiktjien C, de Sonneville L, Vaal J: Callosal size in children with learning disabilities. Behav Brain Res 64:213–218, 1994

O'Neill RE, Horner RH, Albin RW, et al: Functional Analysis of Problem Behavior: A Practical Assessment Guide. Sycamore, IL, Sycamore Press, 1990

Owens D, Dawson JC, Losin S: Alzheimer's disease in Down's syndrome. American Journal of Mental Deficiency 75:606–612, 1971

Pieretti M, Zhang F, Fu Y-H, et al: Absence of expression of the FMR 1 gene in fragile X syndrome. Cell 66:817–822, 1991

Polloway EA, Schewel R, Patton JR: Learning disabilities in adulthood: personal perspectives. Journal of Learning Disabilities 25:520–522, 1992

Previc FH: Assessing the legacy of the CBG model. Brain Cogn 26:174–180, 1994

Pueschel SM, Pueschel JK: Biomedical Concerns in Persons With Down Syndrome. Baltimore, MD, Brookes Publishing, 1992

Rademacher J, Caviness VS Jr, Steinmetz H, et al: Topographical variation of the human primary cortices: implications for neuroimaging, brain mapping, and neurobiology. Cereb Cortex 3:313–329, 1993

Reiss AL, Hagerman RJ, Vinogradov S, et al: Psychiatric disability in female carriers of the fragile X syndrome. Arch Gen Psychiatry 45:25–30, 1988

Reiss AL, Freund L, Vinogradov S, et al: Parental inheritance and psychological disability in fragile X females. Am J Hum Genet 45:697–705, 1989

Reiss S, Benson B: Awareness of negative social conditions among mentally retarded, emotionally disturbed outpatients. Am J Psychiatry 141:88–90, 1984

Reiss S, Levitan G, McNally RJ: Emotionally disturbed mentally retarded people: an underserved population. Am Psychol 37:361–367, 1982a

Reiss S, Levitan G, Szysko J: Emotional disturbance and mental retardation: diagnostic overshadowing. American Journal of Mental Deficiency 86:567–574, 1982b

Repp AC, Singh NN, Olinger E, et al: The use of functional analyses to test causes of self-injurious behavior: rationale, current status and future directions. Journal of Mental Deficiency Research 34:95–105, 1990

Resnick TJ, Rapin I: Language disorders in childhood. Psychiatric Annals 21:709–716, 1991

Rodden PJR: Beyond the Skinner box: a values based approach to behavioral intervention, in Handbook of Mental Health Care for Persons With Developmental Disabilities. Edited by Ryan R. Denver, CO, Mariah Press, 1996

Rosen M: In search of the behavioral phenotype: a methodological note. Ment Retard 31:177–178, 1993

Ross CA, McInnis MG, Margolis RL, et al: Genes with triplet repeats: candidate mediators of neuropsychiatric disorder. Trends Neurosci 16:254–160, 1993

Rousseas F, Heitz D, Bian-Calan V, et al: Direct diagnosis by DNA analysis of the fragile-X syndrome of mental retardation. N Engl J Med 325:1673–1681, 1991

Rumsey JM, Casanova M, Mannheim GB, et al: Corpus callosum morphology, as measured with MRI, in dyslexic men. Biol Psychiatry 39:769–775, 1996

Ryan RM: Treatment resistant chronic mental illness: is it Asperger's syndrome? Hospital and Community Psychiatry 43:807–811, 1992

Ryan RM: Tourette syndrome in persons with developmental disabilities: an underdiagnosed condition? National Association for the Dually Diagnosed Conference Synopsis. Kingston, NY, National Association for the Dually Diagnosed, 1993

Ryan RM: Asperger's syndrome. The Habilitative Mental Healthcare Newsletter 13:1–6, 1994a

Ryan RM: Posttraumatic stress disorder in persons with developmental disabilities. Community Ment Health J 30:45–54, 1994b

Ryan RM, Sunada K: Medical evaluation of persons with mental retardation referred for psychiatric assessment. Gen Hosp Psychiatry 19:274–280, 1997

Ryan RM, Sunada K: Medical assessment of persons with developmental disabilities and mental health needs, in The Colorado Handbook: Providing Services to Persons With Developmental Disabilities and Mental Health Needs. Edited by Ryan R. Denver, CO, Colorado Developmental Disabilities Planning Council, 1994, pp 1–176

Ryan RM, Rodden PJR, Sunada K: A model for interdisciplinary on-site evaluation of people who have "dual diagnosis." The NADD Newsletter 8:1–4, 1991

Schaefer GB, Sheth RD, Bodensteiner JB: Cerebral dysgenesis: an overview. Neurol Clin 12:773–788, 1994

Schultz RT, Cho NK, Staib LH, et al: Brain morphology in normal and dyslexic children: the influence of sex and age. Ann Neurol 35:732–742, 1994

Silverthorn KH, Hornak JE: Beneficial effects of exercise on aerobic capacity and body composition in adults with Prader-Willi syndrome. Am J Ment Retard 97:634–638, 1994

Singer R, Irvin J: Human rights review of intrusive behavioral treatment for students with severe handicaps. Exceptional Children 54:46–52, 1987

Smith RC, Davis JM: Behavioral evidence for supersensitivity after chronic administration of haloperidol, clozapine, and thioridazine. Life Sci 19:725–732, 1976

Sobsey D: Violence and Abuse in the Lives of People With Disabilities: The End of Silent Acceptance? Baltimore, MD, Brookes Publishing, 1994

Sovner R, Hurley AD: Ten diagnostic principles for recognizing psychiatric disorders in mentally retarded people. Psychiatric Aspects of Mental Retardation Reviews 8:9–14, 1989

Sovner R, Hurley AD: Assessment tools which facilitate psychiatric evaluations and treatment. The Habilitative Mental Healthcare Newsletter 9:91–98, 1990

Sovner R, Lowry MA: A behavioral methodology for diagnosing affective disorders in individuals with mental retardation. The Habilitative Mental Healthcare Newsletter 7:55–61, 1990

Sovner R, Hurley AD, Labrie R: Is mania incompatible with Down's syndrome? Br J Psychiatry 146:319–320, 1985

Sprague JR, Flannery KB, O'Neill RE: Effective Consultation: Supporting the Implementation of Positive Behavior Support Plans. Report from the University of Oregon, Eugene, OR, 1992

Spreen O: The relationship between learning disability, emotional disorders, and neuropsychology: some results and observations. J Clin Exp Neuropsychol 11:117–140, 1989

Stark JA, Menolascino FJ, Albarelli MH, et al: Mental Retardation and Mental Health: Classification, Diagnosis, Treatment, Services. New York, Springer, 1988

Stavrakaki C, Klein J: Psychotherapies with the mentally retarded. Psychiatr Clin North Am 9:733–743, 1986

Stein DJ, Keating J, Zar HJ, et al: A survey of the phenomenology and pharmacotherapy of compulsive and impulsive-aggressive symptoms in Prader-Willi syndrome. J Neuropsychiatry Clin Neurosci 6:23–29, 1994

Sunada K: Syndromes: do they make a difference? National Association of the Dually Diagnosed 10th Annual Meeting Synopsis. Kingston, NY, National Association of the Dually Diagnosed, 1993

Swaab DF, Purba JS, Hofman MA: Alterations in the hypothalamic paraventricular nucleus and its oxytocin neurons (putative satiety cells) in Prader-Willi syndrome: a study of five cases. J Clin Endocrinol Metab 80:573–579, 1995

Szymanski LS: Psychiatric diagnostic evaluation of mentally retarded individuals. Journal of the American Academy of Child Psychiatry 16:67–87, 1977

Szymanski L, Madow L, Mallory G, et al: Report of the Task Force on Psychiatric Services to Adult Mentally Retarded and Developmentally Disabled Persons. Washington, DC, American Psychiatric Press, 1991

Teicher MH, Glod CA, Surrey J, et al: Early childhood abuse and limbic system ratings in adult psychiatric outpatients. J Neuropsychiatry Clin Neurosci 5:301–306, 1993

Thase ME: The relationship between Down syndrome and Alzheimer's disease, in The Psychobiology of Down Syndrome. Edited by Nadel L. Cambridge, MA, MIT Press, 1988, p 299

Tinnessen FE, Likken A, Hien T, et al: Dyslexia, left-handedness, and immune disorders. Arch Neurol 50:411–416, 1993

Tu J: A survey of psychotropic medication in mental retardation facilities. J Clin Psychiatry 26:125–128, 1979

U.S. Commission on Civil Rights: Medical Discrimination Against Children With Disabilities. Washington, DC, U.S. Commission on Civil Rights, 1989

Voeller KKS: Social-emotional learning disabilities. Psychiatric Annals 21:735–741, 1991

Voeller KKS, Hanson J: Facial affect recognition in children: a comparison of the performance of children with right- and left-hemisphere lesions (abstract). International Neuropsychological Society Programs and Abstracts, 16th Annual Meeting, 36, 1988, pp 3–6

Wagstaff J, Knoll JHM, Fleming J, et al: Localization of the gene encoding the GABA-A receptor beta-3 subunit to the Angelman/Prader-Willi region of human chromosome 15. Am J Hum Genet 49:330–337, 1991

Warren AC, Holroyd S, Folstein MF: Major depression in Down's syndrome. Br J Psychiatry 155:202–205, 1989

Webb TP, Thake AI, Bundey SE, et al: A cytogenetic study of a mentally retarded school-age population with special reference to fragile sites. Journal of Mental Deficiency Research 31:61–71, 1987

Wilson GN: The child with birth defects: medical diagnosis and parental counseling. Resident and Staff Physician 33:96–102, 1987

Wing L: Asperger's syndrome: a clinical account. Psychol Med 11:115–129, 1981

Wolff PH, Gardner J, Lappen J, et al: Variable expression of the fragile X syndrome in heterozygous females of normal intelligence (abstract). Am J Med Genet 30:213–225, 1988

Yu S, Pritchard M, Kremer E, et al: Fragile X genotype characterized by an unstable region of DNA. Science 252:1179–1181, 1991

CHAPTER 10

Neuropsychiatry of Late-Onset Psychosis and Depression

Ira M. Lesser, M.D.
J. Randolph Swartz, M.D.

Over the last decade, interest has increased significantly regarding the psychiatric problems of our older population. This increased interest has been accompanied by specialized evaluation and treatment programs for older patients, more research, and increasing opportunities for training in geriatric psychiatry. Nonetheless, the range of services available for older patients with psychiatric disorders lags behind that available for younger adult patients, particularly in the public health setting. This is troublesome because psychiatric services for the elderly in the public health setting will likely assume increasing importance for several reasons: the increase in the older population; the lengthening of the life-span, with accompanying increase of comorbid medical and psychiatric problems; the decreasing impact of the nuclear family and the increasing isolation of the older population; the economic burdens of living longer on fixed incomes; and the cost of medical and long-term care.

In this chapter, we focus on two major psychiatric problems of the elderly: depression and psychosis. We have learned considerably more about these problems in the last decade, including how their presentation may differ from that in younger patients, the role of medical illness in their etiology, their course, neuroimaging and cognitive evaluation of patients with these disorders, and their treatment. For reasons discussed in this chapter, many such patients will have their care provided in public health settings: acute care public hospitals, longer-term state hospital settings, day hospitals, Veterans Administration hospitals, and nursing homes. We focus our discussion on epidemiology; clinical characteristics; medical, neuroimaging, and cognitive evaluations; and treatment considerations. The overlap of both psychosis and depression in late life with dementia is discussed; dementia is discussed at length in Chapter 4. Comprehensive reviews of these topics can be found in a book edited by Schneider et al. (1994) and a recent volume of the *Schizophrenia Bulletin* edited by Jeste (1993).

Underlying these general principles of care for the older patient is the need to recognize that patients seeking care in the public health setting typically have not had the level of routine medical care available to patients with more resources. This implies that care for the public patient occurs when the illness is more severe and that the patient is likely to have developed comorbid conditions. Added to this are the accompanying problems of poor nutrition, possibility of head trauma, higher rates of drug and alcohol abuse, and social isolation. All these factors make these patients at high risk for the development of chronic illness with considerable morbidity and even mortality.

Epidemiology

Both the absolute number of older persons living and the percentage of the population who are in the older age groups have markedly increased. In 1990, there were over 31 million people over the age of 65 living in the United States, compared with 3 million in 1900. More than 12% of the population is over the age of 65 years (compared with 4% in 1900); estimates are that by the year 2030 those over age 65 years will make up more than 20% of the population. Among those over 65 years, the most rapidly increasing segment comprises those over age 85 (Day 1992; Taueber 1992).

Over the next 50 years, the ethnic composition of the older population also will undergo considerable change. It is estimated that the proportion of nonwhite persons over age 65 years will double, to more than 20%, by 2050. The largest increase will occur among Asians and Pacific Islanders, followed by Hispanics and African Americans (Day 1992). In 1991, 20% of people over age 65 lived below or near the poverty level (U.S. Bureau of the Census 1992); 13% of men and 34% of women lived alone (Saluter 1992). Estimates are that 40% of those over 65 years of age will spend some time in a nursing home, although at any given time only 5% are residing in long-term care facilities (Butler et al. 1991). The risk of living in poverty is associated with increasing age and (nonwhite) ethnicity. Given the statistics above, it seems likely that in the future we will be seeing more of our older population having fewer resources and relying on the public sector for more of their care.

It is well known that the deinstitutionalization process decreased the number of patients residing in state hospitals. Deinstitutionalization affected older as well as younger patients. It was estimated that in 1987 there were more than 20,000 elderly residents of state and county mental hospitals (approximately one-fifth of the total), with costs of their care estimated to be over $1 billion annually (American Psychiatric Association 1993).

In general, psychiatric disorders, with the exception of cognitive decline, decrease in prevalence among the older groups in the population. Multiple epidemiologic studies show this to be true about depression, particularly depression that meets full syndrome criteria. The Epidemiologic Catchment Area (ECA) study reported the 1-year prevalence of major depression in those over 65 years of age to be 0.6% in men and 1.5% in women (Robins and Regier 1991). It has been theorized that depressive symptoms not severe or frequent enough to meet major depression criteria are much more prevalent than the full syndrome of depression in the older population (Blazer 1994; Meyers 1994). Despite the subsyndromal nature of these symptoms, they do cause considerable morbidity and loss of function. Furthermore, depression in the older population often is comorbid with significant medical problems, with such comorbidity adding to diagnostic dilemmas. The rates of depression seen in residents of nursing homes are much higher than those seen in community residents. Prevalence rates for major depression range from 12% to about 33% of residents with no dementia, with approximately an equal number having depression accompanying a dementia (Ames 1990; Katz and Parmelee 1994; Rovner 1993).

Epidemiologic data sets regarding the prevalence of late-life psychoses are difficult to assess because of a number of factors. One difficulty in ascertaining prevalence rates of late-onset disorders is determining age at onset with any degree of accuracy. The population of older patients with psychoses is made up of those who developed the psychosis earlier in their life and those in whom there has been a late onset. Psychotic symptoms can be found in the diagnoses of schizophrenic disorder, delusional disorder, and mood disorder and as part of medical disorders and dementias. Formal diagnostic criteria and changing nomenclature have added to the problem. Given these caveats, it has been estimated that 3% of patients with schizophrenic disorders begin to have symptoms after age 60 years, up to 4% of the older population have some degree of paranoid thinking, and about one-third of patients with Alzheimer's disease or vascular dementia have some psychotic symptoms

(Devanand et al. 1997; Lacro et al. 1993; Levy et al. 1996; Rockwell et al. 1994; Sultzer et al. 1993). Other investigators have reported an even higher incidence. By using operationalized criteria for schizophrenic disorders, Castle and Murray (1993) reported that in 12% of their sample, the onset of a schizophrenic disorder occurred after the age of 64. The prevalence of late-onset psychosis in a specialized geriatric psychiatry inpatient unit has been reported to be 8% (Leuchter and Spar 1985).

Although the actual prevalence rates of depression and psychosis might be low (and there are methodological problems with how these data were obtained), the number of individuals affected is considerable and expected to increase exponentially over the coming decades. Interestingly, because of a variety of medical and economic factors, over the last two decades the diagnoses of older individuals in state hospitals have shifted. In 1972, about 45% of elders in state hospitals received a diagnosis of "organic brain syndrome" (presumably dementias), and 37% received a diagnosis of schizophrenia. In 1987, those with organic brain syndromes had decreased to 29%, and those with schizophrenic disorders increased to 43% (American Psychiatric Association 1993).

Clinical Picture of Late-Onset Depression

The criteria used to diagnose late-onset depression are the same as those used to diagnose depression at the younger ages and are detailed in DSM-IV (American Psychiatric Association 1994). For a diagnosis of major depressive episode (MDE), in addition to the presence of depressed mood (feeling of sadness, being "down" or "blue") expressed or observed by others and/or a marked loss of interest or getting pleasure in usual activities, one must present with four additional symptoms. Many of these symptoms involve physical changes, for example, appetite change with weight gain or loss, sleep disturbance, and fatigue or loss of energy. Because of the high degree of medical illness in the older person, care needs to be taken to assess these symptoms. Are they part of a medical illness, part of a depression, or both?

These symptoms must be present most of the time for a minimum of 2 weeks, must represent a change from previous function, and must cause significant distress or impairment in social, occupational, or other areas of function. For some elderly, this distinction may be difficult if they were not living particularly active lives. The presence of a specific precipitant, though not considered as a diagnostic criterion, is important to elicit for treatment purposes. Older people are more likely to have suffered multiple losses, and the consequence of these losses may well be depression.

The major risk factors for developing depression in older age groups are being a woman, being unmarried (particularly widowed), having stressful life events, lacking a supportive network, and having medical illnesses. In general, data support an increased risk for depression and a poorer prognosis for recovery associated with the following: lower socioeconomic status, lower occupational achievement, childhood deprivations (poverty, sexual assault), widowhood, social isolation, chronic physical illness, chronic financial problems, and being a caregiver to older adults (especially for women). Not all of these apply equally to older depressed patients, but chronic financial and medical problems, widowhood, and social isolation all appear to be serious problems in the older population (George 1994). In addition, being poor leads to many of these adverse consequences. Hence, it would seem that older patients receiving care in public facilities would be most at risk for depression. Unfortunately, few data address this hypothesis.

After the presence of an MDE is established, it is important to ascertain if there are psychotic symptoms. Questions relating to delusional thoughts, particularly somatic delusions, and to auditory hallucinations must be asked. Data conflict regarding whether rates of psychotic depression are higher in late-onset versus earlier-onset depression (Baldwin 1995; Meyers and Greenberg 1986; Nelson et al. 1989).

Although mania relatively rarely has its onset late in life, establishing its presence has important treatment implications. Late onset of mania may more often be associated with brain injury than is mania in younger people (Shulman et al. 1992; Starkstein et al. 1988). This has relevance to the population discussed in this chapter who are at risk for stroke, trauma, tumors, and so forth.

It also is important to establish whether comorbid psychiatric symptoms or diagnoses are present. Alcohol abuse, sedative/hypnotic abuse, and anxiety disorders all can be present with depression. Alcohol abuse is particularly significant and often is overlooked in evaluating older patients. The prevalence rates of alcoholism are related to lower socioeconomic status, less education, and unemployment, all factors present in the population seeking care in public facilities.

Most studies have found few, if any, meaningful clinical differences between young and older patients with depression. Even the much discussed increase in cognitive impairment seen in older depressed patients has been questioned and may relate more to comorbid medical problems seen in the older population than to the depression per se (Caine et al. 1994).

The problem of medical comorbidity is particularly germane to depression in the older population. Not only can medical illness (e.g., hypothyroidism, stroke, Parkinson's disease, viral syndromes) directly produce depression, but reactions to any medical illness can cause or exacerbate a depressive episode. For older patients, using DSM-IV terminology, the diagnosis major depression due to a general medical condition may be difficult to distinguish from major depression. It takes vigilance on the part of clinical personnel, both medical and psychiatric, to keep a high index of suspicion and evaluate patients from both perspectives. Appropriate screening methods are discussed in Chapter 2.

The course and prognosis of late-life depression vary. Clearly, however, chronicity and deterioration are not necessarily the norm. A recent review of studies regarding prognosis found that approximately 60% of patients had recovered from an initial episode of depression and remained well or relapsed at a later date, whereas up to 25% remained continuously ill (Cole and Bellavance 1997). Physical illness, cognitive impairment, and severity of depression were related to poor prognosis. It is important to keep in mind that the suicide rate, particularly in men, continues to rise with advancing age and that older depressed men are at high risk (Meehan et al. 1991).

Clinical Picture of Late-Life Psychosis

A long and rich literature describes the phenomenon of psychosis presenting in the elderly. Much of this literature refers to the entity *late paraphrenia*, which was described by Roth, Kay, and others (Herbert and Jacobson 1967; Kay 1963; Roth 1959). This term was used to describe the condition of older patients who developed delusions of a rather fixed nature, had relative preservation of personality, and did not necessarily suffer clinical deterioration. Throughout this literature and continuing into the present are references that psychosis in the older population may have more admixtures of affective illness and that in a significant number of cases the psychosis progresses to deteriorating cognitive illness.

Using more modern terminology, investigators have compared the clinical characteristics of patients with early- and late-onset schizophrenia. In general, the earlier clinical descriptions have been corroborated (Harris and Jeste 1988; Howard et al. 1993; Jeste et al. 1995; Pearlson et al. 1989). The patients with schizophrenia of late onset had primary delusions (usually of a paranoid flavor); they may or may not have had hallucinations. There was preservation of personality function, and the patients demonstrated less formal thought disorder and negative symptoms than seen in patients with schizophrenia of early onset. Throughout this literature is the suggestion that patients with late-onset schizophrenia have more sensory deficits (hearing, visual) compared with age-matched patients with schizophrenia of earlier onset (reviewed by Prager and Jeste 1993).

In sum, late-life schizophrenia and schizophrenia of early onset, although in some ways clinically different, are similar enough that the same criteria are used for formal diagnosis. Despite this, classification of the late-onset psychoses remains somewhat unclear, with different terms often used interchangeably (Almeida et al. 1992; Flint et al. 1991; Munro 1991; Riecher-Rössler et al. 1995).

As is the case with depression, many medical illnesses, medications, and drug-drug interactions can cause psychotic behavior. Such behavior may or may not occur along with a change in consciousness; if it does, a diagnosis of delirium should be considered. Prevalent conditions that can lead to psychosis in the older population include polypharmacy, which occurs commonly; toxic reactions to what appear to be normal dosages of drugs (but in reality are much too high for the older patient, whose metabolism of drugs often is slowed); confusional states with psychotic features accompanying medical hospitalization; electrolyte imbalances; and poor oxygenation secondary to respiratory conditions or anemia. All of these are important factors to consider in the differential diagnosis of new-onset psychosis.

The older literature painted a bleak picture of the prognosis of patients with late-life psychosis. However, good controlled studies performed in the era of vigorous medication usage and psychosocial interventions have been rare. Hymas et al. (1989) reported that on follow-up, no patient in their sample of 42 patients with "late paraphrenia" required long-term hospitalization, with about 60% being relatively symptom-free. However, almost one-half showed a decline in cognitive performance, and a large number of patients also demonstrated motor abnormalities. More recently, it has been shown that even if there is not a continual downward course, psychosis in the older population has a substantial impact on health-related quality of life (Patterson et al. 1996).

Differential Diagnosis From Medical Illnesses and Cognitive Disorders

The distinction of both late-onset depression and late-life psychosis from degenerative dementias and other neurological diseases often is blurred. Clarification of these diagnoses is crucial to public sector institutions, particularly state hospitals and nursing homes, where the care for patients with chronic dementias often occurs. There is no need to institutionalize all older patients who present with cognitive decline. Some older patients may suffer from new-onset depression or psychosis and could potentially respond to antidepressants or antipsychotics. These patients possibly could continue leading healthy lives in the community. Although some who initially present with depression or psychosis ultimately do deteriorate to more severe dementia, even these patients may be responsive to medications for a limited time, allowing them more independent functioning in the community and a higher quality of life. Thus, it is in the best interests of the individual patient as well as the publicly funded facility to clarify as much as possible the diagnosis and potential treatments in either inpatient or outpatient settings.

Degenerative cortical dementias, such as Alzheimer's disease or frontotemporal degeneration, can present with depression and/or psychosis as an early symptom. Estimates for the prevalence of depression among Alzheimer's disease patients range from 10% to 50% depending on the stringency of the criteria (Bungener et al. 1996; Cummings and Victoroff 1990; Devanand et al. 1997; Forsell et al. 1993). In frontotemporal degeneration, the depression may occur even in the absence of memory impairment and be the only obvious symptom for months or even years (Miller et al. 1991a, 1994). Frontal lobe injury may lead to states of apathy and withdrawal that mimic depression; if the degenerative process begins frontally, these may be the only symptoms for a period of time.

Degenerative dementias also can present with psychosis as an early manifestation (Cummings and Victoroff 1990; Hymas et al. 1989; Lesser et al. 1989). Cummings and Victoroff (1990) reported that delusions occur in about 50% of Alzheimer's disease patients, whereas hallucinations are present in up to 28% of these patients. A somewhat fluctuating course, in which psychiatric symptoms may appear at various stages of the illness, seems to be the most common pattern, with several studies reporting that the most prevalent noncognitive symptoms in patients with Alzheimer's disease were misidentification, wandering, and agitation (Devanand et al. 1997; Levy et al. 1996). We have reported results from a preliminary study that indicate that attention to the types and patterns of noncognitive behavioral manifestations may actually help in classifying the type of dementia that a patient has (Swartz et al. 1997). Estimates of the percentage of patients with late-life psychosis who go on to develop dementia have ranged from 37% (Holden 1987) to 67% (Craig and Bregman 1988).

Subcortical dementias, such as Parkinson's disease and Huntington's disease, also can present with depression. About 50% of patients with Parkinson's disease will also have a depression some time during the course of their illness (Dooneief et al. 1992; Mayeux 1982); this often is characterized by psychomotor retardation and cognitive slowing (*bradyphrenia*). Interestingly, depression is already present in about one-third of Parkinson's disease patients on diagnosis. The depression of Parkinson's disease is usually mild to moderate, with suicide occurring rarely. Although there are suggestions that the depression is not a reaction to the motor symptoms but a component of the illness itself related to disorders of neurotransmission, this is not entirely clear (Gotham et al. 1986; Mayeux 1982). In comparison, psychosis is rare in Parkinson's disease. Psychotic symptoms, if present, usually are a side effect of medications (e.g., L-dopa, bromocriptine) that are used to treat Parkinson's disease and that have dopamine agonist properties. Visual hallucinations, occurring with a prevalence of 20%, are the most common of the medication-induced psychotic side effects. Delusions occur with all types of medication used to treat Parkinson's disease, with a reported prevalence ranging from 3% to 30%. These delusions are rarely associated with disordered thought processes and are most likely to occur in older Parkinson's disease patients with an accompanying dementia. Medication-induced psychosis among patients with Parkinson's disease may respond well to the novel antipsychotic clozapine without a worsening of parkinsonism (Koller and Megaffin, 1994); this also may be true for risperidone and olanzapine. Huntington's disease often presents with personality and behavioral changes, including irritability, apathy, depression, mood lability, decreased work performance, violence, and impulsive behavior. Over one-third of Huntington's disease patients suffer from an affective disorder (Wojcieszek and Lang 1994), with depression the most common. Mania develops in about 10% of Huntington's disease patients. Suicide in not uncommon, with one study reporting that 25% of Huntington's disease patients attempt suicide at least once, and suicide accounted for 5% of all deaths among these patients (Farrer 1986). Psychosis is rare among Huntington's disease patients.

Conversely, major depression can present with real cognitive deficits that may or may not resolve after successful treatment of the depression. Cognitive deficits associated with depression have been referred to by various names, including pseudodementia (Kiloh 1961), dementia syndrome of depression (Folstein and McHugh 1978), depression-induced organic mental disorder (McAllister 1983), and depression-related cognitive dysfunction (Stoudemire et al. 1989). The results of neuropsychological testing in patients with late-life depression have been inconsistent; they have included mildly impaired naming; impaired attention and immediate memory but intact retention of new material; normal primacy effects on memory tasks; normal learning curve on list learning tasks; normal retrieval and recognition of material; and intact visuospatial processing (Boone et al. 1995; Nussbaum 1994). The boundaries between dementia and pseudodementia are not as clearly defined as was once thought, and the entire concept of pseudodementia has been called into question. Some investigators believe that the major contributor to cognitive decline in older depressed patients is comorbid medical illness or an early stage of a degenerative dementia (Caine et al. 1993; Lesser et al. 1996; Nussbaum et al. 1995). Evidence suggests that when depression is accompanied by severe cognitive decline, even if the depression improves, a large number of these patients go on to develop dementia (Alexopoulos et al. 1993). Furthermore, it has been reported that patients with Alzheimer's disease and concomitant depression were more likely to have had previous episodes of major depression earlier in their lives (Zubenko et al. 1996).

Both late-life depression and psychosis can be a manifestation of other neurological disorders. Common conditions that also should be considered include stroke, vascular dementia, and head trauma. The poststroke depression syndrome is a common phenomenon, particularly following strokes of the frontal lobes (perhaps more commonly left-sided than right-sided) (House 1996; Morris et al. 1996; Robinson et al. 1984). As noted above, the late onset of mania is particularly rare and, when it occurs, may be related to structural brain pathology (Shulman et al. 1992; Starkstein et al. 1988). The prevalence of depression in patients with vascular dementia has been reported to be 19%–27% (Fischer et al. 1990). Depressive symptoms are not uncommon following traumatic brain injury, with the prevalence of depression increasing with severity of the injury (Silver et al. 1992).

Non-neurological conditions associated with depression also should be considered. Cardiovascular disease increases mortality among depressed older patients. One prospective study found that 75% of older depressed patients who were deceased after 1 year had had some type of cardiovascular disease (Rabins et al. 1985). Endocrine disorders, such as hypothyroidism, Cushing's disease, and Addison's disease, also can result in depression. Electrolyte imbalances (such as hypocalcemia, hypercalcemia, and hypoglycemia), as well as vitamin B_{12} and folate deficiencies, also are associated with depression.

Evaluation

Given what has been said thus far in this chapter, it is clear that a thorough evaluation is needed to clarify a patient's diagnosis before decisions regarding treatment and placement are made. Although no guidelines have been studied from a cost-effectiveness perspective, we outline a diagnostic workup that, in our clinical experience, is both comprehensive and practical (Table 10–1).

A detailed history should address issues pertinent to the psychiatric history of depression (e.g., any history of depression, suicide attempts, family history of mood disorder, and feelings of guilt/worthlessness/suicide) and psychosis (e.g., history of early-onset psychosis, visual or auditory impairment, family history of schizophrenia), and a good medical history that includes medical risk factors and medications should be performed. A mental status examination should include questions relating to mood; interest in activities; abnormal perceptions or unusual beliefs, with specific questions relating to auditory and visual hallucinations; and fears or suspiciousness. Information from collateral sources is crucial to supplement the direct examination of the patient. The Mini-Mental State Exam (Folstein et al. 1975) also is helpful in identifying cognitive deficits, particularly of Alzheimer's disease. A careful physical examination, including full neurological testing and evaluation of movement disorders, should be conducted. Laboratory tests should include complete blood count, electrolytes, glucose, calcium, magnesium, liver and renal panels, vitamin B_{12} and folate, thyroid function tests (at least a thyroid-stimulating hormone [TSH] test), fluorescein treponema an-

---

TABLE 10–1. Suggested workup for late-life depression and psychosis

Tests all patients should receive
  In-depth psychiatric history
  In-depth medical history (including medication history)
  Physical and neurological examination
  Screening test for dementia
  Assessment of functional capacities
  Complete blood count
  Electrolytes, calcium, glucose, liver, and renal panels
  FTA
  Thyroid function tests (if depressed)
  Vitamin B_{12} and folate (if depressed)
  Electrocardiogram
  CT or MRI
Tests to consider if certain conditions are present
  Comprehensive neuropsychological evaluation
  Lumbar puncture
  Electroencephalogram

Note. CT = computed tomography; FTA = fluorescent treponema antibody (test); MRI = magnetic resonance imaging.

tibody test (FTA), urinalysis, chest X ray, and electrocardiogram; HIV testing should be considered depending on the clinical situation. Lumbar puncture may also be included if there is any concern about infection.

Neuroimaging tests play an increasingly important role in clarifying diagnosis. Structural imaging (computed tomography [CT], magnetic resonance imaging [MRI]) and functional imaging (single photon emission computed tomography [SPECT], positron-emission tomography [PET]) are now often routinely included in a complete workup of the older patient in many academic medical centers. Their use, however, in public facilities is more limited by availability and cost.

Structural neuroimaging reveals helpful information regarding abnormalities of brain structure, atrophy, ventricle-to-brain ratio (VBR), and subcortical white-matter hyperintensities (WMH) (best seen on T2-weighted images from MRI). A number of studies have reported that a substantial subgroup of patients with late-life psychosis and depression demonstrate abnormalities on CT or MRI consisting of tumors, other mass lesions, and strokes (Breitner et al. 1990; Coffey et al. 1990; Galasko et al. 1988; Howard et al. 1994; Lesser et al. 1991, 1992; Miller and Lesser 1988; Miller et al. 1986, 1991b). For example, Miller et al. (1986) described five patients with the onset of a schizophrenia-like picture after the age of 60. Study with CT showed that three had areas of brain infarction and one had evidence of normal pressure hydrocephalus. This study emphasized the need to perform careful neuroimaging studies in patients with late-onset psychotic symptoms. In many of the reported cases, abnormalities were in brain areas that did not cause any focal neurological symptoms or did not interfere with speech. Howard et al. (1994) showed that patients with late onset of psychosis had larger lateral and third ventricle volumes than control subjects. Although the causal nature of these abnormalities in the production of the behavior cannot be proven with certainty, the likelihood that they were incidental findings in such large numbers seems remote (Cummings 1992; Lesser et al. 1993a; Miller et al. 1986).

An interesting, yet somewhat nonspecific, finding has been that patients with late-life psychiatric disorders have greater amounts of WMH, seen on MRI, than age-matched control subjects (Baldwin 1993; Breitner et al. 1990; Coffey et al. 1990; Keshavan et al. 1996; Lesser et al. 1991, 1992, 1993a, 1993b, 1996; Miller and Lesser 1988; Miller et al. 1991b). Our group (Miller et al. 1991b) reported that in 24 patients with late-onset psychosis in whom WMH were quantified, the mean computer-measured amount of temporal lobe WMH was six times greater in patients than in controls and about four times greater in frontal and occipital areas. Breitner et al. (1990) noted that all 8 late-onset paranoid patients studied had significant WMH, and 7 of 8 also had other vascular lesions in either the pons or basal ganglia. Flint et al. (1991) reported CT data on 16 patients diagnosed as having either late-onset paranoia or paraphrenia. Five of 16 patients had clinically unsuspected ("silent") cerebral infarction: all 5 had subcortical (mostly basal ganglia) or frontal lobe infarctions, with 1 patient also having a parieto-occipital infarct. Lesser et al. (1992) found that 6 of 12 patients with psychotic disorder not otherwise specified (NOS) showed large and confluent areas of WMH. Keshavan et al. (1996) found that older schizophrenic patients showed more WMH (particularly in the right posterior region) than did either late-life depressed patients or control subjects. On the other hand, Krull et al. (1991) did not find an increased mean amount of white-matter disease in 9 late-onset schizophrenic patients compared with control subjects; as the authors noted, this number of subjects may be too small to detect a subgroup with more white matter disease.

Similarly, for both late-onset psychotic (Lesser et al. 1991) and nonpsychotic depressed patients (Coffey et al. 1990; Kumar et al. 1997; Lesser et al. 1996), significantly greater numbers of these patients have WMH when compared with control subjects. Coffey et al. reported that all 51 depressed patients over the age of 60 who had been referred for electroconvulsive therapy (ECT) had some WMH on MRI. All had periventricular WMH, and 86% had deep WMH. Furthermore, the WMH frequently were associated with other structural brain abnormalities (e.g., basal ganglia and thalamic lesions, cortical atrophy). Eighty percent of the patients developed their depression after the age of 60, and all patients with "severe" periventricular or deep WMH had onset of depression after 60. We, too, have noted that patients with the later onset of depression have more WMH than patients with an earlier onset. This association of WMH and late-life depression has recently been reviewed, with increasing attention being paid to comorbid cerebrovascular disease as an additional risk factor (Baldwin 1993; Greenwald et al. 1996; Hickie et al. 1995; Kumar et al. 1997; O'Brien et al. 1996; Salloway et al. 1996).

The prevalence, distribution, pathology, and significance of WMH are not clearly defined. Bradley et al. (1984) estimated that up to 30% of elderly patients had white-matter abnormalities on MRI. Our own data (Boone et al. 1992) suggest that although approximately 25% of healthy older patients have some WMH, only approximately 6% have extensive involvement. This is in contrast to the studies noted above, which showed a significantly higher prevalence of large WMH in patient groups. The contribution that both atrophy and increasing medical burden have in the development of WMH has recently been stressed (Kumar et al. 1997); this may have particular relevance for patients in the public health setting, who are known to have increased medical comorbidities. This relationship between vascular-related medical illness and depression has led to proposals to denote an entity of "vascular depression" (Alexopoulos et al. 1997; Krishnan et al. 1997).

These white-matter changes may be secondary to disseminated atherosclerosis and in some cases may represent small white-matter infarctions. At postmortem examinations, large confluent areas of WMH demonstrated by MRI showed large areas of myelin pallor with sparing of U fibers. Microscopically, these lesions demonstrated vacuolization and glial cell loss. The etiology for the large WMH was hypothesized to be oligodendrocyte injury from leakage of serum proteins into white matter from brain capillaries; this could have been the result of hypertension (Munoz et al. 1993). In several studies, hypertension has been shown to be an important risk factor in the development of WMH. Conversely, the multiple small patchy areas of hyperintensity may represent dilated Virchow-Robin spaces (spaces surrounding blood vessels in the brain).

The significance of WMH has been debated. Some suggest that WMH are asymptomatic, whereas others state that they correlate with impaired cognition or dementia or are associated with psychiatric disorders. As noted, in cross-sectional studies, investigators have described associations between WMH, cortical atrophy, and depression, particularly in patients with late-onset depression. We have reported what we believe to be the only longitudinal study of one patient who initially was studied as a control subject 2 years before the onset of depression and then studied a second time when he experienced his first MDE. In the course of these 2 years, and temporally coincident with the onset of his depression, his total amount of WMH had more than doubled (Lesser et al. 1993a). This may indicate a vascular etiology in some cases of new-onset depression in older patients, as more recently suggested by others (Alexopoulos et al. 1997; Krishnan et al. 1997).

Although the association of WMH with late-life psychiatric disorders is fairly well established, our understanding of its significance and whether it has any relationship to treatment outcome is not clear. Because there is overlap between patients and control subjects, and because many patients do not show WMH, it is not useful to assess WMH as a screening diagnostic test. We hypothesize that WMH would be increased in patients from lower socioeconomic groups because of the lack of adequate medical care during their lifetime. Studies are currently under way to assess whether WMH affect response to treatment. Interestingly, there are preliminary data to suggest that WMH are associated with worse performance on both instrumental and physical activities of daily living (Cahn et al. 1996), suggesting that their presence may not be benign. Irrespective of the use of structural imaging to assess WMH, we believe that its use is justified for all older patients presenting for the first time with a change in behavior severe enough to meet criteria for a depression or psychosis. These studies would evaluate for mass lesions, strokes, and degree of atrophy and serve as a baseline for future studies if the clinical condition deteriorates.

Functional neuroimaging is complementary to the structural imaging described above. It often shows abnormalities when MRI is normal (Miller et al. 1992). Studies of cerebral blood flow (CBF) may be particularly helpful in distinguishing among different diagnoses of dementia. Blood flow studies in Alzheimer's disease, for example, often reveal a pattern of parietal and posterotemporal hypoperfusion, whereas in frontotemporal degeneration the pattern is of frontotemporal and anterotemporal hypoperfusion (Jagust et al. 1989; Miller et al. 1994). However, there is not absolute specificity in these patterns. Similar patterns also can be found among patients with late-onset depression and psychosis, although the CBF declines seen among our patients with frontotemporal degeneration seem to be more severe compared with the CBF changes seen among our nondemented depressed and psychotic patients. Careful comparisons of the frontotemporal CBF changes displayed by these conditions would be helpful to establish the sensitivity and specificity of these CBF changes.

Our evaluation of 20 older patients presenting with late-life psychosis showed 15 abnormal SPECT scans, most commonly frontotemporal hypoperfusion (Miller et al. 1992). In comparison, 26 of 30 age-matched control subjects had normal SPECT scans. This group of patients also had a higher prevalence of large WMH areas (18%) compared with age-matched control subjects (6%). Among other patients whom we studied with SPECT, we identified a pattern of right frontotemporal hypoperfusion in patients who presented with psychosis, compulsions, and behavioral disinhibition (Miller et al. 1993). Their Mini-Mental State Exam results were not necessarily in the range indicative of dementia, although tests such as word generation and formal memory testing typically indicated impairment. However, on follow-up, a much more marked global dementia was apparent. Indeed, our longitudinal studies of patients with late-life psychosis have shown that significant numbers of these patients presenting with minimal cognitive deficits but with abnormal CBF eventually develop a degenerative dementia (Lesser et al. 1989; Miller et al. 1991a, 1991b). Not all patients show this type of deterioration, and this suggests heterogeneous etiologies for the late-life psychosis presentation.

Our SPECT studies of patients with late-life depression have shown decreased global CBF, with regional hypoperfusion in the frontal (right more severe than left) and temporal lobes (Lesser et al. 1994). The finding of reduced CBF in the frontal regions has been seen by other groups as well, though not necessarily with the lateralized findings that we reported (Bench et al. 1995; Mayberg 1994; Vasile et al. 1996). We and others also have found more significant CBF declines among older depressed men than those found among women. Once again, however, the significance of this finding and the predictive value of a SPECT scan in determining a course of treatment or a prognosis have not been established. Because of cost and practical considerations and the lack of specificity of these studies, we do not recommend functional imaging as a routine part of the evaluation of these patients.

A third neuroimaging technology, functional MRI, has been developed recently and could potentially become more desirable than either PET or SPECT. Functional MRI can measure CBF by producing images of hemoglobin as it circulates through the brain. This technology is becoming increasingly available, but it is not currently routinely used in the public health setting.

Neuropsychological testing can be helpful in clarifying syndromes that are associated with specific profiles of test impairment. The typical profile of deficits in Alzheimer's disease shows impaired recent memory; intrusion errors on list learning tasks; poor performance on memory recognition and retention measures; impaired naming; visuospatial processing deficits; general intellectual decline; apraxia; and agnosia (in the advanced stage). The profile for frontotemporal dementia (FLD) includes executive functioning deficits (perseveration, impaired planning, stimulus boundedness, impaired synthesis, impaired mental flexibility); reduced fluency (verbal and nonverbal); impaired insight; impaired selective attention; and relatively preserved memory. These profiles, though not absolutely specific for any given condition, are in contrast to the deficits described above for depression and may be of help in the differential diagnosis of these conditions. As mentioned above, patterns of behavioral abnormalities may augment the information from neuropsychological testing to aid in the differential diagnosis (Swartz et al. 1997). Patients with subcortical dementias such as those associated with Parkinson's disease and Huntington's disease present with psychomotor slowing, prominent memory impairment, speech or motor-system difficulties, impaired concept formation and mental flexibility, impaired insight, and depression. Patients with vascular dementia present with a "patchy" deficit pattern depending on the location of infarcts (may be lateralized) and general intellectual decline over time with a stepwise decline in cognitive functioning (Lovell and Nussbaum 1994).

Of particular importance in the evaluation of elderly individuals, particularly the frail elderly, is the assessment of skills of daily living. This evaluation of functional capacity to manage money, cook, and take care of grooming and medical needs (including taking medication) is crucial if any independent living is planned. Although we cannot discuss evaluation and treatment of nursing home residents in any detail, it is crucial to understand the magnitude of the problem of disability in the elderly and the importance of assessing its causes. The estimates of syndromal depression among nursing home residents vary from 12% to 22%, with an additional 15%–30% having subsyndromal but significant depressive symptomatology. For psychosis or other severe behavioral disturbances, the rates are around 50% (Emerson Lombardo et al. 1996). Barriers to effective recognition of these problems include a shortage of mental health professionals working in these settings, lack of training and knowledge of staff, and difficulty with reimbursements, which, in turn, leads to having few well-trained geriatric psychiatrists working in nursing homes. Because the population of nursing home residents is expected to increase over the next decades, this is an important area to which resources need to be channeled.

Treatment of Late-Life Depression and Psychosis: Public Health Setting Issues

Complete clinical reviews of pharmacological treatments of these disorders are available elsewhere (Hay et al. 1997; Jeste et al. 1996; Lacro et al. 1996; Preskorn 1993; Salzman 1998); they are not repeated here. Rather, we review some basic concerns regarding pharmacological treatment and raise some questions particularly germane to the public health setting. As detailed above, a complete medical evaluation and assessment of medication side effects and interactions must precede pharmacological treatment of these disorders. Clinicians should keep in mind the decline in liver functioning and decrease in albumin that accompany the aging process. Thus, initial doses for treating older patients should be decreased by about 50% below those suggested for younger adults. In addition, doses should be increased more gradually. The increase in half-life will prolong the time needed to reach steady-state in the blood, potentially delaying clinical response. Another issue is the increased sensitivity of older patients to anticholinergic and antiadrenergic side effects. Older patients are extremely sensitive to anticholinergic delirium, constipation, and urinary retention. They also are highly susceptible to falls resulting from orthostatic hypotension and are at increased risk to develop tardive dyskinesia and parkinsonism. Thus, although one need not deny medications to older patients, considerable care should be used in prescribing and monitoring the use of medications (Salzman 1998).

The following specific issues need to be considered when addressing questions of pharmacoeconomics in the public mental health system. Newer medications for treatment of depression (e.g., selective serotonin reuptake inhibitors [SSRIs], bupropion, nefazodone, venlafaxine) and psychosis (clozapine, olanzapine, risperidone, quetiapine) have side-effect profiles that are particularly attractive when treating older patients, but they are more expensive than older medications of the same class. SSRIs have much lower anticholinergic and antiadrenergic side effects compared with tricyclic antidepressants (especially the tertiary amines). Within the group of SSRIs, sertraline and paroxetine have half-lives of only about 1 day, compared with about 1 week for fluoxetine, and this allows them to be cleared from the body more rapidly. Such rapid clearance may be helpful in clinical care of older patients. The role that the cytochrome P450 enzyme system has in mediating metabolism and drug interactions in older patients has recently been discussed (Nemeroff et al. 1996; Preskorn 1993; Riesenman 1995). In vitro studies have shown that some SSRIs and other psychotropics are potent inhibitors of the hepatic isoenzyme p450 2D6, whereas others inhibit 3/4A. Each of these enzymes also metabolizes other compounds, so use of an SSRI may lead to toxic interactions when the patient is also taking another medication metabolized through the same enzyme system. For the medically ill depressed patient who is prescribed multiple medications, awareness of these potential drug interactions is necessary.

The treatment of serious depressions and/or delusional depression in the older patient often is difficult because of the patient's inability to tolerate medications or, in the case of delusional depression, the combination of antidepressants and antipsychotics. In some of these cases, ECT may be the treatment of choice. Despite the negative publicity—and, in some states, legislative action against it—ECT remains a viable and effective treatment modality for these conditions. Newer methods of administering ECT lead to less memory impairment, and in some cases outpatient ECT can be accomplished.

Much has been written on the use of antipsychotics in older patients, although less on the use of novel antipsychotics in this population (Jeste et al. 1996; Lacro et al. 1996). What is new is that recently available novel antipsychotics such as risperidone and olanzapine have been shown to be effective and, in some populations, to have a broader spectrum of activity (e.g., on negative symptoms) compared with that of the older agents. The newer agents also have significantly less anticholinergic effects than do either conventional low-potency antipsychotics or the atypical antipsychotic agent clozapine. Clinically, risperidone has virtually no anticholinergic effects, whereas olanzapine has mild ones (Casey 1997). Both are α-adrenergic antagonists, resulting in a risk of orthostatic hypotension. This risk may be somewhat higher in older patients because of their increased sensitivity to orthostasis.

Risperidone may be less likely to cause extrapyramidal symptoms (e.g., parkinsonism) in some patients than are the conventional high-potency antipsychotics. In addition, switching from a traditional antipsychotic to risperidone may be associated with a decline in tardive dyskinesia severity (Chouinard et al. 1993). Olanzapine and clozapine may be associated with even lower risks of extrapyramidal symptoms or tardive dyskinesia than is risperidone (Casey 1997). In spite of encouraging early studies, it remains unknown whether risperidone or olanzapine will produce tardive dyskinesia after long-term use.

Tardive dyskinesia is of particular concern when treating older patients because of the increased risk associated with increasing age. Tardive dyskinesia must be distinguished from other movement disorder causes, such as schizophrenia, Huntington's disease, basal ganglia infarcts, dyskinesias resulting from medications, spontaneous dyskinesias, dentures that cause oral dyskinesias, and cerebellar vermis lesions. Although the choreoathetoid movements of tardive dyskinesia are similar to those of Huntington's disease, tardive dyskinesia is more likely to involve oral movements, truncal rocking, stereotyped movements, or marching in place (Wojcieszek and Lang 1994). The problem of tardive dyskinesia is comprehensively discussed in Chapter 12.

Many questions regarding the use of these new medications in the public health setting remain unanswered. Despite equal effectiveness of the old and new agents, will an improved side-effect profile translate into improved medication compliance and improved treatment response? If treatment response improves, would this translate into decreased hospitalizations? If so, would the money saved on decreased inpatient admissions justify the increased cost of these new medications? Does an improved side-effect profile on its own justify public funding for significantly more expensive medications? And finally, do ageist attitudes translate into reluctance to use these expensive treatments in the older public patient? Preliminary data comparing the overall costs of treatment (including direct and indirect costs, rehospitalizations, etc.) of the newer versus older medications have shown some advantages to the newer medications; these studies have not been done in older patients or in the public health setting.

Psychosocial therapies are essential elements of a comprehensive treatment plan in the care of patients with late-life depression and psychoses. These therapies, such as individual supportive or cognitive-behavioral therapy, group therapy for patients as well as caregivers, and family therapy, may help lower relapse rates and improve patients' social adjustment outside the hospital. Therapists treating patients with late-onset depression often focus on issues of lost loved ones, loss of health, and loneliness. Therapy for patients with late-life psychosis often focuses on socialization issues and problem solving for tasks of daily living. Consideration must be given to issues such as social isolation, proper nutrition, transportation, activity groups, and finances. The treatment team must take an active role in addressing these concerns and implementing action plans.

Conclusion and Suggestions

There are significant barriers to providing optimal care to older patients with mood and psychotic disorders. Among these are barriers that exist in relation to all older patients: ageism and feelings of hopelessness on the part of providers; lack of training of providers; lack of resources, including a lack of range of services; and economic disincentives. When older patients present with more medically understandable symptoms such as memory loss, the families and caregivers may find the symptoms "more acceptable," the symptoms may be more easily recognized as an illness, and the patients may be more likely to receive adequate medical evaluation than when the behavior is disruptive, frightening, or dangerous (to the patient or to the family). Receiving an appropriate and comprehensive evaluation when these latter behaviors are the presenting ones often is difficult.

When patients are brought to mental health professionals, broad-based knowledge needed to evaluate the medical problems can be lacking; conversely, primary care providers may not grasp that depression and psychosis can begin late in life and are treatable disorders. This all points to the need for a multidisciplinary approach to the treatment of these patients. Such an approach may present problems in traditional public mental health settings, such as state hospitals, where the medical care may not be adequate. A typical way this has been handled is to transfer patients to more acute care facilities for medical problems, but this interrupts continuity of care.

A task force of the American Psychiatric Association (1993) made recommendations regarding the care of older patients in state hospitals. Among the many recommendations were establishment of linkages between state hospitals and academic medical centers, suggestions for recruitment and training of staffs, and establishment of a geriatric assessment team or another similar model to better integrate medical and psychiatric approaches. We are in agreement with these recommendations. Similar ideas could be implemented for the care given to these patients in general hospital psychiatric wards or other public health settings. Specialists in geriatric psychiatry and/or in geriatric medicine should be consultants if a dedicated geriatric ward is not feasible. Other social issues regarding treatment of these patients include improved initial access to the public mental health system, establishment of continuity of care between inpatient and outpatient services, and access to a greater range of innovative services.

We further believe that the technology and assessment strategies often used with younger patients need to be available to older patients as well. This includes access to neuroimaging evaluations when appropriate. The question of cost always arises when one suggests the use of these technologies. It is our opinion that all patients who present with depression or psychosis should have the benefit of CT or MRI to rule out structural brain disease. The possibility of finding a mass lesion, tumor, or stroke is significant enough and might drastically affect the choice of a treatment plan. The use of blood flow studies (PET or SPECT) is not justified on a routine basis, although these can be helpful in trying to differentiate between frontal lobe degenerations and other causes of behavioral and cognitive impairment and might be used in those patients who are treatment refractory. Neuropsychological testing and evaluation of activities of daily living and skills are both extremely helpful as part of comprehensive treatment planning. Again, the circumstances of the patient will dictate how much in-depth evaluation of cognition is necessary. At the very least, a brief but formal assessment of cognition should be performed.

Finally, we wish to emphasize that the older patient in the public mental health system must not be seen as any less worthy of our attention, expertise, and resources than any other patient. The illnesses he or she suffers can be devastating to the person and to the family. Results of their treatment often are positive and can be long-lasting.

References

Alexopoulos G, Meyers BS, Young RC, et al: The course of geriatric depression with "reversible dementia": a controlled study. Am J Psychiatry 150:1693–1699, 1993

Alexopoulos G, Meyers BS, Young RC, et al: Clinically defined vascular depression. Am J Psychiatry 154:562–565, 1997

Almeida OP, Howard R, Förstl H, et al: Should the diagnosis of late paraphrenia be abandoned? Psychol Med 22:11–14, 1992

American Psychiatric Association: State Mental Hospitals and the Elderly (Task Force Report). Washington, DC, American Psychiatric Association, 1993

American Psychiatric Association: Diagnostic and Statistical Manual of Mental Disorders, 4th Edition. Washington, DC, American Psychiatric Association, 1994

Ames D: Depression among elderly residents of local-authority residential homes. Br J Psychiatry 156:667–675, 1990

Baldwin RC: Late life depression and structural brain changes: a review of recent magnetic resonance imaging research. Int J Geriatr Psychiatry 8:115–123, 1993

Baldwin RC: Delusional depression in elderly patients: characteristics and relationship to age at onset. Int J Geriatr Psychiatry 10:981–985, 1995

Bench CJ, Frackowiak RSJ, Dolan RJ: Changes in regional cerebral blood flow on recovery from depression. Psychol Med 25:247–251, 1995

Blazer DG: Is depression more frequent in late life? An honest look at the evidence. Am J Geriatr Psychiatry 2:193–198, 1994

Boone KB, Miller BL, Lesser IM, et al: Neuropsychological correlates of white matter lesions in normal elderly: a threshold effect. Arch Neurol 49:549–554, 1992

Boone KB, Lesser IM, Miller BL, et al: Cognitive functioning in older depressed outpatients: relationship of presence and severity of depression to neuropsychological test scores. Neuropsychology 3:390–398, 1995

Bradley WG, Waluch V, Brant-Zawadzki M, et al: Patchy, periventricular white matter lesions in the elderly: a common observation during NMR imaging. Noninvasive Medical Imaging 1:35–41, 1984

Breitner JCS, Husain MM, Figiel GS, et al: Cerebral white matter disease in late-onset paranoid psychosis. Biol Psychiatry 28:266–274, 1990

Bungener C, Jouvent R, Derouesné C: Affective disturbances in Alzheimer's disease. J Am Geriatr Soc 44:1066–1071, 1996

Butler RN, Lewis MI, Sunderland T: Aging and Mental Health: Positive Psychosocial and Biomedical Approaches, 4th Edition. New York, Macmillan, 1991

Cahn DA, Malloy PF, Salloway S, et al: Subcortical hyperintensities on MRI and activities of daily living in geriatric depression. J Neuropsychiatry Clin Neurosci 8:404–411, 1996

Caine ED, Lyness JM, King DA: Reconsidering depression in the elderly. Am J Geriatr Psychiatry 1:4–20, 1993

Caine ED, Lyness JM, King DA, et al: Clinical and etiological heterogeneity of mood disorders in elderly patients, in Diagnosis and Treatment of Depression in Late Life: Results of the NIH Development Conference. Edited by Schneider LS, Reynolds CF, Lebowitz BD, et al. Washington, DC, American Psychiatric Press, 1994, pp 23–53

Casey DE: How antipsychotic drug pharmacology relates to side effects. Journal of Clinical Psychiatry Monograph 15:30–33, 1997

Castle DJ, Murray RM: The epidemiology of late-onset schizophrenia. Schizophr Bull 19:691–700, 1993

Chouinard G, Jones B, Remington G, et al: A Canadian multicenter placebo-controlled study of fixed doses of risperidone and haloperidol in the treatment of chronic schizophrenic patients. J Clin Psychopharmacol 13:25–40, 1993

Coffey CE, Figiel GS, Djang WT, et al: Subcortical hyperintensity on magnetic resonance imaging: a comparison of normal and depressed elderly subjects. Am J Psychiatry 47:187–189, 1990

Cole MG, Bellavance F: The prognosis of depression in old age. Am J Geriatr Psychiatry 5:4–14, 1997

Craig TJ, Bregman Z: Late onset schizophrenia-like illness. J Am Geriatr Soc 36:104–107, 1988

Cummings JL: Psychosis in neurologic disease: neurobiology and pathogenesis. Neuropsychiatry Neuropsychol Behav Neurol 5:144–150, 1992

Cummings JL, Victoroff JI: Noncognitive neuropsychiatric syndromes in Alzheimer's disease. Neuropsychiatry Neuropsychol Behav Neurol 3:140–158, 1990

Day JC: Population projections of the United States by age, sex, race, and Hispanic origin: 1992 to 2050 (U.S. Bureau of the Census, Current Population Reports, Series P-25, No 1092). Washington, DC, U.S. Government Printing Office, 1992

Devanand DP, Jacobs DM, Tang MX, et al: The course of psychopathologic features in mild to moderate Alzheimer disease. Arch Gen Psychiatry 54:257–263, 1997

Dooneief G, Mirabello E, Bell K, et al: An estimate of the incidence of depression in idiopathic Parkinson's disease. Arch Neurol 4:305–307, 1992

Emerson Lombardo NB, Fogel BS, Robinson GK, et al: Achieving Mental Health of Nursing Home Residents: Overcoming Barriers to Mental Health Care. Policy Brief. Hebrew Rehabilitation Center for Aged, Boston, MA, 1996

Farrer LA: Suicide and attempted suicide in Huntington disease: implications for preclinical testing of persons at risk. Am J Med Genet 24:305–311, 1986

Fischer P, Simamyi M, Danielczyk W: Depression in dementia of the Alzheimer type and in multi-infarct dementia. Am J Psychiatry 147:1484–1487, 1990

Flint AJ, Rifat SL, Eastwood MR: Late-onset paranoia: distinct from paraphrenia? Int J Geriatr Psychiatry 6:103–109, 1991

Folstein MF, McHugh PR: Dementia syndrome of depression, in Alzheimer's Disease: Senile Dementia and Related Disorders. Edited by Katzman R, Terry RD, Bick KL. New York, Raven, 1978, pp 281–289

Folstein MF, Folstein SE, McHugh PR: Mini-Mental State: a practical method for grading the cognitive state of patients for the clinician. J Psychiatr Res 12:189–198, 1975

Forsell Y, Jorm AF, Fratiglioni L, et al: Application of DSM-III-R criteria for major depressive episode to elderly subjects with and without dementia. Am J Psychiatry 150:1199–1202, 1993

Galasko D, Kwo-On-Yuen PF, Thal T: Intracranial mass lesions associated with late-onset psychosis and depression. Psychiatr Clin North Am 11:151–166, 1988

George LK: Social factors and depression in late life, in Diagnosis and Treatment of Depression in Late Life: Results of the NIH Development Conference. Edited by Schneider LS, Reynolds CF, Lebowitz BD, et al. Washington, DC, American Psychiatric Press, 1994, pp 131–153

Gotham A-M, Brown RG, Marsden CD: Depression in Parkinson's disease: a quantitative and qualitative analysis. J Neurol Neurosurg Psychiatry 49:381–389, 1986

Greenwald BS, Kramer-Ginsberg E, Krishnan RR, et al: MRI signal hyperintensities in geriatric depression. Am J Psychiatry 153:1212–1215, 1996

Harris MJ, Jeste DV: Late-onset schizophrenia: an overview. Schizophr Bull 14:39–55, 1988

Hay DP, Renner J, Franson KL, et al: Use of the newer antidepressants in the elderly. Nursing Home Medicine 5:28–40, 1997

Herbert ME, Jacobson S: Late paraphrenia. Br J Psychiatry 134:461–469, 1967

Hickie I, Scott E, Mitchell P, et al: Subcortical hyperintensities on magnetic resonance imaging: clinical correlates and prognostic significance in patients with severe depression. Biol Psychiatry 37:151–160, 1995

Holden NL: Late paraphrenia or the paraphrenias? a descriptive study with a 10 year follow-up. Br J Psychiatry 150:635–639, 1987

House A: Depression associated with stroke. J Neuropsychiatry Clin Neurosci 8:453–457, 1996

Howard R, Castle D, Wessely S, et al: A comparative study of 470 cases of early-onset and late-onset schizophrenia. Br J Psychiatry 163:352–357, 1993

Howard RJ, Almeida O, Levy R, et al: Quantitative magnetic resonance imaging volumetry distinguishes delusional disorder from late-onset schizophrenia. Br J Psychiatry 165:474–480, 1994

Hymas N, Naguib M, Levy R: Late paraphrenia—a follow-up study. Int J Geriatr Psychiatry 4:23–29, 1989

Jagust WJ, Reed BR, Seab JP, et al: Clinical-physiological correlates of Alzheimer's disease and frontal lobe dementia. American Journal of Physiological Imaging 4:89–96, 1989

Jeste DV: Late-life schizophrenia. Schizophr Bull 19:687–690, 1993

Jeste DV, Harris MJ, Krull AJ, et al: Clinical and neuropsychological characteristics of patients with late-onset schizophrenia. Am J Psychiatry 152:722–730, 1995

Jeste DV, Eastham JH, Lacro JP, et al: Management of late-life psychosis. J Clin Psychiatry 57 (suppl 3):39–45, 1996

Katz IR, Parmelee PA: Depression in elderly patients in residential care settings, in Diagnosis and Treatment of Depression in Late Life: Results of the NIH Development Conference. Edited by Schneider LS, Reynolds CF, Lebowitz BD, et al. Washington, DC, American Psychiatric Press, 1994, pp 437–461

Kay DWK: Late paraphrenia and its bearing on the aetiology of schizophrenia. Acta Psychiatr Scand 39:159–169, 1963

Keshavan MS, Mulsant BH, Sweet RA, et al: MRI changes in schizophrenia in late life: a preliminary controlled study. Psychiatry Res 60:117–123, 1996

Kiloh LG: Pseudo-dementia. Acta Psychiatr Scand 37:336–351, 1961

Koller WC, Megaffin BB: Parkinson's disease and parkinsonism, in Textbook of Geriatric Neuropsychiatry. Edited by Coffey CE, Cummings JL. Washington, DC, American Psychiatric Press, 1994, pp 433–456

Krishnan KRR, Hays JC, Blazer DG: MRI-defined vascular depression. Am J Psychiatry 154:497–501, 1997

Krull AJ, Press G, Dupont R, et al: Brain imaging in late-onset schizophrenia and related psychoses. Int J Geriatr Psychiatry 6:651–658, 1991

Kumar A, Miller D, Ewbank D, et al: Quantitative anatomic measures and comorbid medical illness in late-life major depression. Am J Geriatr Psychiatry 5:15–25, 1997

Lacro JP, Harris MJ, Jeste DV: Late life psychosis. Int J Geriatr Psychiatry 8:49–57, 1993

Lacro JP, Eastham JH, Jeste DV, et al: Newer antipsychotics and antidepressants for elderly people. Current Opinion in Psychiatry 9:290–293, 1996

Lesser IM, Miller BL, Boone KB, et al: Psychosis as the first manifestation of degenerative dementia. Bulletin of Clinical Neuroscience 54:59–63, 1989

Lesser IM, Miller BL, Boone KB, et al: Brain injury and cognitive function in late-onset psychotic depression. J Neuropsychiatry Clin Neurosci 3:33–40, 1991

Lesser IM, Jeste DV, Boone KB, et al: Late-onset psychotic disorder, not otherwise specified (NOS): clinical and neuroimaging findings. Biol Psychiatry 31:419–423, 1992

Lesser IM, Hill-Gutierrez E, Miller BL, et al: Late-onset depression and white matter lesions: a case report. Psychosomatics 34:364–367, 1993a

Lesser IM, Miller BL, Swartz JR, et al: Brain imaging in late-life schizophrenia and related psychoses. Schizophr Bull 19:773–782, 1993b

Lesser IM, Mena I, Boone KB, et al: Reduction of cerebral blood flow in older depressed patients. Arch Gen Psychiatry 51:677–686, 1994

Lesser IM, Boone KB, Mehringer MC, et al: Cognition and white matter hyperintensities in older depressed patients. Am J Psychiatry 153:1280–1287, 1996

Leuchter AF, Spar JE: The late-onset psychoses: clinical and diagnostic features. J Nerv Ment Dis 173:488–494, 1985

Levy M, Cummings JL, Fairbanks LA, et al: Longitudinal assessment of symptoms of depression, agitation, and psychosis in 181 patients with Alzheimer's disease. Am J Psychiatry 153:1438–1443, 1996

Lovell MR, Nussbaum PD: Neuropsychological assessment, in Textbook of Geriatric Neuropsychiatry. Edited by Coffey CE, Cummings JL. Washington, DC, American Psychiatric Press, 1994, pp 129–144

Mayberg HS: Frontal lobe dysfunction in secondary depression. J Neuropsychiatry Clin Neurosci 6:428–442, 1994

Mayeux R: Depression and dementia in Parkinson's disease, in Movement Disorders. Edited by Marsden CO, Fahn S. London, Butterworth, 1982, pp 75–95

McAllister TW: Overview: pseudodementia. Am J Psychiatry 140:528–533, 1983

Meehan PJ, Saltzman LE, Sattin RW: Suicides among older United States residents: epidemiologic characteristics and trends. Am J Public Health 81:1198–1200, 1991

Meyers BS: Epidemiology and clinical meaning of "significant" depressive symptoms in later life: the question of subsyndromal depression. Am J Geriatr Psychiatry 2:188–192, 1994

Meyers BS, Greenberg R: Late-life delusional depression. J Affect Disord 11: 133–137, 1986

Miller BL, Lesser IM: Late-life psychosis and modern neuroimaging. Psychiatr Clin North Am 11:33–46, 1988

Miller BL, Benson F, Cummings JL, et al: Late-life paraphrenia: an organic delusional syndrome. J Clin Psychiatry 47:204–207, 1986

Miller BL, Cummings JL, Villanueva-Meyer J, et al: Frontal lobe degeneration: clinical, neuropsychological, MRI and SPECT characteristics. Neurology 41:1374–1382, 1991a

Miller BL, Lesser IM, Boone KB, et al: Brain lesions and cognitive function in late-life psychosis. Br J Psychiatry 158:76–82, 1991b

Miller BL, Lesser IM, Mena I, et al: Regional cerebral blood flow in late-life-onset psychosis. Neuropsychiatry Neuropsychol Behav Neurol 5:132–137, 1992

Miller BL, Chang L, Mena I, et al: Progressive right frontotemporal degeneration: clinical, neuropsychological and SPECT characteristics. Dementia 4:204–213, 1993

Miller BL, Chang L, Oropilla G, et al: Alzheimer's disease and frontal lobe dementias, in Textbook of Geriatric Neuropsychiatry. Edited by Coffey CE, Cummings JL. Washington, DC, American Psychiatric Press, 1994, pp 389–404

Morris PLP, Robinson RG, Raphael B, et al: Lesion location and poststroke depression. J Neuropsychiatry Clin Neurosci 8:399–403, 1996

Munoz DG, Hastak SM, Harper B, et al: Pathologic correlates of increased signals of the centrum ovale on magnetic resonance imaging. Arch Neurol 50:492–497, 1993

Munro A: A plea for paraphrenia. Can J Psychiatry 36:667–672, 1991

Nelson JC, Conwell Y, Kim K, et al: Age at onset in late-life delusional depression. Am J Psychiatry 146:785–786, 1989

Nemeroff CB, DeVane CL, Pollock BG: Newer antidepressants and the cytochrome P450 system. Am J Psychiatry 153:311–320, 1996

Nussbaum PD: Pseudodementia: a slow death. Neuropsychol Rev 4:71–90, 1994

Nussbaum PD, Kaszniak AW, Allender J, et al: Depression and cognitive decline in the elderly: a follow-up study. Clinical Neuropsychologist 9:101–111, 1995

O'Brien J, Ames D, Schwietzer I: White matter changes in depression and Alzheimer's disease: a review of magnetic resonance imaging studies. Int J Geriatr Psychiatry 11:681–694, 1996

Patterson TL, Kaplan RM, Grant I, et al: Quality of well-being in late-life psychosis. Psychiatry Res 63:169–181, 1996

Pearlson GD, Kreger L, Rabins PV, et al: A chart review study of late-onset and early-onset schizophrenia. Am J Psychiatry 146:1568–1574, 1989

Prager S, Jeste DV: Sensory impairment in late-life schizophrenia. Schizophr Bull 19:755–772, 1993

Preskorn SH: Recent pharmacologic advances in antidepressant therapy for the elderly. Am J Med 94 (suppl 5A):2S–12S, 1993

Rabins PV, Harvis K, Koven S: High fatality rates of late-life depression associated with cardiovascular disease. J Affect Disord 9:165–167, 1985

Riecher-Rössler A, Rössler W, Förstl H, et al: Late-onset schizophrenia and late paraphrenia. Schizophr Bull 21:345–354, 1995

Riesenman C: Antidepressant drug interactions and the cytochrome P450 system: a critical appraisal. Pharmacotherapy 15(suppl):84S–99S, 1995

Robins LN, Regier DA: Psychiatric Disorders in America: The Epidemiologic Catchment Area Study. New York, Free Press, 1991

Robinson RG, Kubos KL, Starr LB, et al: Mood disorders in stroke patients: importance of location of lesion. Brain 107:81–93, 1984

Rockwell E, Jackson E, Vilke G, et al: A study of delusions in a large cohort of Alzheimer's disease patients. Am J Geriatr Psychiatry 2:157–164, 1994

Roth M: The natural history of mental disorder in old age. Journal of Mental Science 101:281–301, 1959

Rovner BW: Depression and increased risk of mortality in the nursing home patient. Am J Med 94 (suppl 5A):19S–23S, 1993

Salloway S, Malloy P, Kohn R, et al: MRI and neuropsychological differences in early and late-life-onset geriatric depression. Neurology 46:1567–1574, 1996

Saluter AF: Marital status and living arrangements: March 1991 (U.S. Bureau of the Census, Current Population Reports, Series P-20, No 461). Washington, DC, U.S. Government Printing Office, 1992

Salzman C: Clinical Geriatric Psychopharmacology, 3rd Edition. Baltimore, Williams & Wilkins, 1998

Schneider LS, Reynolds CF, Lebowitz BD, et al (eds): Diagnosis and Treatment of Depression in Late Life: Results of the NIH Development Conference. Washington, DC, American Psychiatric Press, 1994

Shulman KI, Tohen M, Satlin A, et al: Mania compared with unipolar depression in old age. Am J Psychiatry 149:341–345, 1992

Silver JM, Hales RE, Yudofsky SC: Neuropsychiatric aspects of traumatic brain injury, in Textbook of Neuropsychiatry, 2nd Edition. Edited by Yudofsky SC, Hales RE. Washington, DC, American Psychiatric Press, 1992, pp 363–395

Starkstein SE, Boston JD, Robinson RG: Mechanisms of mania after brain injury. J Nerv Ment Dis 176:87–100, 1988

Stoudemire A, Hill C, Gulley LR, et al: Neuropsychological and biomedical assessment of depression-dementia syndromes. J Neuropsychiatry Clin Neurosci 1:347–361, 1989

Sultzer DL, Levin HS, Mahler ME, et al: A comparison of psychiatric symptoms in vascular dementia and Alzheimer's disease. Am J Psychiatry 150:1806–1812, 1993

Swartz JR, Miller BL, Lesser IM, et al: Behavioral phenomenology in Alzheimer's disease, frontotemporal dementia, and late-life depression: a retrospective analysis. J Geriatr Psychiatry Neurol 10:67–74, 1997

Taueber C: Sixty-five plus in America (U.S. Bureau of the Census, Current Population Reports, Special Studies, 23–178). Washington, DC, U.S. Government Printing Office, 1992

U.S. Bureau of the Census: Poverty in the United States: 1991 (Current Population Reports, Series P-60, No 181). Washington, DC, U.S. Government Printing Office, 1992

Vasile RG, Schwartz RB, Garada B, et al: Focal cerebral perfusion defects demonstrated by ^{99m}Tc-hexamethylpropyleneamine oxime SPECT in elderly depressed patients. Psychiatry Res Neuroimaging 67:59–70, 1996

Wojcieszek JM, Lang AE: Hyperkinetic movement disorders, in Textbook of Geriatric Neuropsychiatry. Edited by Coffey CE, Cummings JL. Washington, DC, American Psychiatric Press, 1994, pp 405–431

Zubenko GS, Hind Rifai A, Mulsant BH, et al: Premorbid history of major depression and depressive syndrome of Alzheimer's disease. Am J Geriatr Psychiatry 4:85–90, 1996

CHAPTER 11

Neuropsychiatry and the Homeless

Jonathan M. Silver, M.D.
Alan Felix, M.D.

Epidemiology of Homelessness

It has been estimated that there are from 250,000 to 2,000,000 homeless individuals in the United States (Caton 1990). Methodological limitations have made more precise counts impossible. Most studies estimated the homeless population at only one point in time. However, a recent study examined 5-year and lifetime prevalences of "literal homelessness" (i.e., living on the street, in a shelter, or in other public spaces, but not doubling up with others) in a sample representative of the U.S. population (Link et al. 1994). The study found a lifetime prevalence of homelessness of 7.4% (13.5 million people) and a 5-year prevalence of 3.1% (5.7 million people). These findings suggest that the extent of homelessness may be greater than that suggested by earlier surveys.

Neuropsychiatric disorders are common in the homeless population; some disorders have resulted in homelessness, whereas others are a result of homelessness. Approximately 30% of homeless individuals have serious mental illness; 25%–33% of these individuals have a history of psychiatric hospitalization (Caton 1990). The homeless population has a high prevalence of substance abuse disorders and chronic physical ailments, often in combination. In a survey of New York City shelters, Cuomo (1992) found that 53% of a sample population self-reported a history of mental illness or substance abuse and 21% reported having a chronic health problem. The rate of schizophrenia (10%–13%) is more than 10 times that of the overall population; 21%–29%

have affective disorders; 14%–20% have antisocial personality disorder; and 2%–3% have dementia (Fischer and Breakey 1991). Unfortunately, these disorders can occur in combination with each other. There is a high incidence of "triple disorder" (e.g., schizophrenia, substance abuse, and antisocial personality) in the chronically mentally ill homeless (Caton et al. 1994). Approximately 10%–20% of the homeless have coexisting severe mental illness and substance abuse disorders (Drake et al. 1991).

The multiple medical conditions found in the homeless individual can result in neuropsychiatric disabilities. Chronic health problems are common and occur in 21% of this population (17% of men and 41% of women). The homeless are especially at risk for trauma-related disorders, infectious diseases (acquired immunodeficiency syndrome [AIDS], tuberculosis [TB], sexually transmitted diseases), untreated diabetes and hypertension, and peripheral vascular disease (Drapkin 1990). Furthermore, in a survey of New York City shelters using structured interviews, Struening and Padgett (1990) discovered that homeless adults with the heaviest use of drugs and alcohol and/or histories of mental illness also had the highest rates of poor physical health. All of these disorders can adversely affect neuropsychological functioning.

In this chapter, we review the neuropsychiatric sequelae of some disorders that commonly occur in the homeless and the several studies that have specifically addressed neuropsychiatric disorders in the homeless. We then discuss the implications for assessment and treatment of this population.

Neuropsychiatric Sequelae of Specific Disorders Found in the Homeless

Substance Abuse

Alcohol abuse is a problem in 58%–68% of the homeless, a rate that is six to seven times that in the general population (Fischer and Breakey 1991). Chronic abuse of substances such as alcohol or cocaine may result in neuropsychiatric impairment even in the absence of acute intoxication. Psychotic disorders and affective disorders may result from the long-term use of many substances. Chronic alcohol use may lead to hallucinations (alcoholic hallucinosis), retrograde and anterograde amnesia (alcohol amnestic disorder or Korsakoff's psychosis), or cognitive impairment, including dementia and Wernicke's syndrome (Charness et al. 1989). Computed tomography (CT) shows cortical shrinkage in those with chronic alcohol abuse (Cala and

Mastaglia 1981). Other neurological complications from alcohol abuse include alcoholic polyneuropathy, hepatic encephalopathy, acquired hepatocerebral degeneration, acute and chronic subdural hematomas, and cerebellar degeneration (Franklin and Frances 1992).

Cocaine intoxication and abuse may result in affective changes, perceptual dysfunction, or ideational distortions. Common symptoms include grandiosity, paranoid delusions, euphoria, and impaired judgment. Neurological complications of cocaine use include transient ischemic attacks (TIAs), stroke, seizures, and headaches (Jacobs et al. 1989). Seizures may occur more frequently with the use of crack or intravenous cocaine (Pascual-Levine et al. 1990). A detailed discussion of substance abuse in the homeless is found in Chapter 5.

Acquired Immunodeficiency Syndrome

AIDS and human immunodeficiency virus (HIV) infection are associated with multiple neuropsychiatric symptoms. HIV infection may result in dementia. In addition, some individuals with asymptomatic HIV infection may develop mild cognitive problems, including apathy, mental slowing, forgetfulness, lethargy, social withdrawal, and changes in personality (Markowitz and Perry 1992). In addition, depression, anxiety, and psychosis may occur. Secondary infections in individuals with AIDS may result in encephalitis and mental status changes.

Traumatic Brain Injury

Each year in the United States, more than three million people sustain a traumatic brain injury (TBI). Those at highest risk are men in the young adult age group, and the majority of the homeless are males in this age group. Patients may have difficulties in many vital areas of functioning, including family, interpersonal, work, school, and recreational activities. Many have severe personality changes. Unfortunately, the psychiatric impairments caused by TBI often go unrecognized. We believe that the homeless population is at increased risk for TBI because of victimization; risk-taking behaviors, including substance abuse; and the presence of antisocial personality disorder.

The neuropsychiatric sequelae of TBI are affected by the extent and type of injury, in addition to the unique history, temperament, and psychosocial status of the person who became injured (Silver et al. 1994). A history of depression is more common among those patients who become depressed after TBI (Robinson and Jorge 1994). Intoxication at the time of the accident is associated with longer periods of hospitalization, longer periods of posttraumatic agitation, more impaired cognition at the time of discharge, and increased mortality after the injury (Sparadeo et al. 1990). Unfortunately, many people sustain more than one brain injury. This group of TBI victims experience more symptoms and have a poorer outcome than those who sustain a single injury only (Carlsson et al. 1987).

Typical personality changes include problems with judgment, sense of self, and childishness. The brain-injured individual may lose the ability to reflect on planned actions and their effects on others. An increase in impulsivity is accompanied by poor social judgment. Damage to specific areas of the frontal lobe may result in characteristic personality changes. Injury to the orbital frontal surface is characterized by impulsivity, disinhibition, hyperactivity, distractibility, and lability. In contrast, lack of initiation, slowness, and perseveration are caused by dorsolateral frontal lobe damage. When there is injury to the orbital surface of the frontal lobe or the anterotemporal lobe, intermittent violent outbursts frequently result (Taylor and Price 1994). Personality changes may persist indefinitely after moderate and severe brain injuries. In DSM-IV (American Psychiatric Association 1994), these changes are diagnosed as "Personality Change Due to Traumatic Brain Injury" and are subtyped as labile, disinhibited, apathetic, aggressive, mixed, or other type.

Cognitive changes, including problems with arousal, attention, memory, abstraction, language, and perception, are obvious in patients with more severe TBI but may also be present in patients with mild brain injury. Executive functioning, which includes abilities to set goals, assess one's own strengths and weaknesses, plan and/or direct activity, initiate and/or inhibit behavior, monitor current activity, and evaluate the results of actions, can be impaired.

Depression is common after TBI. Robinson and Jorge (1994) found that 42% of a group of 66 hospitalized patients who had acute TBI developed depression during the first year after injury. Mania, although less common, also can occur subsequent to TBI. Although many patients have signs and symptoms that fulfill the diagnostic criteria for major depressive disorder, others have mood lability, with frequent shifts from euthymia to tearfulness. Other patients become sad as an appropriate reaction to the losses that invariably accompany brain injury.

Psychosis that occurs long after trauma is more difficult to diagnose and to treat. Many patients with schizophrenia have sustained brain injury that will remain undetected unless the clinician carefully elicits a history specific for the occurrence of brain trauma. Smeltzer and co-workers (1994) reviewed the scientific literature regarding the presence of posttraumatic psychosis in patients with TBI. Schizophrenia-like symptoms of many patients appear after TBI, and the psychotic symptoms may persist despite improvement in the cognitive deficits caused by trauma. Davison and Bagley (1969) found that 1%–15% of schizophrenic inpatients had histories of brain injury, and patients who had sustained brain injury had a two- to threefold increase in the incidence of schizophrenia. Wilcox and Nasrallah (1987) found that a group of patients whose condition had been diagnosed as schizophrenia more commonly had a history of brain injury with loss of consciousness before the age of 10 than did those patients with mania or depression or who were hospitalized for surgery.

The postconcussive syndrome (PCS), often called *minor brain injury*, occurs when loss of consciousness is less than 20 minutes and posttraumatic amnesia lasts for less than 24 hours. The patient may appear stunned or dazed and is often disoriented after the accident. Several symptoms are common subsequent to minor injury and include cognitive complaints (impaired attention or concentration), somatic complaints (fatigue, headache, dizziness, sensitivity to noise or light), and behavioral changes (irritability, anxiety, or depression).

Irritability and aggression are common after brain injury. During the acute phase after TBI, 35%–96% of patients exhibit agitated behaviors. These behaviors continue long after the trauma. Studies have shown that 31%–71% of patients after severe TBI are chronically agitated or irritable (Silver and Yudofsky 1994a).

Medical Disorders

Medical disorders such as diabetes and hypertension are often untreated in the homeless and result in neuropsychiatric symptoms. Diabetes is associated with an increased prevalence of depression and anxiety (Lustman et al. 1986), as well as painful neuropathies. Hypoglycemia or hyperglycemia can present as disorientation, lethargy, and confusion. Vascular disease and strokes are long-term complications of diabetes. Poorly controlled hypertension increases the risk for cerebrovascular disease, including vascular dementia (multi-infarct dementia). The relationship between stroke and affective disorders has been well described by Starkstein and Robinson (1992). Because the homeless may develop malnutrition, they are subject to the resultant impairments in memory, mood, and thinking.

Tuberculosis

Although TB does not usually result in brain pathology, it does cause general physical deterioration and weakness. Those who are homeless, in addition to being at risk for AIDS, are at increased risk for TB (Susser et al. 1993).

Schizophrenia

Because more than 10% of the homeless population have schizophrenia (Fischer and Breakey 1991), it is important to recognize the neuropsychiatric problems that are part of this disorder. Several abnormalities have been demonstrated with brain imaging of patients with schizophrenia, including dilation of the cerebral ventricles, smaller midsagittal craniums and cerebrums, sulcal widening, cerebellar vermis atrophy, and reversed cerebral asymmetries (Nasrallah 1992). Functional imaging studies, such as those using positron-emission tomography (PET), have revealed "hypofrontality" and dysfunction of the dorsolateral prefrontal cortex (Weinberger et al. 1986). In addition to the presence of neurological "soft signs," cognitive impairment may be present in the areas of attention, memory, abstraction, and ability to plan (Granholm and Jeste 1994).

Epilepsy

Brief episodic psychoses may occur with epilepsy; about 7% of patients with epilepsy have persistent psychoses (McKenna et al. 1985). These psychoses exhibit a number of atypical features, including confusion and rapid fluctuations in mood. Psychiatric evaluation of 101 patients with epilepsy revealed that 8% had organic delusional disorder that, at times, was difficult to differentiate symptomatically from schizophrenia (Garyfallos et al. 1988). Other emotional changes can occur, including depression and panic attacks. A personality change characterized by emotional lability, impairment of impulse control, and suspiciousness has been described in patients with temporal lobe seizure foci (Garyfallos et al. 1988).

Neuropsychiatric Problems Among the Homeless

Few studies have directly explored the neuropsychiatric sequelae of the disorders that occur in a homeless population. This oversight in the medical and psychiatric literature might stem from clinicians' reluctance to work with homeless patients (Kass and Silver 1990). Checklist surveys found only a 3%–8% incidence of cognitive impairment among the homeless (Farr et al. 1986; Fischer et al. 1986; Koegel et al. 1988). We believe this is an underestimate, because more formal cognitive assessment is more sensitive in detecting deficits.

Strain and co-workers (1992) explored the possible relationship between cognitive impairment and homelessness. They performed a chart review of consecutive admissions to a day hospital over the course of 1 year, examining 145 cases for the prevalence of "triply diagnosed" patients (i.e., patients with major mental illness, substance abuse, and cognitive impairment) (Strain et al. 1992). (Note that the triple diagnosis in these patients differs from the triple diagnosis in the patients described by Caton et al. 1994.) This population, which was 59% women and 77% white, had an average age of 43.2 years. Cognitive impairment was defined as an IQ less than 84; a diagnosis of mental retardation, borderline intellectual functioning, or dementia; delayed developmental milestones; or a physician's notation of cognitive impairment in the chart. Those who were triply diagnosed (26% of the patient population) had significantly higher rates of legal problems, inpatient psychiatric treatment, and substance abuse treatment. In addition, there was a trend toward higher rates of homelessness among these individuals. Although this study suggests a correlation between cognitive disorders and homelessness, it does not clarify the causal relationships between mental illness, substance abuse, cognitive impairment, and homelessness.

Kass et al. (1989) performed a neuropsychiatric evaluation of 13 chronically mentally ill men living in a large municipal shelter. The average age of the subjects was 31.6 years. Eleven were African American, and 2 were Latino. All had histories of psychiatric hospitalization, and none had current substance abuse diagnoses, although several had histories of drug or alcohol abuse. The evaluation included a psychiatric evaluation, medical assessment (which included physical examination, electrocardiogram, blood work, chest X ray, TB test, and optional HIV test), and a neurological examination. A neuropsychologist performed a 2- to 3-hour battery of tests measuring intelligence; reading, writing, and arithmetic skills; memory; language skills; and set-shifting.

The most common medical problems were mild anemia, inactive TB, early syphilis, gonorrhea, lice, venous stasis, and cellulitis. Interestingly, six men had a history of significant TBI, usually predating the onset of homelessness. High rates of neurological soft signs, usually dysarthria and poor fine finger movements, were found. One patient had central nervous system sarcoidosis. One patient had AIDS.

On neuropsychological evaluation, the mean Wechsler Full Scale IQ was 77.7, with three of the patients scoring below 70 (in the range of mild mental retardation). Achievement tests revealed illiteracy and poor arithmetic skills in almost all of the men (11 subjects scored at or below the 2nd percentile in oral reading comprehension). Virtually none of the men understood full written sentences. Testing of memory revealed that 8 men scored in the impaired range. Naming deficits were demonstrated in 12 men. Consistent with research findings on deficits in the Wisconsin Card Sorting Test (Heaton 1985), 8 men demonstrated impairment. Not surprisingly, most low neuropsychological scores correlated with history of TBI with loss of consciousness.

The authors conceded that their data were inconclusive because of the small sample size, confounding variables, and possible cultural bias in neuropsychological testing. It is difficult to sort out, for example, whether cognitive impairment is a risk factor for homelessness and poverty or caused by them. It is similarly difficult to determine the role of mental illness versus other factors, such as head trauma or other illness, in causing cognitive impairment in the homeless mentally ill. However, there was a great likelihood of finding significant medical, neurological, and cognitive impairment in the homeless mentally ill sample studied.

In a case-control study of homeless mentally ill persons in Boston, neuropsychological testing was performed at baseline (while homeless) and 15 months into housing (Goldfinger et al. 1994). The sample of 118 individuals was 71% male and 40.7% African American; the average age was 37.5 years. More than 67% had a high school diploma or its equivalent. A history of psychiatric hospitalization was found in 92.4%. The most common diagnoses were schizophrenia (45.3%), followed by schizoaffective disorder (17.1%), bipolar disorder (13.7%), major depression (12.8%), and other psychotic disorders (9.3%). Preliminary findings (two-thirds of the cases have had follow-up testing at 15 months) show improvement during the time in housing, but, according to the investigators, the group "remains significantly impaired compared to the general population." Areas of impairment include attention, reasoning, abstraction, visual-perceptual ability, school-based achievement, and IQ. In the last two areas, subjects scored lower than hospitalized patients with schizophrenia. The researchers plan to analyze the follow-up data to determine the effects of medication, housing, and long-term substance abuse on cognitive performance.

Silver et al. (1993) evaluated 200 men and 200 women who were diagnosed as having schizophrenia or schizoaffective disorder for the occurrence of TBI. One-half of this group was homeless. In the group of men, 36 who were homeless and 19 who were domiciled had a history of TBI ($P = 0.01$). In the group of women, 16 of the homeless and 19 of those domiciled had had a TBI. Premorbid adjustment was significantly better in the men, but not the women, in the TBI group. No differences were found in positive and negative symptoms for those individuals with and without brain injury. For many patients, the TBI had occurred within 1 year prior to the onset of psychosis.

These data suggest that TBI occurs at a higher rate than would be expected for this socioeconomic group. The higher prevalence of TBI among homeless schizophrenic men underscores the vulnerability of this patient group and their need for treatment and support services.

A case presentation illustrates the clinical challenges and complexities of treating a homeless mentally ill patient with significant cognitive impairment. A model for comprehensive day treatment is also described.

Case History: "Right Between the Eyes"

Mr. A is a 42-year-old single African American man who had been living in a large municipal shelter for 2 years before shelter staff asked the psychiatrist to examine him because of his poor hygiene. The first interaction between Mr. A and the psychiatrist took place in the shelter hallway: The psychiatrist was trying, in vain, to convince Mr. A to take a shower. Mr. A became so annoyed that he began to mumble barely comprehensible threats to kill someone. It was clear that he was holding a conversation with himself and probably was experiencing auditory hallucinations. In the psychiatrist's judgment, Mr. A was a danger to himself and others and required involuntary commitment to a psychiatric hospital. On evaluation in the emergency room, Mr. A was found to have gastrointestinal bleeding. He was admitted to a medical unit at the hospital. It was determined that his gastrointestinal bleeding was not significant.

Mr. A was raised in the inner city by both parents until their deaths, approximately 2 years apart, when he was a teenager. He then lived with his godmother and dropped out of school during the 11th grade. Unemployed, Mr. A began to steal and sell drugs. He spent a good deal of time in prison but lived with his godmother for many years. When she decided to move, Mr. A entered the shelter system.

As a teen, Mr. A started drinking and using marijuana, but he purports to have stopped many years ago. He later used cocaine for several years but claimed to be abstinent for the 6 years before his presentation. He reports having a long history of a "nervous condition" but denies any psychiatric hospitalizations. However, he does not seem capable of giving a wholly accurate history.

According to Mr. A, he was shot "by a friend" for no apparent reason. He laughingly states that he took a .22 "right between the eyes." The bullet lodged in his frontal lobe and was removed by surgery. He has a scar from the bullet entry between his eyes and a surgical scar over his right frontal region.

After psychiatric consultation, he was restarted on 300 mg of phenytoin for a long-standing seizure disorder stemming from a bullet wound to the head 25 years earlier. He was diagnosed as having chronic paranoid schizophrenia (which improved with 5 mg of haloperidol bid), mild dementia (probably related to the bullet wound or to past alcohol abuse), and a history of antisocial behavior before the onset of his schizophrenia.

When Mr. A returned to the shelter from his hospitalization, he was more organized and less paranoid, and his hygiene improved. He continued to talk to himself at times but denied hearing voices. He also revealed a long-standing delusion that the Federal Bureau of Investigation destroyed his records because they mixed him up with a famous gangster who shares the patient's nickname. In addition, Mr. A had some gaps in his remote memory, and he did not know the correct date. On discharge, he entered the Critical Time Intervention Mental Health Program, or CTI (Susser et al. 1997), where he has received day treatment in the shelter for the past 18 months.

In contrast to his past attitude, Mr. A was amenable to attending a mental health program after stabilization in the hospital. His dosage of haloperidol was increased gradually to a maximum of 20 mg/day in an attempt to control what appeared to be hallucinatory behavior (talking to himself). However, the patient had repeated oculogyric crises despite high doses of benztropine. He was switched to perphenazine, up to 40 mg/day, but again experienced dystonic reactions without optimal therapeutic response.

Fourteen months into his treatment in the shelter, Mr. A was admitted to the psychiatric service at the hospital because of threatening and agitated behavior. He was stabilized on 3 mg of risperidone bid, and his dosage of phenytoin was lowered from 300 mg to 200 mg/day because the higher dosage was a slightly toxic level. Since his discharge 3 months ago, the patient has been stable. The current plan is to apply for supportive housing with community-based intensive treatment. As part of the CTI program, he will receive follow-up in the community by his shelter treatment team until a solid network of supports is developed.

The case of Mr. A illustrates some of the complexities of treating homeless mentally ill persons. Although it is unlikely that all of Mr. A's psychiatric symptoms can be attributed to brain injury resulting from both the bullet wound and alcoholism, these organic factors probably play a role in Mr. A's inability to recover further.

In the presence of substance abuse and organic factors, the physician must be especially aware of the potential for medication side effects. For example, Mr. A's head injury complicated treatment by making him especially vulnerable to extrapyramidal side effects of neuroleptics, as well as to the potentially impairing effects on cognition of phenytoin and benztropine (Silver and Yudofsky 1994b).

Medication is just one aspect of treating homeless patients. Treatment for a patient such as Mr. A must be continuous, comprehensive, and highly supportive. The goal should be to maximize independence, but with realistic expectations for someone with multiple areas of impairment. His case is a good argument for assertive, multidisciplinary teams, such as the CTI program or the model of care now known as Assertive Community Treatment (ACT) (Stein and Test 1980).

The CTI model, developed at Columbia-Presbyterian Medical Center, provides continuous treatment during the transition from shelter to community living. Treatment is built around a case-management relationship but includes access to medical care, psychiatric services, housing, and other social services. The intervention focuses on the clinical areas that present the greatest risk of relapse for the homeless mentally ill. These include medication compliance, substance abuse treatment, money management, and housing-related crises. The overriding aim of CTI is to prevent homelessness through a time-limited (9-month) intervention during a period of vulnerability (moving from the shelter to the community).

Similarly, ACT teams provide assertive treatment wherever the patient goes; they are interdisciplinary, client-centered, and comprehensive. However, ACT teams are usually not time-limited and have somewhat broader explicit aims than does CTI, such as the prevention of hospitalization and the improvement of quality of life.

Conclusion

Generally, adequate neuropsychiatric assessment and treatment are lacking for the homeless. We therefore concur with the recommendations of Kass et al. (1989) that with a high-risk population, such as the homeless mentally ill, comprehensive neuropsychological testing and careful neurological assessment should be standard tools in our efforts to serve these most challenging individuals. The most important information is obtained through a thorough history that includes past and present trauma and substance use. Laboratory evaluation of sexually transmitted diseases and anemia appears particularly important. A cognitive evaluation of memory and basic literacy and math skills may have the greatest implication for rehabilitation and functioning in the community with the greatest possible degree of independence. Treatment approaches must be comprehensive and provide access to all necessary services.

As a group, the homeless present a formidable challenge to the clinician who wishes to obtain a thorough history. Patient-centered obstacles to the offering of accurate historical data include cognitive deficits resulting from neuropsychiatric disorders, distrust of providers based on actual past experiences, paranoia, poor education, and lack of collaborating sources.

Provider-centered obstacles include countertransference reactions and biases against the homeless (especially beliefs that the homeless are hopeless or unworthy of treatment), cultural or language barriers, and lack of adequate time to obtain necessary history. The last mentioned is often the result of funding policies that limit the role of physicians to part-time or even volunteer positions, a situation that leads to unmanageably high patient-physician ratios.

A clinician often must rely on a longitudinal view of a homeless patient before a definitive diagnosis and treatment plan can be formulated. By emphasizing the formation of a trusting relationship over the attainment of history, the history will usually unfold gradually and the patient will reveal other sources, such as family and previous providers.

On the institutional level, there must be adequate staffing and funding to allow the necessary work to be done to foster a treatment alliance with the patient. Toward this end, we argue for the role of full-time psychiatrists (Felix 1994) and physicians in clinical settings that serve the homeless. Furthermore, institutions generally can improve access to medical records. With the wide prevalence of fax machines and computer networks, information can be exchanged efficiently. Outdated modes of medical record keeping must be replaced.

Nonpharmacological interventions that directly address cognitive problems include educational programs, vocational training, and skills training (Liberman et al. 1985). Of course, the formation of a strong treatment alliance, discussed above with reference to history taking, is an essential step leading to the provision of biological therapies, especially in the difficult-to-reach homeless population.

References

American Psychiatric Association: Diagnostic and Statistical Manual of Mental Disorders, 4th Edition. Washington, DC, American Psychiatric Association, 1994

Cala LA, Mastaglia FL: Computerized tomography in chronic alcoholics. Alcoholism (NY) 5:283–294, 1981

Carlsson GS, Svardsudd K, Welin L: Long-term effects of head injuries sustained during life in three male populations. J Neurosurg 67:197–205, 1987

Caton CLM: Homeless in America. New York, Oxford University Press, 1990

Caton CLM, Shrout PE, Eagle PF, et al: Correlates of co-disorders in homeless and never-homeless indigent schizophrenic men. Psychol Med 24:681–688, 1994

Charness ME, Simon RP, Greenberg DA: Ethanol and the nervous system. N Engl J Med 312:442–454, 1989

Cuomo A: The Way Home. Report of the New York City Commission of the Homeless, 1992

Davison K, Bagley CR: Schizophrenic-like psychoses associated with organic disorders of the central nervous system: a review of the literature, in Current Problems in Neuropsychiatry: Schizophrenia, Epilepsy, the Temporal Lobe. Edited by Herrington RN. Br J Psychiatry (Special Publ No 4), 1969, pp 113–184

Drake RE, Osher FC, Wallach MA: Homelessness and dual diagnosis. Am Psychol 46:1149–1158, 1991

Drapkin A: Medical problems of the homeless, in Homeless in America. Edited by Caton CLM. New York, Oxford University Press, 1990, pp 59–109

Farr RK, Koegel P, Burnam A: A study of homelessness and mental illness in the skid row area of Los Angeles. Los Angeles, CA, Los Angeles County Department of Mental Health, 1986

Felix A: The role of a full-time psychiatrist in the treatment of mentally ill men in a shelter. Symposium: The Homeless Mentally Ill: Role of the Psychiatrist. Paper presented at the annual meeting of the American Psychiatric Association, May 1994

Fischer PJ, Breakey WR: The epidemiology of alcohol, drug, and mental disorders among homeless persons. Am Psychol 46:1115–1128, 1991

Fischer PJ, Shapiro S, Breakey WR, et al: Mental health and social characteristics of the homeless. Am J Public Health 76:519–524, 1986

Franklin JE Jr, Frances RJ: Alcohol-induced organic mental disorders, in American Psychiatric Press Textbook of Neuropsychiatry, 2nd Edition. Edited by Yudofsky SC, Hales RE. Washington, DC, American Psychiatric Press, 1992, pp 563–583

Garyfallos G, Manos N, Adamopoulou A: Psychopathology and personality characteristics of epileptic patients: epilepsy, psychopathology, and personality. Acta Psychiatr Scand 78:87–95, 1988

Goldfinger SM, Dickey B, Hellman S, et al: Promoting housing stability and consumer empowerment, in Making a Difference: Interim Status Report of the McKinney Research Demonstration Program for Homeless Mentally Ill Adults. Rockville, MD, Center for Mental Health Services, 1994, pp 43–61

Granholm E, Jeste DV: Cognitive impairment in schizophrenia. Psychiatric Annals 24:484–490, 1994

Heaton RK: Wisconsin Card Sorting Test. Odessa, FL, Psychological Assessment Resources, 1985

Jacobs IG, Roszler MH, Kelly JK, et al: Cocaine abuse: neurovascular complications. Radiology 170:223–227, 1989

Kass F, Silver JM: Neuropsychiatry and the homeless. J Neuropsychiatry Clin Neurosci 2:15–19, 1990

Kass FI, Kahn DA, Felix A: Day treatment in a shelter: a setting for assessment and treatment, in Treating the Homeless Mentally Ill. Washington, DC, American Psychiatric Association, 1989, pp 263–277

Koegel P, Burnam MA, Farr RK: The prevalence of specific psychiatric disorders among homeless individuals in the inner city of Los Angeles. Arch Gen Psychiatry 45:1085–1092, 1988

Liberman RP, Massel HK, Mosk M, et al: Social skills training for chronic mental patients. Hospital and Community Psychiatry 36:396–403, 1985

Link BG, Susser E, Stueve A, et al: Lifetime and five-year prevalence of homelessness in the United States. Am J Public Health 84:1907–1912, 1994

Lustman PJ, Griffith LS, Clouse RE, et al: Psychiatric illness in diabetes mellitus: relationship to symptoms and glucose control. J Nerv Ment Dis 174:736–742, 1986

Markowitz JC, Perry SW: Effects of human immunodeficiency virus on the central nervous system, in American Psychiatric Press Textbook of Neuropsychiatry, 2nd Edition. Edited by Yudofsky SC, Hales RE. Washington, DC, American Psychiatric Press, 1992, pp 499–518

McKenna PJ, Kane JM, Parrish K: Psychotic syndromes in epilepsy. Am J Psychiatry 142:895–904, 1985

Nasrallah HA: The neuropsychiatry of schizophrenia, in American Psychiatric Press Textbook of Neuropsychiatry, 2nd Edition. Edited by Yudofsky SC, Hales RE. Washington, DC, American Psychiatric Press, 1992, pp 621–638

Pascual-Levine A, Dhuna A, Altafullah I, et al: Cocaine-induced seizures. Neurology 40:404–407, 1990

Robinson RG, Jorge R: Mood disorders, in Neuropsychiatry of Traumatic Brain Injury. Edited by Silver JM, Yudofsky SC, Hales RE. Washington, DC, American Psychiatric Press, 1994, pp 219–250

Silver JM, Yudofsky SC: Aggressive disorders, in Neuropsychiatry of Traumatic Brain Injury. Edited by Silver JM, Yudofsky SC, Hales RE. Washington, DC, American Psychiatric Press, 1994a, pp 313–353

Silver JM, Yudofsky SC: Psychopharmacology, in Neuropsychiatry of Traumatic Brain Injury. Edited by Silver JM, Yudofsky SC, Hales RE. Washington, DC, American Psychiatric Press, 1994b, pp 631–670

Silver JM, Caton CM, Shrout PE, et al: Traumatic brain injury and schizophrenia. Presented at the 146th annual meeting of the American Psychiatric Association, May 22–27, 1993, San Francisco, CA

Silver JM, Yudofsky SC, Hales RE (eds): Neuropsychiatry of Traumatic Brain Injury. Washington, DC, American Psychiatric Press, 1994

Smeltzer DJ, Nasrallah HA, Miller SC: Psychotic disorders, in Neuropsychiatry of Traumatic Brain Injury. Edited by Silver JM, Yudofsky SC, Hales RE. Washington, DC, American Psychiatric Press, 1994, pp 251–283

Sparadeo FR, Strauss D, Barth JT: The incidence, impact, and treatment of substance abuse in head trauma rehabilitation. Journal of Head Trauma and Rehabilitation 5(3):1–8, 1990

Starkstein SE, Robinson RG: Neuropsychiatric aspects of cerebral vascular disorders, in American Psychiatric Press Textbook of Neuropsychiatry, 2nd Edition. Edited by Yudofsky SC, Hales RE. Washington, DC, American Psychiatric Press, 1992, pp 449–472

Stein LI, Test MA: Alternative to mental hospital treatment. Arch Gen Psychiatry 37:392–397, 1980

Strain EC, Buccino DL, Brooner RK, et al: The triply diagnosed: patients with major mental illness, cognitive impairment, and substance abuse. Am J Psychiatry 149:585–587, 1992

Struening EL, Padgett DK: Physical health status, substance use and abuse, and mental disorders among homeless adults. Journal of Social Issues 46:65–81, 1990

Susser E, Valencia E, Conover S, et al: Preventing recurrent homelessness among mentally ill men: a "critical time" intervention after discharge from a shelter. Am J Public Health 87:256–262, 1997

Taylor CA, Price TRP: Neuropsychiatric assessment, in Neuropsychiatry of Traumatic Brain Injury. Edited by Silver JM, Yudofsky SC, Hales RE. Washington, DC, American Psychiatric Press, 1994, pp 81–132

Weinberger DR, Berman KF, Zec RF: Physiologic dysfunction of dorsolateral prefrontal cortex in schizophrenia, I: regional cerebral blood flow evidence. Arch Gen Psychiatry 43:114–124, 1986

Wilcox JA, Nasrallah HA: Childhood head trauma and psychosis. Psychiatry Res 21:303–306, 1987

CHAPTER 12

Neuropsychiatric and Mental Health Services Aspects of Tardive Dyskinesia

Dilip V. Jeste, M.D.
David Naimark, M.D.
Maureen C. Halpain, M.S.
Brian Cuffel, Ph.D.

Tardive dyskinesia (TD) is an important iatrogenic disorder of movement that is induced by long-term use of neuroleptic medication. It is an example of a disease that pertains to both psychiatry and neurology. Optimal management may require an interdisciplinary approach between the two fields. Although psychiatrists are more likely than other physicians to see patients with TD, they may seek neurological consultation in occasional cases in which TD is difficult to distinguish from neurological movement disorders such as Sydenham's chorea. TD represents a particular challenge for clinicians working in the public health setting, be-

This work was supported in part by the National Institute of Mental Health (Grants MH43693, MH45131, MH49671, and MH51459) and by the Department of Veterans Affairs.

cause it is in this context that many of the patients with psychopathology requiring the use of neuroleptic medication are treated. It is ironic that challenging conditions such as TD are often seen by clinicians who may, because of institutional demands, have the least amount of time available to diagnose and treat the problem adequately.

TD is a relatively common condition, with a prevalence of nearly 25% in patients treated with neuroleptics (Jeste and Wyatt 1981). It persists for 3 months or longer in approximately 60% of patients whether or not neuroleptics are continued (Jeste and Wyatt 1982). No effective treatment exists for persistent TD. Furthermore, recent years have seen a dramatic increase in the malpractice litigation initiated against physicians and hospitals by patients with TD (Tancredi 1988).

The clinical relevance of TD is underscored by the formation of two American Psychiatric Association task forces reporting on TD since 1980 (Baldessarini et al. 1980; Kane et al. 1992). In 1994, for the first time, TD was included in the *Diagnostic and Statistical Manual of Mental Disorders* (American Psychiatric Association 1994), reflecting a recognition by the profession that TD nomenclature must be standardized to prevent underdiagnosis and inadequate documentation of the disorder by practitioners.

TD was first reported in 1957 by Schonecker in France (Schonecker 1957). Since then, an extensive research effort has been aimed at unraveling the intricacies of this perplexing disorder. There is now consensus that neuroleptic-induced TD is a valid clinical entity. Advances in research have led to improved knowledge of the epidemiology, phenomenology, risk factors, and course of the disorder. The pathophysiology of TD, as well as satisfactory treatment interventions for this syndrome, remains elusive, however.

Our goal in this chapter is to provide updated and clinically relevant information on TD for mental health professionals in the public health setting. We refer the reader to the appropriate research literature so that the basis of the clinical recommendations may be further explored.

Clinical Features

TD is a neuroleptic-induced disorder that consists of abnormal, involuntary movements. The movements are mainly choreiform (rapid, jerky), athetoid (slow, sinuous), or rhythmic (stereotypical) (American Psychiatric Association 1994). The orofacial region and the upper extremities are most commonly involved. Less commonly affected areas include the lower extremities and trunk. The least frequently affected areas are the muscles of respiration and the muscles involved in swallowing.

The most common orofacial features of TD are involuntary movements of the tongue (including thrusting, protrusion, and vermicular motions), jaw opening and closing, lip smacking, blinking, grimacing, and repetitive frowning. Upper extremity movements include writhing finger and thumb movements as well as flexion and extension of the wrist. Foot stamping, side-to-side foot movements, and up-and-down movements of the great toe can be seen in the lower extremity. Truncal motions include rocking and twisting of the trunk and neck as well as shoulder shrugging. Pharyngeal-laryngeal dyskinesias and diaphragmatic, intercostal, and abdominal muscle contractions are rarely seen but can cause severe complications, including respiratory and gastrointestinal disorders (Lohr and Jeste 1988).

TD can be seen at any age and has a variable pattern of appearance. The earliest symptoms typically involve buccolingual-masticatory movements but may occasionally appear in the upper extremities and other areas. TD can occasionally become severe and manifest as impaired gait, striking of the body with the limbs, and damage to the oral mucosa. Severe TD differs from mild TD in the frequency and amplitude of the movements (Gardos and Cole 1992). In children, TD is not uncommon and is phenomenologically similar to that in adults, with a predominantly orofacial distribution.

TD is exacerbated by stimulants, short-term withdrawal of neuroleptics, stress, anticholinergic medication, arousal, and voluntary movements of other parts of the body. It is relieved by sleep, increased dose of neuroleptics, relaxation, and voluntary movement of the involved parts of the body (American Psychiatric Association 1994).

TD usually develops over several months and then remains fairly stable over a period of several years (though some patients seem to get worse and some better during this period). It is not known how to predict which patients may develop severe TD, but there is some indication that severe TD may be relatively more common in patients with diagnoses other than schizophrenia (Gardos and Cole 1983). A recent longitudinal prospective study in older patients found, however, that the best predictor of severe TD was cumulative neuroleptic amount (Caligiuri et al. 1997).

If neuroleptic medication is discontinued, one-third of patients will experience remission of TD within 3 months, and one-half of patients experience improvement in symptoms within 12–18 months. When neuroleptic medication must be continued, TD remains unchanged in approximately one-half of patients, improves spontaneously in about one-third, and worsens in the rest. When neuroleptic medication is discontinued, certain patients may experience an immediate improvement in TD symptoms, whereas a substantial proportion experience an initial, short-lived exacerbation of movements.

This exacerbation (or, sometimes, first appearance of dyskinesia) is referred to as *neuroleptic-withdrawal emergent dyskinesia* and may become noticeable in the absence of preexisting TD. This condition, by definition, disappears within 1–4 weeks of neuroleptic discontinuation, but when it persists longer, the diagnosis of TD should be made.

Time may, in general, be the most important factor in determining the outcome of TD. When patients are followed for longer than 5 years, TD seems to improve or remain stable in a majority of patients with or without further neuroleptic treatment. TD is now accepted to be a syndrome rather than one specific disease entity, and it is likely that different variants of the disorder follow different courses. Several subclassification schemes have been proposed on the basis of the topographical distribution of movements, such as limb-truncal versus orofacial (Kidger et al. 1980), but the validity of these classification schemes has not been sufficiently established.

Both common and rare complications of moderate-to-severe TD occur. Common physical complications include dental and denture problems, oral mucosal ulceration, and dysarthria (Yassa and Jones 1985). Common psychosocial complications include social stigmatization with resultant embarrassment and social withdrawal. Depression and anxiety may be seen. Less common complications include temporomandibular joint disease, respiratory disturbances, dysphagia and vomiting, weight loss, and injuries from falls resulting from gait disturbance (Lohr and Jeste 1988). Suicidal ideation and some successful suicides related to TD have been reported, though the actual cause-and-effect relationship is difficult to establish because of the underlying psychopathology.

Epidemiology and Risk Factors

The prevalence of TD reported in the literature varies widely. The reasons for this variation include differences in methodology, TD criteria, and patient populations. A special difficulty with TD assessment relates to the paradoxical ability of neuroleptics to suppress TD symptoms at least temporarily. There are, therefore, a number of false negative values in any prevalence study. In a recent review (Yassa and Jeste 1992), the overall prevalence of TD in approximately 40,000 neuroleptic-treated patients was 24.2%, and the prevalence was much higher (50% or greater) in older patients.

Reported incidence of TD shows similar variability with respect to age. A large prospective study of young adults by Kane et al. (1988) showed an incidence after cumulative exposure to neuroleptics of 18.5% after 4 years, 40%

after 8 years, and 44% after 10 years. These figures assume special importance for clinicians working in the public health setting, where patients often require neuroleptic maintenance for long periods of time. A much higher incidence is reported in the older population. Jeste et al. (1995) found an alarmingly high (26.1%) cumulative annual incidence among psychiatric outpatients with a mean age of 65.5 years who were being treated with low doses of neuroleptics (an average of 150 mg of chlorpromazine equivalents). This rate is approximately five to six times greater than that reported among younger adults.

Despite years of research, the risk factors for TD are incompletely understood. Aging has been thought to be the most important risk factor for the development of TD (Kane et al. 1992). The relationship between age and TD prevalence, however, appears to be curvilinear, not linear, with prevalence increasing until age 70 and then decreasing, especially in men. Mood disorders have also been associated with an increased risk of TD (Casey 1988). More recent studies (Jeste et al. 1995; Saltz et al. 1991), however, did not find psychiatric diagnosis to be a significant risk factor for TD.

Female gender has been thought to be related to TD risk (Yassa and Jeste 1992). Meta-analysis of the available literature showed a prevalence of 26.6% in women and 21.6% in men, but it is unclear if this difference could also be accounted for by neuroleptic treatment–related factors. Furthermore, other investigators have demonstrated a greater incidence of TD in older men compared with older women (Saltz et al. 1991).

"Organic" brain dysfunction may or may not be a risk factor for TD. Yassa et al. (1984) found evidence that central nervous system damage was a risk factor for TD, but Gold et al. (1991) were not able to support such an association. Investigations designed to determine the specific relationship between brain damage and TD have demonstrated variable results (Paulsen et al. 1994).

A history of alcohol abuse or dependence has been found to be a significant predictor of the risk of TD in a multivariable analysis of 266 patients (Jeste et al. 1995). This finding was previously noted by Olivera et al. (1990) and Dixon et al. (1992). The mechanism of this alcohol-induced propensity to TD development is currently unknown. Smoking has been reported by Yassa et al. (1987) to be associated with increased prevalence of TD in psychiatric outpatients. However, replication of this finding has been inconsistent.

The relationship of ethnicity to TD is confusing in the assessment of risk factors for TD. No significant differences in the prevalence of TD were found among African Americans, whites, and Asians in a study of 491 chronic psychiatric patients (Sramek et al. 1991), but Lacro and Jeste (1997) found a nonsignificantly higher incidence of TD in African Americans compared with whites. Morgenstern and Glazer (1993) observed greater risk of TD in African Americans than in whites. Yassa and Jeste (1992) found that the lowest reported prevalence of TD appeared to be in the continent of Asia. Confounding effects of differences in treatment make it difficult to interpret the observed ethnic differences in the frequency of TD.

The presence of extrapyramidal side effects (EPS) (particularly parkinsonism or akathisia) early on in the course of neuroleptic treatment has been associated with an increased risk for TD development (Kane et al. 1988; Saltz et al. 1991). Jeste et al. (1995) found that the presence of preexisting tremor on instrumental assessment was a significant predictor of TD development. In this study, clinical ratings of EPS were not significant predictors of TD development. Subclinical motor abnormalities may, therefore, define TD risk more accurately. In addition, a positive (>0) global score on the Abnormal Involuntary Movement Scale (AIMS) (National Institute of Mental Health 1975) in the absence of clinically significant TD was found to place a patient at high risk to be subsequently diagnosed with TD. This finding points to the importance of early screening for TD, even in the absence of overt clinical symptoms, because some treatments such as vitamin E have been found to be effective mostly in patients with TD of relatively short duration (Lohr and Caligiuri 1996; Lohr et al. 1988).

Jeste et al. (1995) found that both baseline duration of neuroleptic use and cumulative neuroleptic amount were highly significant predictors of TD risk. Furthermore, cumulative high-potency (but not low-potency) neuroleptic amount seemed to be a predictor for TD onset. This finding might be explained by the tendency of clinicians to prescribe higher doses of high-potency neuroleptics. In recent years, there has been a growing clinical practice to use higher doses of high-potency neuroleptics as compared with doses of low-potency neuroleptics (Baldessarini et al. 1984; Reardon et al. 1989). Independent of this practice pattern, a possibility remains that high-potency neuroleptics may be more likely to cause TD in some patients. As mentioned above, early EPS have been reported as a possible risk factor for TD. This finding must be considered in the context of the possibility that patients with early EPS are more likely to have been taking high-potency neuroleptics, which would be more likely to produce clinically significant EPS.

The "atypical" antipsychotic clozapine appears to have a lower propensity to cause TD and may be an effective treatment for some cases of established TD (Kane et al. 1993). Clozapine acts in a pharmacologically novel fashion, different from the "typical" neuroleptics, and it may be this distinct action that results in the decreased incidence of TD. The incidence of TD with the newer serotonin-dopamine antagonists such as risperidone and olanzapine is currently unknown.

It has been speculated that the use of anticholinergic medication may promote the development of TD, but current findings do not support such an effect. In a multivariable analysis, no unique contribution of anticholinergic use to the risk of TD could be found other than that which could be explained by its association with other predictors of TD risk, in particular cumulative high-potency neuroleptic amount (Jeste et al. 1995). Anticholinergic medications should nonetheless be kept to a minimum because they appear to worsen the symptoms of preexisting TD and have other deleterious side effects such as confusion, disorientation, and urinary retention, especially in the older population.

Differential Diagnosis

Making a differential diagnosis between TD and other motor disorders can be difficult. Though choreoathetoid movements are most characteristic of TD, nearly every type of hyperkinetic movement has been reported to occur as part of TD. TD is also known to coexist with other neuroleptic-induced movement disorders. The differential diagnosis of TD is best approached by the clinician in a systematic fashion. The importance of an early differential diagnosis becomes obvious in view of the lack of effective treatments for persistent TD. Therefore, TD should be considered early in the process of evaluating a new-onset movement disorder. Three questions may be useful to guide the investigation (Jeste and Wyatt 1982): 1) Does the patient have dyskinesia? 2) Does another disorder explain the dyskinesia? 3) If the dyskinesia is related to neuroleptic use, is it TD?

Does the Patient Have Dyskinesia?

Many nondyskinetic movement disorders can be difficult to distinguish from TD, and many of these conditions may coexist with TD. Tremor may be easily confused with TD, especially the tremor of neuroleptic-induced parkinsonism, rabbit syndrome, cerebellar disease, dystonias, and drug-induced akathisia. These conditions are considered in more detail below.

Several studies have reported the coexistence of TD and neuroleptic-induced parkinsonism in 12%–18% of patients treated with neuroleptics

(Bitton and Melamed 1984; Caligiuri et al. 1991; Crane 1972; Richardson and Craig 1982). Distinguishing between these two conditions is essential because they require different treatment approaches. The tremor of TD in the fingers (2 cycles/second or less) is generally slower in frequency than the tremor of parkinsonism in the fingers (4–7 cycles/second) (Lohr and Jeste 1988). The lack of orofacial and extremity dyskinesias, as well as the improvement in neuroleptic-induced parkinsonism with anticholinergic medication, can also be used to help differentiate between neuroleptic- induced parkinsonism and TD.

Rabbit syndrome is a parkinsonian tremor in the orofacial area notable for fine, rhythmic movements of the lips, tongue, and jaw in a manner that resembles the movements that a rabbit makes when chewing. Unlike TD, the rabbit syndrome responds to anticholinergic medication and is reversible on discontinuation of the neuroleptic.

Cerebellar disease can produce an action tremor of the hands, but it is differentiated from TD by the presence of associated nystagmus, dysarthria, ataxia, and hypotonia. Fine tremors of the hands and fingers are also produced by anxiety, alcoholism, hyperthyroidism, and numerous drugs, including lithium and antidepressants.

Dystonias are disorders of muscle spasm that involve irregular, slow, contorting movements. Dystonia musculorum deformans is a genetically transmitted disorder characterized by progressive dystonia beginning in late childhood or adolescence. The movements in this disorder tend to be more progressive, severe, and dystonic than those of TD. Acute neuroleptic-induced orofacial dystonias may be confused with TD, but such dystonias are typically rapidly responsive to antihistaminic or anticholinergic medication. Idiopathic orofacial dystonia (Meige's disease) typically begins in middle to late life and consists of prolonged, symmetric, spasmodic contractions of orofacial muscles. Tardive dystonia may appear after months to years of neuroleptic exposure and may coexist with choreoathetoid TD. The neck, jaw, limbs, and back seem to be most commonly affected. Unlike TD, tardive dystonia may improve with anticholinergic medication.

Drug-induced akathisia refers to subjective complaints of restlessness or an intensely unpleasant need to move and the behavioral concomitants (e.g., swinging of the legs while sitting, rocking from foot to foot while standing) occurring secondary to drug treatment. Acute akathisia presents with motor restlessness and subjective distress. It tends to occur within the first 4 weeks of initiating or increasing the dose of neuroleptic medication, and it may develop rapidly. Chronic akathisia refers to akathisia that persists for a period longer than 3 months. Tardive akathisia appears late in the course of neuroleptic treatment. The dysphoria that accompanies akathisia of any type is a useful feature in making a differential diagnosis between akathisia and other neuroleptic-induced movement disorders. Although a patient with akathisia tends to be keenly aware of his or her distress, TD is frequently associated with a lack of awareness of having a movement disorder. Also, TD usually involves the face, mouth, and upper extremities, whereas akathisia generally involves the lower extremities.

Does Another Disorder Explain the Dyskinesia?

If it can be determined decisively that a patient has a dyskinesia, the cause of the dyskinesia must be elucidated. Numerous conditions other than neuroleptic treatment may cause dyskinesia. A common condition in a young person with orofacial dyskinesia is the use of illicit drugs, especially amphetamines. Other drugs that have been implicated include antidepressant medications, L-dopa, bromocriptine, antihistamines, anticonvulsants, and antimalarials (Jeste and Wyatt 1982). Except for amphetamines, nonneuroleptic drugs are rarely associated with persistent TD. Two neuroleptics that are commonly used for nonpsychiatric indications have been reported to produce TD. These are metoclopramide and prochlorperazine, used for gastroparesis and emesis, respectively (Sewell and Jeste 1992; Sewell et al. 1994).

Sydenham's (rheumatic) chorea is a delayed reaction to group A streptococcal infection in children or adolescents that is notable for choreiform movements of the limbs, face, and trunk. The diagnosis is established by noting other manifestations of rheumatic fever and elevated antistreptolysin O (ASO) titers.

Tourette syndrome is an interesting condition beginning between ages 2 and 15 years. It is marked by tics of the face and extremities, vocal tics, echolalia (mimicking words), echopraxia (mimicking actions), coprolalia (utterance of obscenities), compulsive behavior, attentional problems, and avoidant behavior. Tourette syndrome can usually be distinguished from TD by its distinctive presentation. In addition, the motor tics of Tourette syndrome tend to be more highly repetitive than the movements of TD. A frequently prescribed treatment for Tourette syndrome is neuroleptic medication. Therefore, it is possible to see TD existing concomitantly with Tourette syndrome, and eliciting the different components may be challenging.

Both conversion disorder and malingering are conditions that, at times, may present with apparently involuntary movements (Jeste and Wyatt 1982; Kane et al. 1992). Such dyskinesias usually involve multiple body parts and tend to be dramatic or bizarre. History taking may reveal a conscious or unconscious motivation for the symptoms. A history of psychosomatic symptoms is common in patients with conversion disorder. Hysterical symptoms may also present as an overlay with true TD.

Wilson's disease is a degenerative central nervous system disorder involving an abnormality in copper metabolism that results in several movement abnormalities, psychiatric symptoms, and systemic organ damage. A coarse "flapping" tremor and rigidity are the two most commonly seen motor signs. This disorder should be ruled out by observation for Kayser-Fleischer rings (brownish red or green crescents in the superior and inferior aspects of the corneoscleral junction) on ophthalmoscopic examination, abnormal liver function tests, and serum ceruloplasmin levels.

Both hyperthyroidism and hypoparathyroidism can produce dyskinesias similar to TD.

Huntington's disease may be difficult to distinguish clinically from TD. Huntington's disease is a hereditary (autosomal dominant mode of inheritance) degenerative disease that is marked by pathological changes in the basal ganglia. Progressive clumsiness and choreoathetoid movements usually begin before age 30. Tics, rigidity, and dystonias may also occur. The dyskinetic movements are not distinguishable from those induced by neuroleptic medication, so clinicians must make the diagnosis of Huntington's disease by focusing on the following characteristics: 1) a positive family history, 2) the presence of dementia, 3) a slowly progressive degenerative course, and 4) atrophy of the caudate on computed tomography (CT) scan or magnetic resonance imaging (MRI). These characteristics, although typical of Huntington's disease, are not generally a part of the picture with TD. Molecular genetic techniques using DNA polymorphisms linked to the disease gene are available (Koroshetz et al. 1992). Similar to Tourette syndrome, TD may develop in a patient with Huntington's disease who is receiving neuroleptics for the psychiatric symptoms of that disorder (which include dementia [89%], affective disorder [42%], and schizophrenia-like psychosis [18%]) (Jeste et al. 1984).

Another genetic disorder characterized by chorea and caudate atrophy is choreoacanthocytosis. This autosomal dominant disease has several additional clinical features such as self-mutilation, myopathy, peripheral neuropathy, and seizures (Feinberg et al. 1991). Peripheral blood smear shows the presence of acanthocytosis. Creatine phosphokinase is elevated, and the electromyelogram (EMG) shows peripheral neuropathy.

In the older patient, denture and dental difficulties, common causes of dyskinesia in the geriatric population, can present with signs remarkably similar to those of TD. Oral examination may be diagnostic of the problem, and dental consultation is warranted to correct the difficulty.

Any lesion of the basal ganglia may result in dyskinesia in the older population. The use of antiparkinsonian medications with dopaminergic properties, such as levodopa, amantadine, and bromocriptine, often causes dyskinesia in the older patient. Levodopa-induced dyskinesia is common, occurring in 40%–80% of levodopa-treated patients, and can be difficult to distinguish from TD. Jeste and Wyatt (1982) reviewed the literature on this subject and concluded that levodopa-induced dyskinesias usually resulted from high-dose therapy and were typically not persistent. The data on manifestations in different body regions are variable, with some, but not all, investigators reporting neuroleptic-induced movements as being more likely to occur in the orofacial region and levodopa-induced dyskinesia being more likely in the neck and extremities.

Spontaneous Dyskinesia

The issue of whether TD is caused by neuroleptic medication or whether it, in part, represents an inherent aspect of schizophrenia has been debated extensively. The presence of abnormal movements (often of a choreoathetoid nature) has been noted in patients with schizophrenia and other disorders. The prevalence of spontaneous dyskinesia is in the range of 4%–7% (Lohr and Jeste 1988). Women, chronically institutionalized patients, older patients, and patients with "organic" mental disorders may be at greater risk for developing these abnormal movements (Casey and Hansen 1984). These movements, although they may resemble TD, are most often mild in severity. Some schizophrenic and manic patients, especially those with catatonia, may have stereotypical movements that are more complex and repetitive than the dyskinetic movements of TD.

A high prevalence (28%) of various forms of movement disorder ("grimace, jerky, and fidgety movements") was noted in nineteenth-century patients with a predominant diagnosis of poor-prognosis chronic schizophrenia (Turner 1992). Some authors have suggested that dyskinesia, of some form, is an intrinsic sign of chronic schizophrenic illness, in line with what Kraepelin called "making faces or grimacing and the fine muscular twitching in the face." Rogers (1985) proposed that the mental and motor disturbances of schizophrenia both might be an expression of a unitary cerebral disorder and that neuroleptics might interact to hasten the appearance of TD in patients who had a likelihood of developing dyskinesia spontaneously as cerebral deterioration progressed. Waddington (1987) reported an association of orofacial (but not limb-truncal) dyskinesia with aging and cognitive impairment.

Fenton et al. (1994) studied risk factors for spontaneous dyskinesias by retrospectively examining a cohort of neuroleptic-naive schizophrenic patients. Of 100 patients, 23% had some form of movement disorder, and 15% had documented orofacial dyskinesia. These patients had lower IQ and more negative symptoms and were more symptomatic at follow-up compared with the others. The investigators proposed that the major risk factor for spontaneous dyskinesia was the deficit syndrome (which included a triad of enduring negative symptoms, cognitive dysfunction, and movement disorder) and that the two might share a common underlying psychopathology.

As Jeste and Wyatt (1982) pointed out previously, there are important differences between Kraepelin's description of motor disturbances and those in TD. Kraepelin's descriptions appear more similar to dystonias than to TD. The patients described by Kraepelin had chronic poor-prognosis schizophrenia. There is no evidence that all TD patients have schizophrenia with a worse prognosis than nondyskinetic patients. TD is reported in outpatients with schizophrenia as well as in patients with other psychiatric (e.g., affective) disorders. The symptom complex that constitutes TD is several times more common in neuroleptic-treated patients than in comparable populations not treated with neuroleptics.

Our recent study (Jeste et al. 1995) found that psychiatric diagnosis was not a significant predictor of TD on either univariable or multivariable analysis, and this suggested that the apparently increased risk of TD in patients with schizophrenia was likely to be secondary to the use of neuroleptics for longer periods and in higher amounts in this group. When a multivariable model was used, neither age nor diagnosis contributed to TD risk, a finding which suggested that these patient-related variables were less important than neuroleptic-related ones. That TD occurred with comparable frequency in patients with schizophrenia as in those without schizophrenia suggests that TD is not merely a symptom of the psychosis.

There is no argument that some patients with schizophrenic disorders manifest spontaneous dyskinesias with similar characteristics to neuroleptic-induced TD. The more important issue, from our standpoint, is that many more cases of TD in psychiatric patients are clearly the result of neuroleptic treatment. One can draw an analogy with cigarette smoking and lung cancer. Lung cancer certainly occurs in the absence of cigarette smoking, but many more cases occur in the context of cigarette smoke exposure. Likewise, TD-like spontaneous dyskinesias may occur in the absence of neuroleptic medication, but the majority of TD cases result from neuroleptic exposure.

If the Dyskinesia Is Related to Neuroleptic Use, Is It TD?

When it is established by a careful process of exclusion that neuroleptic medication is responsible for the dyskinesia, it must be determined whether the dyskinesia is indeed TD. Acute dyskinesias occurring early in the course of neuroleptic treatment have been well described and respond to administration of antihistaminic or anticholinergic medication in a similar fashion to the other acute neuroleptic-induced movement disorders. Withdrawal-emergent dyskinesia (in which dyskinetic movements are initiated or worsened when neuroleptic medication is withdrawn) is also well documented in the literature and is probably more common in children. This dyskinesia, by definition, resolves within 1–4 weeks of its onset but may herald the development of persistent TD in some patients.

Management Strategies

Despite an intense effort by investigators over the last three decades, there is no reliable therapy for TD. Therefore, the cornerstone of clinical effort must be toward prevention of the disorder.

The only method to guarantee success at TD prevention is complete avoidance of neuroleptic medication. This approach is neither feasible nor desirable in clinical psychiatric practice because neuroleptics represent the key to effective treatment of psychosis. However, it is important that neuroleptics be used only for appropriate indications. Before initiation of medication, the clinician should be certain that the psychiatric diagnosis is correct. If there is doubt, consultation should be obtained or standardized diagnostic instruments should be employed for clarification. At present, neuroleptics are considered the medication of first choice exclusively for psychotic disorders or psychotic symptoms resulting from other disorders. When a clinician uses neuroleptics for other indications (such as violent behavior, severe anxiety, or insomnia), the door is opened to clinical and legal difficulties. This is particularly important in the public health setting, where continuity of care may be compromised as a result of a patient's being seen by multiple clinicians over time. It is inadvisable to continue a neuroleptic prescribed by another physician without clarifying the clinical need.

Once the clinician is certain that a neuroleptic is warranted, a process of patient education and informed consent must be initiated. This discussion must be open and should be viewed as an *ongoing dialogue* with the patient and the patient's family (if appropriate). The physician must present the risks and benefits of treatment in a way that is commensurate with the patient's and family's level of understanding and medical sophistication. The ongoing discussions should be noted in the medical record. However, documentation, although important, does not relieve the clinician of the responsibility to ensure that the verbal communication is adequate. Viewing informed consent as an ongoing process, rather than a one-time event, is helpful for the public health clinician as well as the patient. It is unfortunate that the informed consent process has come to be viewed by many clinicians as an adversarial event between physician and patient. Learning to view the process as a shared responsibility between the two parties makes for a better physician-patient relationship as well as a sense of increased control and satisfaction for both parties. Once the neuroleptic has been initiated, the clinician must continue to assess whether there is sufficient clinical evidence to demonstrate that the benefits of continued treatment outweigh the potential risk of TD.

The finding by Jeste et al. (1995) that the Abnormal Involuntary Movement Scale (AIMS; National Institute of Mental Health 1975) global score and tremor on instrumental assessment were both significant predictors for TD lends weight to the assertion that patients requiring neuroleptic treatment over protracted periods should have periodic evaluations to assess for TD symptoms. Although instrumental assessment is probably not clinically feasible currently for most facilities, the AIMS is easily administered and has fairly good interrater reliability. The patient in the public health setting may see different clinicians over time, and the AIMS provides a method for consistently tracking a patient's symptoms. A positive score (≥ 0) on the AIMS indicates that TD may be impending even in the absence of overt physical symptoms. Although the length of time between screenings is a matter of clinical discretion, TD assessment can be quickly and reliably completed and should not represent an overwhelming, time-consuming burden.

Once new-onset TD is suspected or diagnosed, the first step is a medical workup including a complete history and physical examination (with attention to drug and toxin exposure, rheumatic fever, Sydenham's chorea, Huntington's disease, etc.). Laboratory workup, such as a CT scan, thyroid function tests, serum copper and ceruloplasmin levels, urine drug screen, and ASO titer, may be undertaken depending on diagnostic considerations in individual cases but is not necessarily indicated in every patient with suspected TD. If there is any suspicion of Wilson's disease, slit-lamp examination is strongly recommended in view of the confusing psychiatric picture of Wilson's disease, its treatability if diagnosed early, and the fatality associated with the disease if untreated. A referral to an expert in movement disorders or to a neurologist may be useful in patients with a difficult differential diagnosis.

When the medical workup is complete, an assessment of the patient's psychiatric stability must be made. A risk-benefit analysis of neuroleptic withdrawal versus neuroleptic maintenance should be undertaken with the patient and patient's family. (The risks of neuroleptic maintenance pertain primarily to side effects such as TD.) Any anticholinergic medications should be tapered (if possible) because these medications can worsen the symptoms of TD.

If neuroleptic taper is unsuccessful or is not thought to be appropriate, the "atypical" antipsychotic clozapine may deserve consideration. A recent review (Lieberman et al. 1991) indicated that clozapine was helpful in decreasing TD symptoms in 43% of patients. The advantage of clozapine as a TD treatment is that it is an effective treatment for psychosis. The implication, therefore, is that some patients who must be maintained on neuroleptic medication can potentially receive treatment for both psychosis and TD with one medication. The disadvantages of clozapine are its high expense and its range of unpleasant and dangerous side effects (the most serious being the 1% incidence of life-threatening agranulocytosis). The decision to start clozapine cannot be taken lightly. It is unknown whether the newer serotonin-dopamine antagonists such as risperidone (Marder and Meibach 1994) have a lower incidence of TD than "typical" neuroleptics, nor is it known if they possess treatment efficacy against established TD.

If clozapine is deemed an unsuitable alternative for a given patient, any one of a number of experimental treatment strategies can be tried. All of these treatment approaches have met with inconsistent results, as reported in the available literature (Jeste et al. 1988). Possibilities include dopamine antagonists, cholinergic agonists, γ-aminobutyric acid agonists, benzodiazepines, and miscellaneous other drugs. The reader is referred to an article by Jeste et al. (1988) for details. One treatment that has shown some degree of promise has been the use of the antioxidant vitamin E (α-tocopherol). Dosages are in the range of 400–1,200 mg/day. This is a reasonably safe treatment approach and may be especially useful for patients with recently diagnosed TD.

TD is a serious problem that presents the public health physician with clinical challenges and legal concerns. Because there is currently no reliably effective treatment for TD, and accurate prediction of who will develop TD is not possible, clinicians must focus on prevention of the condition. We can only hope that psychopharmacological research will develop new anti-

psychotic agents that do not cause TD and have less drastic side-effect profiles than that of clozapine. It is worth reemphasizing the value of an active
process of informed consent and patient education. This will foster a more
satisfying and productive relationship between doctor and patient and will
undoubtedly reduce the risk of malpractice litigation in the event of an unfa-
vorable outcome.

Health Services Aspects

The NIMH national plan for mental health services research, as outlined in
Caring for People With Severe Mental Disorders, calls for an expanded study
of the outcomes and effectiveness of treatments for persons with schizophrenia and other disabling mental disorders, including such potentially disabling
and unintended outcomes as TD (National Institute of Mental Health 1991).
Although TD is widely recognized as an important and prevalent complication
of neuroleptic treatment with clinical and legal implications for mental health
providers (Mills and Eth 1987), a review of the literature indicates that little
empirical research exists on 1) functional impairment (i.e., effects of TD on
patients' lives, including disability, quality of life, patient distress, and life satisfaction), and 2) screening and treatment strategies (i.e., responses of mental
health providers and mental health service systems to TD).

Functional Impairment

Except for clinical case studies, little research has been done on the functional
impairment, disability, and quality-of-life deficits associated with TD in
schizophrenia. Most clinical reports indicate that the functional impairments
resulting from severe TD may be pronounced and have profound implications
for patients' lives (Yassa and Jones 1985).

In a study of 22 patients consecutively referred to a movement disorder
clinic, several categories of functional impairment were identified, including
gait and postural impairments, speech and eating impediments, suicidal
ideation, and a variety of psychosocial impairments (Yassa and Jones 1985).
Severe limb and axial impairments contributed to problems in mobility, frequent falls, and discomfort in a variety of postures (6 of 22 cases). Speech
problems were observed to result from abnormal movements in 5 of 22 patients. A variety of psychosocial problems, including suicidal ideation, were
noted in half of all patients studied. Frequently noted were problems with
embarrassment and social stigmatization in work, school, and home settings,

leading to isolative behavior and difficulties in effectively integrating into community settings. Individual coping responses to TD, functional impairment with TD, and social responses to TD may contribute to treatment outcome in schizophrenia (Yassa and Jeste 1988). However, the functional impairments, disabilities, and quality-of-life deficits resulting from TD have received insufficient empirical attention in the literature.

Perhaps obscuring the need for systematic studies of these deficits associated with TD has been the often replicated finding that persons with TD are rarely aware of their abnormal movements in contrast with persons with Parkinson's disease (Sandyk et al. 1991). Studies of lack of awareness indicate that between 55% and 82% of patients with TD are unaware of abnormal movements. Attempts to increase subjective awareness of abnormal involuntary movements using verbal and visual feedback have shown immediate increases in awareness that are not sustained at 2-week follow-up (Decina et al. 1990). Although increased severity of TD is associated with greater awareness of abnormal involuntary movements, the presence of abnormal tongue and lip movements is generally not recognized by patients and is less likely to be associated with subjective distress in the patients (Sandyk et al. 1991). If persons with TD are unaware of abnormal movements, their ability to participate in early detection and prevention efforts may be limited (Sandyk et al. 1991).

Of particular interest is the possibility, as yet untested, that the pathogenesis of TD is heterogeneous, yielding subtypes that may vary in their effects on functional impairment, disability, and quality of life. The effect of TD on clinical outcomes is likely to be multifaceted, varying with the type and severity of TD. Factor analytic studies suggest that the pattern of correlation observed on multiarea ratings of abnormal involuntary movements in persons with TD varies according to the localization of TD: 1) lip and tongue movements, 2) trunk and limb movements, and 3) facial movements (Brown and White 1992; Glazer and Morgenstern 1988). The second factor, measuring abnormal trunk and limb movements, was more pronounced in males and was associated with higher cognitive impairment as measured by the Mini-Mental State Exam (Folstein et al. 1975) and by higher rates of negative symptoms such as affective blunting and alogia (Brown and White 1992). It has been proposed that persons with TD movements are more often aware of their limb-axial dyskinesias and that such movements produce higher levels of subjective distress.

At least one study showed that negative symptoms were associated with orofacial, but not trunk and limb, dyskinesia (Liddle et al. 1993). This suggests that the clinical and psychosocial consequences of TD may vary according to type of the disorder. In contrast, the association between TD movements and type II schizophrenia, or deficit syndrome, has not been consistently established even when subtypes of TD were taken into account.

Screening and Treatment Strategies

The advent of TD as a risk associated with neuroleptic treatment has created a great deal of concern in the psychiatric community regarding methods of best practice in the treatment of schizophrenia (Glazer et al. 1994). Two related questions are of interest regarding TD and the mental health service systems for persons with severe and persistent mental illness. First, do mental health providers recognize the occurrence of TD in routine clinical care, and does this recognition affect the typical course of treatment? Second, to what extent is the patient care affected by the treatment of TD?

Screening Strategies

The American Psychiatric Association's two task force reports (Baldessarini et al. 1980; Kane et al. 1992) on TD emphasize the importance of prevention and early detection of TD, particularly through regular screening. Screening is particularly important in the public health setting (e.g., community mental health centers and public hospitals). These entities have the predominant responsibility for treating patients with chronic mental illness who are at high risk for developing TD.

Several questions need to be answered in regard to screening. How often is screening currently performed? How often *should* screening be performed? What instrument should be used? And who should perform the screening? The ultimate question, from a clinician's point of view, may be, What are the potential consequences of not screening for TD?

Few data indicate how often screening for TD is actually performed. A study conducted by Benjamin and Munetz (1994) found that nearly 93% of the community mental health centers they surveyed screened patients for TD. Forty-one percent of these community mental health centers had a formal policy on TD screening, and 43% had actual TD screening programs. There were no data on how often the screening was performed. Little information is available on how frequently patients in other settings (public hospitals, private practice, etc.) are screened for TD.

The APA recommends screening for TD at least semiannually and more frequently when dosages or medications are being adjusted (Kane et al. 1992). Patients with chronic mental illness whose conditions have been stabilized are often seen once in 6 months in the public health setting to refill their medications. Screening or observations should be conducted and carefully recorded in the patient's chart to provide documentation of the presence or absence of TD at these visits.

A limited number of instruments have been used for screening for TD. These include the Dyskinesia Identification System—Coldwater (DIS-CO; Sprague et al. 1984); the St. Hans Rating Scale (Gerlach 1979; Gerlach et al. 1993); the Rockland Tardive Dyskinesia Rating Scale (Simpson et al. 1979); and the widely used AIMS (National Institute of Mental Health 1991). The DIS-CO is a 34-item instrument that was designed and used initially for individuals with mental retardation. This scale has been used with psychiatric patients, too. The St. Hans Rating Scale for Extrapyramidal Syndromes is a multidimensional scale that evaluates neuroleptic-induced hyperkinesia, parkinsonism, akathisia, and dystonia. The scale was developed around the same time as the AIMS; however, it is not used as widely. It has been shown to be both reliable and valid for the assessment of TD. The Rockland Tardive Dyskinesia Rating Scale, developed by Simpson and co-workers (1979), has both a longer and an abbreviated version. The abbreviated version has been used more frequently. The Rockland Scale is probably the second most commonly used scale after the AIMS. The most widely employed scale for TD appears to be the AIMS (Figure 12–1). A recent survey found that nearly two-thirds of community health centers that screened for TD used the AIMS; moreover, among the clinics having a formal policy on TD screening, more than 80% used this scale (Benjamin and Munetz 1994). The AIMS is designed to rate the severity of abnormal involuntary movements in seven different body areas. It is not intended to be a diagnostic tool in and of itself. The AIMS takes approximately 10 minutes to administer. This scale is also used widely in research on TD.

Although there are some instrumental measures that rate TD (Caligiuri et al. 1993), these are not currently widely available and are therefore not yet a practical means of assessing TD in the public health setting.

Who should perform the screening? The AIMS, like other scales, can be administered by a psychiatrist or other mental health professional. Appropriate training is important in determining who can administer the scale. In a community mental health center, nonphysicians should be encouraged to learn and administer the scale as a cost-savings measure. Time and financial resources are limited, and no evidence suggests that only psychiatrists are qualified to administer movement disorder scales. Often in the community mental health setting, psychologists, psychiatric nurses, social workers, and case managers administer the TD screenings.

The ultimate question, from a clinician's point of view, may concern the

ABNORMAL INVOLUNTARY MOVEMENT SCALE (AIMS)
Examination Procedure

Either before or after completing the examination procedure, observe the patient unobtrusively at rest (e.g., in waiting room).

The chair to be used in this examination should be a hard, firm one without arms.

1. Ask patient whether there is anything in mouth (gum, candy, etc.), and if there is, to remove it.
2. Ask patient about the *current* condition of his or her teeth. Ask if patient wears dentures. Do teeth or denture bother patient *now?*
3. Ask whether patient notices any movements in mouth, face, hands, or feet. If yes, ask to describe and to what extent they *currently* bother patient or interfere with activities.
4. Have patient sit in chair with hands on knees, legs slightly apart, and feet flat on floor. (Look at entire body for movements while patient is in this position.)
5. Ask patient to sit with hands hanging unsupported—if male, between legs; if female and wearing a dress, hanging over knees. (Observe hands and other body areas.)
6. Ask patient to open mouth. (Observe tongue at rest within mouth.) Do this twice.
7. Ask patient to protrude tongue. (Observe abnormalities of tongue movement.) Do this twice.
8. Ask patient to tap thumb, with each finger, as rapidly as possible for 10–15 seconds, first with right hand, then with left hand. (Observe facial and leg movements.)
9. Flex and extend patient's left and right arms (one at a time). (Note any rigidity separately.)
10. Ask patient to stand up. (Observe in profile. Observe all body areas again, hips included.)
11. Ask patient to extend both arms outstretched in front with palms down. (Observe trunk, legs, and mouth.)
12. Have patient walk a few paces, turn, and walk back to chair. (Observe hands and gait.) Do this twice.

(continued)

FIGURE 12–1.   Abnormal Involuntary Movement Scale (AIMS).
Source.   The Abnormal Involuntary Movement Scale was developed by the Psychopharmacology Research Branch, National Institute of Mental Health; Alcohol, Drug Abuse, and Mental Health Administration; Public Health Service; U.S. Department of Health, Education, and Welfare (from *Early Clinical Drug Evaluation Unit Intercom* 4:3–6, 1975).

Department of Health and Human Services
Public Health Services

ABNORMAL INVOLUNTARY
MOVEMENT SCALE (AIMS)

PATIENT'S NAME _____

RATER _____

DATE _____

INSTRUCTIONS: Complete Examination Procedure before making ratings.
MOVEMENT RATINGS: Rate highest severity observed.

Code   0 = None
       1 = Minimal, may be extreme normal
       2 = Mild
       3 = Moderate
       4 = Severe

		(Circle One)	CARD 01 (18-19)
Facial and Oral Movements:	1. **Muscles of facial expression,** e.g., movements of forehead, eyebrows, periorbital area, cheeks: include frowning, blinking, smiling, grimacing	0 1 2 3 4	(20)
	2. **Lips and perioral area,** e.g., puckering, pouting, smacking	0 1 2 3 4	(21)
	3. **Jaw,** e.g., biting, clenching, chewing, mouth opening, lateral movement	0 1 2 3 4	(22)
	4. **Tongue** Rate only increase in movement both in and out of mouth, NOT inability to sustain movement	0 1 2 3 4	(23)
Extremity Movements	5. **Upper (arms, wrists, hands, fingers)** Include choreic movements (i.e., rapid, objectively purposeless, irregular, spontaneous), athetoid movements (i.e., slow, irregular, complex, serpentine). Do NOT include tremor (i.e., repetitive, regular, rhythmic)	0 1 2 3 4	(24)
	6. **Lower (legs, knees, ankles, toes),** e.g., lateral knee movement, foot tapping, heel dropping, foot squirming, inversion and eversion of foot	0 1 2 3 4	(25)
Trunk Movements	7. **Neck, shoulders, hips,** e.g., rocking, twisting, squirming, pelvic gyrations	0 1 2 3 4	(26)

FIGURE 12–1.   Abnormal Involuntary Movement Scale (AIMS). *(continued)*

		(Circle One)	CARD 01 (18-19)
	8. Severity of abnormal movements	None, normal 0 Minimal 1 Mild 2 Moderate 3 Severe 4	(27)
Global Judgments:	9. Incapacitation due to abnormal movements	None, normal 0 Minimal 1 Mild 2 Moderate 3 Severe 4	(28)
	10. Patient's awareness of abnormal movements Rate only patient's report	No awareness 0 Aware, no distress 1 Aware, mild distress 2 Aware, moderate distress 3 Aware, severe distress 4	(29)
Dental Status:	11. Current problems with teeth and/or dentures	No 0 Yes 1	(30)
	12. Does patient usually wear dentures?	No 0 Yes 1	(31)

FIGURE 12-1.   Abnormal Involuntary Movement Scale (AIMS). *(continued)*

potential consequences of not screening for TD. First and foremost, a case of mild TD may go undetected for some time. Some evidence suggests that the earlier TD is noted and "treated" (by lowering dosages or changing medications), the better the outcome (Jeste and Wyatt 1982). This can have a significant impact on a patient's future treatment as well as his or her quality of life. Patients are more likely to continue treatment for their psychoses if they are not experiencing adverse effects from the medications they are receiving. The control of psychotic symptoms is generally the primary concern of most clinicians, and medication maintenance is often the only way to achieve this.

From a clinician's point of view, not screening for TD can have additional ramifications. In our increasingly litigious society, the threat of a lawsuit may have a bearing on the importance of screening for TD. Again, it is important not only to screen but also to document screening for TD. It is also advisable to document the means by which a patient was informed of the presence or absence of TD, the need for neuroleptic use, and the patient's consent for the same.

In summary, screening for TD is an important part of the patient's medical care. Screening is currently performed in a number of community mental health centers either formally or informally. It should be performed a minimum of twice per year, and the results of the screening should be carefully documented. The most widely used screening instrument, the AIMS, can be administered by psychiatrists as well as other mental health professionals with training. Screening for TD has potential benefits for both patient and mental health care provider.

Treatment strategies.   A wide range of clinical and rehabilitation outcomes can be affected directly and indirectly by the disabling influence of abnormal involuntary movements, although data on the clinical effects of such movement disorders are inadequate. TD movements may directly impede progress toward hospital release, community integration, and psychiatric rehabilitation by interfering with patients' role functioning in the community, increasing the social isolation and stigma faced by patients in the community, and, in cases of severe dyskinesia, decreasing the ability of some patients to perform activities of daily living (Yassa and Jeste 1988).

Other potential effects may stem from management of the abnormal movements themselves. Mental health providers, under clinical and legal pressures to assess and manage TD, are now faced with a nearly insoluble set of risks and benefits with regard to the use of neuroleptic agents. Several medication management strategies, including dosage reduction, targeted medication, and intermittent medication trials, designed to limit exposure to neuroleptic agents, have been employed in clinical settings and have received investigation in controlled trials (Gilbert et al. 1995). These studies have generally shown limited benefits from less aggressive management with psychotropic agents in terms of freedom from TD and clinical outcomes even if active community management and family support treatments are provided (N. Schooler, personal communication, October 1996).

The clinical risks of psychotic relapse with dosage reduction strategies should be weighed against potential benefits to patients from reduced risk of TD. Research is needed to identify patients at high risk for the development of TD in order to set guidelines for the clinical management of TD. Equally critical is the development of research that identifies the treatment practices that are associated with "optimal" outcomes in routine clinical settings. This research should consider a wide range of clinical, functional, and quality-of-life outcomes and should assess the subjective preferences of mental health consumers in understanding what is optimally effective. Presently, the best advice to the clinician in the public health setting is to use neuroleptics, when needed, in the lowest effective doses. The cost-benefit ratio of recently approved drugs such as clozapine and risperidone in the public mental health systems should be evaluated carefully.

References

American Psychiatric Association: Diagnostic and Statistical Manual of Mental Disorders, 4th Edition. Washington, DC, American Psychiatric Association, 1994

Baldessarini RJ, Cole JO, Davis JM, et al: Tardive Dyskinesia: A Task Force Report of the American Psychiatric Association. Washington, DC, American Psychiatric Association, 1980

Baldessarini RJ, Katz B, Cotton P: Dissimilar dosing with high-potency and low-potency neuroleptics. Am J Psychiatry 141:748–752, 1984

Benjamin S, Munetz M: CMHC practices related to tardive dyskinesia screening and informed consent for neuroleptic drugs. Hospital and Community Psychiatry 45:343–346, 1994

Bitton V, Melamed E: Coexistence of severe parkinsonism and tardive dyskinesia as side effects of neuroleptic therapy. J Clin Psychiatry 45:28–30, 1984

Brown KW, White T: The influence of topography on the cognitive and psychopathological effects of tardive dyskinesia. Am J Psychiatry 149:1385–1389, 1992

Caligiuri MP, Lohr JB, Bracha HS, et al: Clinical and instrumental assessment of neuroleptic-induced parkinsonism in patients with tardive dyskinesia. Biol Psychiatry 29:139–148, 1991

Caligiuri MP, Lohr JB, Panton D, et al: Extrapyramidal motor abnormalities associated with late-life psychosis. Schizophr Bull 19(4):747–754, 1993

Caligiuri MP, Lacro JP, Rockwell E, et al: Incidence and risk factors for severe tardive dyskinesia in older patients. Br J Psychiatry 171:148–153, 1997

Casey DE: Affective disorders and tardive dyskinesia. L'Encephale 14:221–226, 1988

Casey DE, Hansen TE: Spontaneous dyskinesias, in Neuropsychiatric Movement Disorders. Edited by Jeste DV, Wyatt RJ. Washington, DC, American Psychiatric Press, 1984, pp 67–95

Crane GE: Pseudoparkinsonism and tardive dyskinesia. Arch Neurol 27:426–430, 1972

Decina P, Caracci G, Sandyk R, et al: Cigarette smoking and neuroleptic-induced parkinsonism. Biol Psychiatry 28:502–508, 1990

Dixon L, Weiden PJ, Haas G, et al: Increased tardive dyskinesia in alcohol-abusing schizophrenic patients. Compr Psychiatry 33:121–122, 1992

Feinberg TE, Cianci CD, Morrow JS, et al: Diagnostic tests for choreoacanthocytosis. Neurology 41:1000–1006, 1991

Fenton WS, Wyatt RJ, McGlashan TH: Risk factors for spontaneous dyskinesia in schizophrenia. Arch Gen Psychiatry 51:643–650, 1994

Folstein MF, Folstein SE, McHugh PR: Mini-Mental State: a practical method for grading the cognitive state of patients for the clinician. J Psychiatr Res 12: 189–198, 1975

Gardos G, Cole J: The prognosis of tardive dyskinesia. J Clin Psychiatry 44:177–179, 1983

Gardos G, Cole JO: Severe tardive dyskinesia, in Movement Disorders in Neurology and Neuropsychiatry. Edited by Joseph AB, Young RR. Boston, MA, Blackwell Scientific, 1992, pp 40–45

Gerlach J: Tardive dyskinesia. Dan Med Bull 26:209–245, 1979

Gerlach J, Korsgaard S, Clemmesen P, et al: The St. Hans Rating Scale for extrapyramidal syndromes: reliability and validity. Acta Psychiatr Scand 87:244–252, 1993

Gilbert PL, Harris MJ, McAdams LA, et al: Neuroleptic withdrawal in schizophrenic patients. Arch Gen Psychiatry 52:173–188, 1995

Glazer WM, Morgenstern H: Predictors of occurrence, severity, and course of tardive dyskinesia in an outpatient population. J Clin Psychopharmacol 8(suppl): 10S–16S, 1988

Glazer WM, Morgenstern H, Doucette J: Race and tardive dyskinesia among outpatients at a CMHC. Hospital and Community Psychiatry 45:38–42, 1994

Gold JM, Egan MF, Kirch DG, et al: Tardive dyskinesia: neuropsychological, computerized tomographic, and psychiatric symptom findings. Biol Psychiatry 30: 587–599, 1991

Jeste DV, Wyatt RJ: Changing epidemiology of tardive dyskinesia—an overview. Am J Psychiatry 138:297–309, 1981

Jeste DV, Wyatt RJ: Understanding and Treating Tardive Dyskinesia. New York, Guilford, 1982

Jeste DV, Karson CN, Wyatt RJ: Movement disorder and psychopathology, in Neuropsychiatric Movement Disorders. Edited by Jeste DV, Wyatt RJ. Washington, DC, American Psychiatric Press, 1984, pp 119–150

Jeste DV, Lohr JB, Clark K, et al: Pharmacological treatment of tardive dyskinesia in the 1980s. J Clin Psychopharmacol 8(suppl):38S–48S, 1988

Jeste DV, Caligiuri MP, Paulsen JS, et al: Risk of tardive dyskinesia in older patients: a prospective longitudinal study of 266 patients. Arch Gen Psychiatry 52: 756–765, 1995

Kane JM, Woerner M, Lieberman J: Tardive dyskinesia: prevalence, incidence, and risk factors. J Clin Psychopharmacol 8 (4, suppl):52S–56S, 1988

Kane JM, Jeste DV, Barnes TRE, et al: Tardive Dyskinesia: A Task Force Report of the American Psychiatric Association. Washington, DC, American Psychiatric Association, 1992

Kane JM, Woerner MG, Pollack S, et al: Does clozapine cause tardive dyskinesia? J Clin Psychiatry 54:327–330, 1993

Kidger T, Barnes TRE, Trauer T, et al: Sub-syndromes of tardive dyskinesia. Psychol Med 10:513–520, 1980

Koroshetz WJ, Myers RH, Martin JB: The neurology of Huntington's disease, in Movement Disorders in Neurology and Neuropsychiatry. Edited by Joseph AB, Young RR. Boston, MA, Blackwell Scientific, 1992, pp 167–177

Lacro JP, Jeste DV: The role of ethnicity in the development of tardive dyskinesia, in Neuroleptic-Induced Movement Disorders. Edited by Yassa R, Nair NVP, Jeste DV. New York, Cambridge University Press, 1997, pp 298–310

Liddle PH, Barnes TR, Speller J, et al: Negative symptoms as a risk factor for tardive dyskinesia in schizophrenia. Br J Psychiatry 163:776–780, 1993

Lieberman JA, Saltz BL, Johns CA, et al: The effects of clozapine on tardive dyskinesia. Br J Psychiatry 158:503–510, 1991

Lohr JB, Caligiuri MP: A double-blind placebo-controlled study of vitamin E treatment of tardive dyskinesia. J Clin Psychiatry 57:167–173, 1996

Lohr JB, Jeste DV: Neuroleptic-induced movement disorders: tardive dyskinesia and other tardive syndromes, in Psychiatry, Revised Edition. Edited by Michels R, Cavenar JO Jr, Brodie NKH, et al. Philadelphia, PA, JB Lippincott, 1988, pp 1–17

Lohr JB, Cadet JL, Lohr MA, et al: Vitamin E in the treatment of tardive dyskinesia: the possible involvement of free radical mechanisms. Schizophr Bull 14:291–296, 1988

Marder SR, Meibach RC: Risperidone in the treatment of schizophrenia. Am J Psychiatry 151:825–835, 1994

Mills MJ, Eth S: Legal liability with psychotropic drug use: extrapyramidal syndromes and tardive dyskinesia. J Clin Psychiatry 48 (suppl):28–33, 1987

Morgenstern H, Glazer WM: Identifying risk factors for tardive dyskinesia among long-term outpatients maintained with neuroleptic medications: results of the Yale Tardive Dyskinesia Study. Arch Gen Psychiatry 50:723–733, 1993

National Institute of Mental Health: Abnormal Involuntary Movement Scale (AIMS). Early Clinical Drug Evaluation Unit Intercom 4:3–6, 1975

National Institute of Mental Health: Caring for people with severe mental disorders: a national plan of research to improve services (abstract) (DHHS Publ No ADM-91-1762). Bethesda, MD, National Institute of Mental Health, 1991

Olivera AA, Kiefer MW, Manley NK: Tardive dyskinesia in psychiatric patients with substance use disorders. Am J Drug Alcohol Abuse 16(1–2):57–66, 1990

Paulsen JS, Heaton RK, Jeste DV: Neuropsychological impairment in tardive dyskinesia. Neuropsychology 8:227–241, 1994

Reardon GT, Rifkin A, Schwartz A, et al: Changing patterns of neuroleptic dosage over a decade. Am J Psychiatry 146:726–729, 1989

Richardson MA, Craig TJ: The coexistence of parkinsonism-like symptoms and tardive dyskinesia. Am J Psychiatry 139:341–343, 1982

Rogers D: The motor disorders of severe psychiatric illness: a conflict of paradigms. Br J Psychiatry 147:221–232, 1985

Saltz BL, Woerner MG, Kane JM, et al: Prospective study of tardive dyskinesia incidence in the elderly. JAMA 266:2402–2406, 1991

Sandyk R, Kay SR, Awerbuch GI, et al: Risk factors for neuroleptic-induced movement disorders. Int J Neurosci 61:149–188, 1991

Schonecker M: Ein eigentumliches Syndrom im oralen Bereich bei Megaphen Applikation. Nervenarzt 28:35, 1957

Sewell DD, Jeste DV: Metoclopramide-associated tardive dyskinesia: an analysis of 67 cases. Arch Fam Med 1:271–278, 1992

Sewell DD, Kodsi AB, Caligiuri MP, et al: Metoclopramide and tardive dyskinesia. Biol Psychiatry 36:630–632, 1994

Simpson GM, Lee JH, Zoubok B, et al: A rating scale for tardive dyskinesia. Psychopharmacology (Berl) 64:171–179, 1979

Sprague RL, Kalachmk JE, Bruenig SE, et al: The Dyskinesia Identification System–Coldwater (DIS-CO): a TD rating scale for the developmentally disabled. Psychopharmacol Bull 20:328–338, 1984

Sramek J, Roy S, Ahrens T, et al: Prevalence of tardive dyskinesia among three ethnic groups of chronic psychiatric patients. Hospital and Community Psychiatry 42: 590–592, 1991

Tancredi LR: Malpractice and tardive dyskinesia: a conceptual dilemma. J Clin Psychopharmacol 8(suppl):71S–76S, 1988

Turner TH: A diagnostic analysis of the case books of Ticehurst House Asylum, 1845–1890. Psychological Medicine Monograph Supplement 21:1–70, 1992

Waddington JL: Tardive dyskinesia in schizophrenia and other disorders: associations with aging, cognitive dysfunction and structural brain pathology in relation to neuroleptic exposure. Human Psychopharmacology 2:11–22, 1987

Yassa R, Jeste DV: Tardive dyskinesia 1988: thirty-one years later. J Clin Psychopharmacol 8(4, suppl):1S, 1988

Yassa R, Jeste DV: Gender differences in tardive dyskinesia: a critical review of the literature. Schizophr Bull 18:701–715, 1992

Yassa R, Jones BD: Complications of tardive dyskinesia: a review. Psychosomatics 26:305–313, 1985

Yassa R, Nair V, Schwartz G: Tardive dyskinesia and the primary psychiatric diagnosis. Psychosomatics 25:135–138, 1984

Yassa R, Lal S, Korpassy A, et al: Nicotine exposure and tardive dyskinesia. Biol Psychiatry 22:67–72, 1987

CHAPTER 13

Neuropsychiatry of Sexual Deviations

Jeffrey L. Cummings, M.D.

Sexual deviations are disturbances of behavior in which the individual has recurrent sexual urges involving nonhuman objects, the suffering or humiliation of oneself or one's partner, or children or nonconsenting adults (American Psychiatric Association 1994). Sexual deviations involve institutional neuropsychiatry in two major ways: 1) imposition of one's sexual behavior on a child or nonconsenting person is illegal and may result in arrest or incarceration, and 2) brain diseases may cause aberrant sexual behavior, and institutions with large populations of patients with brain disorders—nursing homes, institutions for the mentally retarded, chronic mental hospitals—will care for individuals with sexually deviant behavior.

This chapter begins with a brief review of the physiology of sexual arousal. Sexual deviations are defined and described, and their prevalence is described. The occurrence of sexual deviations among individuals in the major neuropsychiatric institutions is discussed, and sexually deviant behavior in patients with overt neurological diseases is noted. Evaluation and treatment of sexual deviations are discussed. Although rape is an act of sexual aggression and is not considered a sexual deviation, it is considered at some points

This project was supported by the Department of Veterans Affairs and Grant AG10123 for an Alzheimer's Disease Core Center from the National Institute on Aging.

in this chapter because it is a major type of sexual behavior that results in incarceration and is an important aspect of institutional neuropsychiatry.

Anatomy and Physiology of Sexual Behavior

Human sexual activity can be divided into three phases: attraction to a potential partner, sexual arousal, and intercourse. Each of these phases of sexual behavior—desire, excitement, orgasm—is mediated by separate but related anatomical structures and physiological functions (Kaplan 1979). The anatomy and physiology of desire is the least well understood of the three stages of sexual behavior and is the aspect of sexual behavior that is altered in some of the sexual deviations. Sexual desire is a basic survival drive similar to eating, drinking, and sleeping and shares with these behaviors a complex neural organization that involves both primitive structures of the brain such as the hypothalamus and more recently evolved brain regions such as the temporal and frontal lobes. The object of sexual desire is determined by one's sexual orientation, and orientation is, in turn, a product of one's genetic sex (XX for females, XY for males), hormonal influences on specific hypothalamic nuclei and possibly other brain structures, and early life experiences relevant to erotic behavior (Money 1986). Thus, sexual deviations with sexual urges involving fetishes, children, nonconsenting adults, or humiliation of one's partner or oneself may result from aberrant sexual orientation associated with either abnormal brain function or atypical early life experiences. This model of sexual deviations predicts that some, but not all, individuals manifesting deviant behavior will have evidence of brain dysfunction and that sexual deviations will occur more often in individuals with overt brain disease than in the general population. Substantial evidence supports both of these predictions.

In addition to sexual orientation, the desire phase of sexual life includes libido, the strength or urgency of sexual impulses. Reduced desire for sexual activity (hypoactive sexual desire disorder), although it may be a source of distress for the individual or the individual's mate, does not lead to adverse legal consequences. Increased sexual desire, however, may result in socially provocative behavior that can lead to incarceration or promiscuity. Occasionally, heightened libido can lead to forced sexual behavior or rape. Mania with hypersexuality, hypersexuality associated with brain injury, and idiopathic nymphomania in women and satyriasis in men are the principal clinical disorders with increased sexual activity (Goodman 1981; Gorman and

Cummings 1992; Miller et al. 1986). In some circumstances, altered sexual orientation and hypersexuality co-occur.

Transitional between desire and arousal is the ritual of courtship. Courtship is the process by which, under normal circumstances, the potential partner is attracted. Although educational, social, and cultural influences affect courtship, many aspects of courtship are stereotyped and innate. The timing of courtship, for example, is linked to hormonal status and typically begins in adolescence with the onset of puberty (LeVay 1993). Some types of sexual deviations may be disorders of courtship behavior (Freund 1988). Whereas displays of wealth, power, strength, and sexual prowess are part of typical courtship behavior, exhibitionism, for example, is a disorder of excessive and inappropriate sexual exposure. Likewise, voyeurism may be a perversion of the normal neuropsychological processes involved in sexual attraction in the courtship process. Frotteurism may be a distortion of the normal physical touching that occurs in the course of courtship. In this approach, some types of rape could be seen as the preferential omission or suppression of courtship behaviors. These four types of behavioral disturbances—exhibitionism, voyeurism, frotteurism, and rape—occur in the same individuals with unusual frequency, suggesting that they share common pathophysiological mechanisms. Freund and Lanchard (1986) found that 73.5% of voyeurs have also engaged in exhibitionism, 33.7% were involved in frotteurism, and 18.4% were rapists.

Successful courtship leads to an opportunity for sexual activity. The hallmark of sexual excitement is reflex vasodilation of the genital blood vessels, leading to penile erection in men and engorgement of the labia and the tissues of the vaginal barrel in women (Kaplan 1979). Excitement phase disorders are typically conditions that interfere with normal physiological function and include impotence and dyspareunia. Sexual deviations are not found among disorders of the excitement phase, although sexual photographs and films, erotic literature, sexually explicit discussions (usually on the telephone), and other pornographic material, some of which can be illegal, can induce the excitement phase.

Orgasm is the final phase of the sexual act. A plateau stage of increasing muscular tension, accelerated heart rate, and rising blood pressure precedes orgasm, and the orgasm is followed by a resolution stage in which the anatomical and physiological changes of the excitement and plateau stages reverse (Brackett et al. 1994). Premature ejaculation and retarded ejaculation (in either men or women) are disorders of the orgastic phase of sexual behavior. Table 13–1 provides a summary of disorders of sexual behavior according to which phase of sexual behavior is disturbed.

TABLE 13–1.   Disorders of sexual behavior classified according to the phase of sexual behavior altered

Desire-phase disorders
   Hypoactive sexual desire
   Sexual aversion
   Paraphilias (sexual deviations)
   Nymphomania and satyriasis
Excitement-phase disorders
   Female sexual arousal disorder
   Male erectile disorder (impotence)
Orgasm-phase disorders
   Female orgasmic disorder
   Male orgasmic disorder
   Premature ejaculation

Types of Sexual Deviations

Sexual deviations (also known as paraphilias) are characterized by recurrent intense sexually arousing fantasies, sexual urges, or behaviors generally involving nonhuman objects, the suffering or humiliation of oneself or one's partner, or children or other nonconsenting persons (American Psychiatric Association 1994). Paraphilic behavior may lead to arrest and incarceration when it involves children or nonconsenting adults. Pedophilia, exhibitionism, and voyeurism are the most common sexual deviations for which arrest occurs. Sexual deviations are far more common among men than among women, but with sexual deviations associated with neurological disorders, women are involved approximately as often as men (Cummings and Miller 1994).

An extraordinarily wide variety of paraphilias have been reported, attesting to the diverse array of objects and activities that can be imbued with erotic significance for the paraphilic individual. The most common paraphilias are exhibitionism, fetishism, frotteurism, pedophilia, sexual masochism, sexual sadism, transvestic fetishism, and voyeurism (American Psychiatric Association 1994).

Paraphilias often co-occur. For example, Prentky and colleagues (1989) examined serial sexual murderers and found that 70% had compulsive masturbation, 25% had engaged in indecent exposure, 75% evidenced voyeurism, 71% had fetishism, and 25% engaged in cross-dressing. Rooth (1973) found that among a series of individuals convicted of exhibitionism, 40% had also been involved in frotteurism, 25% had pedophilic experiences, and 17% exhibited voyeurism.

The prevalence of paraphilic disorders in the population is unknown because individuals come to attention only if they violate the law, are distressed by the behavior and seek professional help, or are brought to counseling by a partner. In a recent national survey of 2,765 individuals over age 18 (approximately 50% men and 50% women) from a broad range of socioeconomic backgrounds, 2% of men and 0% of women indicated that they had personal experience with sex with children, 14% of men and 11% of women had personal experience with sadomasochism, 6% of men and 3% of women had personal experience with cross-dressing, 11% of men and 6% of women had personal experience with fetishes, and 6% of men and 4% of women had personal experience with being urinated on to achieve sexual arousal (Janus and Janus 1993). The accuracy of the survey responses cannot be directly verified, but the answers suggest that some degree of paraphilic behavior is not distinctly unusual.

Review of prison populations provides insight into the prevalence of paraphilias sufficiently severe to require incarceration. An investigation of psychiatric disorders among women serving prison sentences in England found that 0.4% had sexual disorders compared with 2.2% of male prisoners (Maden et al. 1994). Among 119,951 felons in California State prisons in 1994, there were 4,989 (4%) whose crime was a paraphilia. Of these, the vast majority involved pedophilic acts (4,752 of the 4,989, or 95%). In addition, there were 3,350 individuals who had been convicted of sexually aggressive actions (2,206 for rape, 690 for oral copulation, 197 for sodomy, and 257 for penetration with an object) (data from the Department of Corrections, State of California, 1994). These figures suggest that pedophilia is the sex-behavior crime most likely to lead to conviction and that it is a far more common reason for incarceration than any other sexual offense including rape.

Rape

Rape is considered separately because it is not classified as a sexual deviation but is an important disorder as it relates to institutional neuropsychiatry. Rape is conventionally defined as vaginal penetration of a nonconsenting female by a male offender. A broader definition of rape subsumes related forms of sexual aggression and forced body contact with unwilling women including forced oral and anal sex (Langevin and Lang 1987).

When examined from a clinical perspective, rape is found to be associated with several psychiatric disorders; data linking rape with paraphilias have been inconsistent. Langevin and Lang (1987) found that approximately 40% of rapists have antisocial personality disorder and the rape is one manifestation of the individual's impulsiveness, recklessness, and disregard for social norms and lawful behaviors. Forty percent of the rapists met criteria for sadism, and the rape was one expression of sadistic behavior. Twenty-five percent of these individuals also engaged in transvestic fetishism (cross-dressing). Both sadistic and nonsadistic rapists had an increased frequency of brain pathology, endocrine disturbances, and substance abuse and a history of physical and sexual abuse and violent socialization. Freund (1988) reported that of patients assessed for rape, 11.5% also manifested voyeurism, 17.3% had engaged in exhibitionism, and 12.8% admitted frotteurism. Henn et al. (1976), however, studied 239 individuals convicted of rape or attempted rape and referred for forensic assessment and found that 48% had antisocial personality disorders, 31% had other personality disorders, 13% had schizophrenia, and the others had schizoaffective disorder, mood disorders, substance abuse, neurological disorders, or mental retardation. No patients with paraphilic disorders were identified in this study. Alcohol use is frequently a contributing factor to rape. Ellis and Brancale (1956) found that alcohol played a role in 38% of forcible rapes and 53% of sexual assaults. Thus, there is a consensus that antisocial personality disorder is the most common psychiatric diagnosis among rapists, but the frequency of paraphilias among rapists and how often rape may be a manifestation of a paraphilia are controversial. Likewise, although neurological disorders are more common among rapists than among control subjects, the specifics of these relationships have not been detailed.

Neurological Disorders With Sexual Deviance

Brain disorders are frequently manifested by changes in behavior, and altered sexual behavior is among the types of behavioral change occasionally observed. Reduced sexual behavior is common in many neurological disorders and is the most frequent change in sexual conduct reported. A few diseases, however, may cause sexual deviations or marked increase in libido (Table 13–2). Exhibitionism and pedophilia are the two types of paraphilic behavior most commonly reported in patients with neurological disorders.

TABLE 13–2.   Sexual deviations reported in patients with neurological disorders

Neurological disorder	Sexual deviation
Alzheimer's disease	Exhibitionism, pedophilia, sexual aggression
Vascular dementia	Exhibitionism
Hydrocephalus	Voyeurism, exhibitionism
Huntington's disease	Exhibitionism
Brainstem tumor	Pedophilia
Anoxic brain injury	Pedophilia
Multiple sclerosis	Fetishism, zoophilia
Parkinson's disease plus treatment	Sadism, masochism
Anterior communicating aneurysm	Exhibitionism
Gilles de la Tourette's syndrome	Exhibitionism
Postencephalitic parkinsonism	Exhibitionism, sadism, pedophilia, zoophilia, sexual aggression
Postencephalitic syndrome following herpes encephalitis	Altered sexual orientation, hypersexuality
Temporal lobe epilepsy	Transvestism, fetishism, exhibitionism, masochism, voyeurism, pedophilia

Brain tumors are one potential cause of sexually deviant behavior. A brainstem tumor that invaded the midbrain and hypothalamus has been associated with late-onset pedophilia (Miller et al. 1986). Regestein and Reich (1978) described a patient with a frontal lobe tumor who exhibited hypersexuality and pedophilia, and Langevin et al. (1988) observed a sexually aggressive patient with a left frontotemporal glioma.

Huntington's disease is associated with paraphilic behaviors. Among 39 patients with Huntington's disease studied by Federoff and colleagues (1994), 19% of men and 8% of women had paraphilias including exhibitionism, transvestic fetishism, pedophilia, and telephone scatophilia. Sexual aggression occurred in some patients. Hypersexuality occurring after onset of Huntington's disease was not uncommon. An association emerged between inhibited orgasm, hypersexuality, and paraphilic behavior.

Multiple sclerosis has occasionally been associated with paraphilic behavior. Hypersexuality and a foot fetish were observed following onset of multiple sclerosis in a man in whom magnetic resonance imaging (MRI) revealed bilateral frontal and temporal lobe lesions (Huws et al. 1991). Ortego and colleagues (1993) reported a 39-year-old woman who manifested multiple paraphilias (zoophilia, exhibitionism, voyeurism, and ephebophilia [arousal by adolescent-age individuals]) in addition to new-onset incest, homosexuality, and hypersexuality after the appearance of symptoms of multiple sclerosis. Despite clear evidence of a neurological disease, the patient was incarcerated for her behavior and died of complications of her illness while in jail. At autopsy, there was widespread cerebral demyelination including the white matter of the frontal lobes.

Patients with dementia rarely exhibit sexually deviant behavior. Rabins et al. (1982) found that families of 1 of 51 patients with dementia identified sexually inappropriate behavior as a problem, and Kumar et al. (1988) reported sexually assaultive or inappropriate behavior in 2 of 49 patients with dementia. Ryden (1988) identified sexual aggression in 18% of 183 patients with dementia living in the community, and Burns et al. (1990) reported sexual disinhibition in 7% of patients with Alzheimer's disease.

Idiopathic Parkinson's disease has not been reported to produce paraphilic behavior, but treatment with dopaminergic agents may lead to sexually deviant behavior. Patients with masochism and sexual sadism following levodopa treatment have been reported (Harvey 1988; Miller et al. 1986). Postencephalitic syndromes (with and without parkinsonism) following von Economo's disease were often complicated by paraphilic behavior. Sexual deviations were particularly common in childhood victims of the disease. Hypersexuality, exhibitionism, sadism, pedophilia, zoophilia, and sexual aggression were observed in postencephalitic patients (Cheyette and Cummings 1995; Poeck and Pilleri 1965).

An unusual number of patients with paraphilias and temporal lobe epilepsy have been reported. The prevalence of sexual deviations among patients with epilepsy is low, but the frequency of such deviations in patients with epilepsy exceeds that in the general population. Exhibitionism, voyeurism, fetishism, sadism, masochism, frotteurism, nymphomania, and pedophilia have been reported in patients with temporal lobe dysfunction and seizures (Erickson 1945; Hooshmand and Brawley 1969; Hunter et al. 1963; Kolarsky et al. 1967; Mitchell et al. 1954).

A variety of other neurological disorders occasionally have been associated with paraphilias. Miller et al. (1986) reported a patient with postencephalitic hydrocephalus who exhibited hypersexuality, frotteurism, exhibitionism, and triolism. Gorman and Cummings (1992) described two patients who developed marked hypersexuality following injury to the septal area incurred in the course of placing ventriculoperitoneal shunts for the treatment of obstructive hydrocephalus. Walinder (1965) described a patient who developed transvestism following a traumatic brain injury. Exhibitionism and telephone scatophilia may occur as manifestations of obsessive-compulsive disorder in Gilles de la Tourette's syndrome (Comings and Comings 1982). Rupture of anterior cerebral artery aneurysms produces injury to the orbitofrontal cortex, which can lead to disinhibited behavior. Patients may exhibit sexually deviant behavior, including exhibitionism, lewd behavior, and frotteurism (Miller et al. 1986).

Hypersexuality can occur with secondary mania, and in some cases the exaggerated sexual behavior is disproportionate to other manic symptoms. Frontal lobe tumors, strokes, or injury to the temporobasal region, perithalamic areas, or caudate nucleus may cause secondary mania and hypersexuality (Miller et al. 1986; Richfield et al. 1987).

Klüver-Bucy syndrome is associated with hypersexuality, hyperorality, placidity, agnosia, and hypermetamorphosis (compulsive exploration of objects in the environment). Fragments of Klüver-Bucy syndrome, including hypersexuality, may be seen in a variety of clinical conditions such as stroke, herpes encephalitis, posttraumatic encephalopathy, paraneoplastic limbic encephalitis, Pick's disease, Alzheimer's disease, hypoglycemia, and toxoplasmic encephalitis (Lilly et al. 1983; Monga et al. 1986). Klüver-Bucy syndrome may account for increased sexual activity in postictal states or after successful epilepsy surgery (Blumer 1970; Miller et al. 1986).

Brain dysfunction associated with chronic or acute substance use is common in patients with paraphilias. Psychoactive substance abuse was present in 46.7% and alcohol abuse in 40% of one large sample (Kafka and Prentsky 1994).

Neurological Dysfunction in Sexual Offenders

Few studies have assessed the prevalence of neurological disorders among sexual offenders. In one of the few studies to address this issue, Henn et al. (1976) reviewed the records of 1,195 individuals referred to a forensic mental health center. Of these, 239 had committed sexual offenses. Organic mental syndromes (OMS) and mental retardation were not uncommon in these individuals: 2.9% of rapists had OMS, and 2.9% had mental retardation; 14.4% of pedophiles had OMS, and 13.5% were mentally handicapped. What proportion of offenders were referred for this type of evaluation was not stated.

Evidence of biological dysfunction is common among individuals with sexual deviations. Berlin (1983) summarized findings in 34 individuals evaluated for paraphilias in a university sexual disorders clinic. He found that 19 had elevated levels of testosterone, luteinizing hormone, or follicle-stimulating hormone; 4 had excessive cortical atrophy or other abnormalities on computed tomography (CT); 2 had dyslexia; 2 had neuro-ophthalmological abnormalities; 4 had Klinefelter's syndrome, and 2 had other chromosomal defects; 1 was nearly blind from brain injury; and 1 had seizures. None were without some evidence of biological dysfunction.

Neuroimaging

Studies with CT have usually revealed more brain abnormalities among sexual offenders than among matched control subjects, although the sample sizes of these studies have been small and the differences have not always reached statistical significance. Focal abnormalities have been detected in 25%–52% of pedophilic individuals, and the abnormalities occur most frequently in the temporal lobes (Raine 1993). Langevin and co-workers (1988) compared CT scans of patients with sexual sadism with scans of nonsadistic sexually aggressive individuals and control subjects. Forty-one percent of the patients with sexual sadism had right temporal horn enlargement consistent with right temporal lobar atrophy, whereas only 11% of nonsadistic sexually aggressive individuals and 13% of control subjects exhibited this phenomenon.

Cerebral blood flow studies of pedophilic individuals have shown reduced blood flow in most brain regions compared with cerebral blood flow in control subjects, but only a few studies have been performed (Raine 1993). Graber and colleagues (1984) found reduced cerebral blood flow in three of six pedophilic individuals: all had more marked reductions involving the left than the right hemisphere, and in one patient right brain blood flow was normal.

Neuropsychological Assessment

Neuropsychological studies reveal a higher prevalence of neuropsychological deficits among sexual offenders than among control subjects, but no specific pattern of deficits has been identified (Raine 1993). Graber et al. (1984) reported that of 6 sexual offenders, 3 had abnormalities on the Luria-Nebraska Neuropsychological Battery. Performance profiles suggested multifocal abnormalities involving the right frontal lobe in two of the patients and right temporal lobe in one. Sexually aggressive offenders were also found by Langevin et al. (1988) to demonstrate more abnormalities on neuropsychological tests than control subjects. Ellis and Brancale (1956) reported that in their study of 300 convicted sex offenders, 55% had scores indicating average or superior intelligence, 27% had scores reflecting intelligence in the dull-normal range, and 18% had scores indicating mental handicap. Low intelligence was most common among those convicted of offenses involving minors and animals.

Electroencephalography

A few studies have used electroencephalography to assess brain function in patients with sexual deviations. One study of transsexual individuals found that 48% had definite and 24% had borderline abnormalities on the electroencephalogram (EEG). Ten had focal changes in the temporal lobes (6 left-sided and 4 right-sided) (Hoenig and Kenna 1979). Walinder (1965) studied 26 individuals with transvestism and found that 14 had normal or probably normal EEGs, 2 had borderline recordings, and 10 had definite abnormalities. EEG disturbances noted included generalized slowing and focal temporal lobe changes. Gilby and colleagues (1989) compared mentally retarded adolescent sex offenders with nonretarded adolescent offenders and found EEG abnormalities in 50% of the former and 10% of the latter.

Neuroendocrinological Investigations

Studies of neuroendocrinological function in patients with paraphilias suggest that many patients have neuroendocrinological disturbances. High resting levels of testosterone, luteinizing hormone, and follicle-stimulating hormone are common (Berlin 1983), and hyperprolactinemia has been reported in pedophilia (Harrison et al. 1989). Pedophilic individuals often have a markedly elevated response of luteinizing hormone to luteinizing hormone–releasing hormone compared with that of control subjects and nonpedophilic paraphilia patients (Gaffney and Berlin 1984).

Aberrant Sexual Behavior in Residents of Noncriminal Institutions

Residents of Mental Hospitals for Long-Term Care

Sexually deviant behavior or increased sexual activity may be observed among the residents of mental hospitals that provide long-term care. In some cases, paraphilic behavior can be part of the mental illness, whereas in others the aberrant sexual activity can result from the marked restriction of opportunities for more normal sexual behavior afforded by institutional life. Hypersexuality is common in the course of manic episodes, occurring in 65% of manic patients (Tsuang 1975). Schizophrenic patients are often hyposexual but may manifest bizarre sexual behavior as part of a delusional disorder. Delusions of sexual metamorphosis, sexual persecution, sexualization of body parts, or pregnancy, as well as sexual hallucinations (visual, olfactory, somatosensory), have been described. Exhibitionism, pedophilia, and sexual masochism have been reported in schizophrenia (Akhtar and Thomson 1980).

Individuals With Mental Retardation

Sexually deviant behavior occurs with increased frequency among people who are mentally retarded. The incidence of sexual offenses has been found to be four to six times that in the general population (Day 1993). Among aberrant sexual acts, indecent assaults, indecent advances, and indecent exposure are the most common sexual acts committed by people who are mentally impaired. Rape and attempted rape account for only 1% of the crimes committed by individuals with mental retardation (Day 1993). Sexual crimes committed by individuals who are mentally retarded are less patterned than those of individuals who are not mentally retarded. Offenses may involve victims of any age or sex, and the offender is likely to know the victim. The acts depend on opportunity more than specific intent and may partially reflect the restricted outlets for sexual behavior available to most individuals who are mentally retarded. Aberrant sexual behavior is the principal reason for institutionalization of women who are mentally retarded, accounting for half or more of the aberrant activities. In many cases, commitment appears to be out of concern for the health and welfare of the individual. Promiscuity, sexual delinquency, and prostitution are the behaviors most often reported (Day 1993).

Residents of Nursing Homes

Dementia is present in 40%–80% of nursing home residents, and, as noted above, 2%–20% of patients with dementia have been reported to exhibit sexual aggression and other inappropriate sexual activity.

Evaluation Strategies for Sexual Offenders

The high rate of neurological abnormalities among patients with sexual deviations, as well as the large number of neurological diseases that can produce sexually deviant behavior, makes a search for neurological dysfunction among institutionalized patients with paraphilic behavior imperative. Table 13–3 provides a guide to the evaluation of the paraphilic patient (see also Chapter 2). Assessment of sexual misconduct in penal settings is typically more comprehensive than evaluations of sexual misconduct in other settings because of the greater severity of behavioral pathology and the greater likelihood of brain disorders. A developmental history will reveal evidence of developmental delay or adverse early life events. Any history of physical abuse, sexual abuse, family violence, and marital discord should be sought. A medical history should include a search for trauma, seizures, neurological symptoms, headaches, or visual changes. Review of the substance abuse history can contribute information regarding addiction and dependency. Alcohol consumption contributes to many sexually aggressive behavioral acts (Ellis and Brancale 1956), and cocaine also appears to activate sexually aggressive behavior. Neurological examination should concentrate on focal neurological signs, extrapyramidal dysfunction, and head size. Mental status examination will elicit information concerning memory function, frontal lobe abnormalities and disinhibition, obsessions and compulsions, psychosis, and mood changes.

Neuropsychological assessment should be routinely performed as part of the evaluation of paraphilic individuals. Evidence of mental retardation, dementia, or focal temporal or frontal lobe dysfunction relevant to understanding the behavioral changes may be identified. Similarly, EEG and neuroimaging (CT or MRI) should be obtained, given the high frequency of abnormalities discovered in studies of paraphilic patients. Neuroendocrine testing may reveal abnormalities in patients with sexually deviant behavior, but the interpretation of these changes is not clear and the results do not provide information that guides treatment. Such assessments are not indicated in patients unless there is evidence of an endocrine disorder on physical examination.

Evaluations that are more specific to assessment of paraphilic urges may have diagnostic and prognostic applications. For example, Freund (1988) found that rapists had greater penile tumescence than did control subjects when exposed to stimulus narratives that depict the protagonist in a voyeuristic situation, and rapists maintained penile tumescence more than did control subjects when narratives depict a fearful woman.

Comprehensive evaluation may reveal a treatable neurological disorder (e.g., epilepsy, brain tumor), may affect the types of intervention considered (e.g., some types of treatment will be less efficacious among patients with mental retardation; substance abuse therapy may be an important aspect of management if intoxication was an important contributor to a sexual of-

TABLE 13–3. Key areas to be explored in the history and examination of individuals with paraphilic behavior to help discover neurological factors contributing to the behavior

Historical information	Neurological condition
Developmental history	
Difficult labor	Birth injury
Delayed acquisition of developmental milestones	Mental retardation
Poor academic performance	Learning disability, mental retardation
Febrile convulsions	Epilepsy
History	
Head trauma	Traumatic brain injury
Convulsions	Epilepsy
Alcohol or other substance abuse	
Chronic	Dementia
Acute (at time of crime)	Intoxication
Temporary numbness or blindness	Multiple sclerosis
Headaches	Brain tumors
Tics	Gilles de la Tourette's syndrome
Excessive movement, fidgeting	Huntington's disease
Sudden onset of neurological dysfunction	Stroke
Memory impairment	Dementia
Delusions	Psychosis
Hyperactivity, grandiosity	Mania
Sadness, hopelessness, worthlessness	Depression
Obsessions, compulsions	Obsessive-compulsive disorder
Neurological examination	
Head circumference	Arrested brain growth (small) or compensated hydrocephalus (large)
Facial asymmetry	Common in temporal lobe epilepsy
Focal neurological signs	Trauma, tumor, stroke
Tics	Gilles de la Tourette's syndrome
Akinesia, rigidity	Parkinsonism
Neurological soft signs	Mild brain dysfunction
Congenital anomalies	Prenatal disorder

(continued)

TABLE 13–3.   Key areas to be explored in the history and examination of individuals with paraphilic behavior to help discover neurological factors contributing to the behavior *(continued)*

Historical information	Neurological condition
Neuropsychological assessment	
Memory disturbances	Amnesia, dementia
Executive dysfunction	Frontal lobe syndrome, dementia
Mental retardation	Prenatal or early-life disorder
Neuropsychiatric assessment	
Mood disorder	Depression, mania
Delusions	Psychosis
Obsessions, compulsions	Obsessive-compulsive disorder
Laboratory assessment	
EEG	Generalized, focal, or epileptic brain dysfunction
CT or MRI	Excessive atrophy, hydrocephalus, brain tumor, stroke, traumatic changes
PET, SPECT	Experimental assessments
Penile tumescence	Experimental evaluation

Note. CT = computed tomography; EEG = electroencephalography; MRI = magnetic resonance imaging; PET = positron-emission tomography; SPECT = single photon emission computed tomography.

fense), and may condition sentencing if the neurological condition that was revealed produced diminished capacity for personal responsibility.

Treatment and Management of Sexual Deviations

Physical treatment (pharmacotherapy, castration, behavioral neurosurgery) of sexual deviations has been fraught with controversy and contradiction. Biological therapies have generally been eschewed in favor of conditioning therapies and incarceration. Controlled studies are virtually nonexistent and results are inconclusive.

Medical Treatment

Medroxyprogesterone acetate (MPA) is the drug most frequently used in the United States for the treatment of paraphilic behavior. It induces testosterone-

A-reductase in the liver, accelerates the metabolism of testosterone, and lowers serum testosterone levels (Bradford 1988). The drug appears to reduce sexual desire, and the relapse rate among patients taking the depot form is approximately 15% per year, which is less than the rate among untreated patients (Berlin 1983). Satyriasis has been suppressed by treatment with MPA (Moore 1980), and sexual aggression in dementia has also been effectively reduced by MPA (Cooper 1987). Oral MPA successfully reduced a variety of types of paraphilic behaviors in six patients by 50%–75% (Gottesman and Schubert 1993). An increased risk of stroke can be found among patients administered MPA (Biller and Saver 1995).

Cyproterone acetate (CPA), an androgen receptor blocker, has also been used to suppress hypersexual and sexually deviant behavior (Mellor et al. 1988). Markedly reduced recidivism has been reported among offenders treated with CPA as long as they continue to take the drug (Bradford 1988).

Leuprolide, a gonadotropin-releasing hormone agonist, has been used to treat exhibitionism in a patient with Huntington's disease (Rich and Ovsiew 1994). In a recent single-case study, leuprolide proved to be more efficacious than CPA (100 or 200 mg/day) in suppressing testosterone levels and sexual arousal (based on self-reports) in a chronic pedophile (Cooper and Cernovsky 1994).

Anecdotal observations indicate that fluoxetine, a selective serotonin reuptake inhibitor, decreases voyeurism and exhibitionism (Bianchi 1990; Emmanuel et al. 1991). Fluoxetine has also been used to relieve depression and paraphilic behavior in patients with depression and sexual masochism or depression and transvestic fetishism (Masand 1993). Clomipramine inhibits the reuptake of both serotonin and norepinephrine and reportedly ameliorates exhibitionism and fetishism (Casals-Ariet and Cullen 1993; Clayton 1993). Similarly, the serotonin reuptake inhibitor fluvoxamine has been observed to reduce exhibitionistic behavior (Zohar et al. 1994).

Castration

Leuprolide, MPA, and CPA produce temporary chemical "castration" through their effects on the hypothalamus. Surgical removal of the testes has a more dramatic and permanent effect. Castration definitely reduces paraphilic behavior, and the recidivism rate among castrated male sexual offenders is substantially less than the rate among uncastrated offenders (Berlin 1983; Bradford 1988). In a study in Switzerland, for example, the recidivism rate among castrated offenders was 5.8% during follow-up of 5–30 years, whereas the recidivism rate among men who were recommended for castration but who refused was 52% (Cornu 1973, quoted in Berlin 1983).

Neurosurgery

Posterior hypothalamotomy has been used with reportedly good success in the treatment of sexual offenders. Schmidt and Schorsch (1981) noted that deviant sexual activity was decreased in 6 of 10 patients who underwent stereotactic hypothalamotomy. The number of patients treated in this way is small, follow-up data are limited, and conclusions regarding the surgery are preliminary (Berlin 1983).

Forensic Issues

Issues regarding personal responsibility, public safety, justice, and punishment of paraphilic individuals have not been resolved. How best to treat repeat sexual offenders, particularly pedophiles, is among the most frustrating challenges for society and the criminal justice system. Recidivism rates are high among sexual offenders. Liability under criminal law depends on several conditions, including proof that the individual committed the act, that the act was performed voluntarily, and that the individual was of sound mind (Baker 1993). Sexually deviant behavior per se is not evidence of an unsound mind, although data indicating that the altered behavior was a product of brain disease would mitigate responsibility. Neuropsychiatric assessment thus contributes to both assessment and sentencing of paraphilic offenders. Reduced responsibility, however, does not improve recidivism or increase public safety. Thus, the emphasis must be on identifying means of reducing recurrent undeniable urges for paraphilic behavior, providing safe nonpunitive containment, and improving medication compliance after release from the institution.

Institutional Issues

Aberrant sexual behavior within institutions may be partially ameliorated by a more enlightened attitude toward the sexuality of institutional residents. Individuals who are mentally retarded often have few social skills and are unable to develop interpersonal relationships that would allow intimacy. Providing social skills training and more opportunity for the development of psychosexual relationships should be encouraged. Similarly, development of social skills for those residing in mental institutions and provision of opportunities for sexual relationships should be facilitated. In nursing homes, conjugal visits may be appropriate for some patients, whereas distracting activities and antiandrogenic treatment may be better for others.

Conclusion

The paraphilias are a diverse group of behaviors that come to clinical or legal attention only when they produce distress or bring the individual into contact with law enforcement personnel. In some cases, the paraphilia is the product of a neurological disease (e.g., exhibitionism as part of a frontal lobe disinhibition syndrome); in others, there may be evidence of neurological dysfunction (e.g., abnormal EEG) but no diagnosable neurological disease. Evidence of brain dysfunction is common in patients with paraphilias. The temporal lobe is the brain region most often found to be abnormal in sexually deviant individuals, but evidence of more widespread dysfunction is present in many patients. Several available agents suppress paraphilic behavior, and more rigorous testing of these and other agents is warranted. Nonpharmacological treatments that preserve the rights of individuals with brain disorder while protecting society are urgently needed.

References

Akhtar S, Thomson JA Jr: Schizophrenia and sexuality: a review and report of twelve unusual cases. J Clin Psychiatry 41:134–142 (part I), 166–174 (part II), 1980

American Psychiatric Association: Diagnostic and Statistical Manual of Mental Disorders, 4th Edition. Washington, DC, American Psychiatric Association, 1994

Baker E: The social and legal framework, in Clinical Approaches to the Mentally Disordered Offender. Edited by Howells K, Hollin CR. New York, Wiley, 1993, pp 9–33

Berlin FS: Sex offenders: a biomedical perspective and a status report on biomedical treatment, in The Sexual Aggressor. Edited by Greer JG, Stuart IR. New York, Van Nostrand Reinhold, 1983, pp 83–123

Bianchi MD: Fluoxetine treatment of exhibitionism. Am J Psychiatry 147: 1089–1090, 1990

Biller J, Saver JL: Ischemic cerebrovascular disease and hormone therapy for infertility and transsexualism. Neurology 45:1611–1613, 1995

Blumer D: Hypersexual episodes in temporal lobe epilepsy. Am J Psychiatry 126: 1099–1106, 1970

Brackett NL, Bloch WE, Abae M: Neurological anatomy and physiology of sexual function, in Sexual Dysfunction. A Neuro-medical Approach. Edited by Singer C, Weiner WJ. Armonk, NY, Futura, 1994, pp 1–43

Bradford JMW: Organic treatment for the male sexual offender. Ann N Y Acad Sci 528:193–202, 1988

Burns A, Jacoby R, Levin R: Psychiatric phenomena in Alzheimer's disease, IV: disorders of behaviour. Br J Psychiatry 157:86–94, 1990

Casals-Ariet C, Cullen K: Exhibitionism treated with clomipramine. Am J Psychiatry 150:1273–1274, 1993

Cheyette S, Cummings JL: Encephalitis lethargica: lessons for contemporary neuropsychiatry. J Neuropsychiatry Clin Neurosci 7:125–134, 1995

Clayton AH: Fetishism and clomipramine. Am J Psychiatry 150:673–674, 1993

Comings DE, Comings BG: A case of familial exhibitionism in Tourette's syndrome successfully treated with haloperidol. Am J Psychiatry 139:913–915, 1982

Cooper AJ: Medroxyprogesterone acetate (MPA) treatment of sexual acting out in men suffering from dementia. J Clin Psychiatry 48:368–370, 1987

Cooper AJ, Cernovsky ZZ: Comparison of cyproterone acetate (CPA) and leuprolide acetate (LHRH agonist) in a chronic pedophile: a clinical case study. Biol Psychiatry 36:269–271, 1994

Cummings JL, Miller B: Disorders of sexual behavior in neurological disease, in Sexual Dysfunction. A Neuro-medical Approach. Edited by Singer C, Weiner WJ. Armonk, NY, Futura, 1994, pp 199–218

Day K: Crime and mental retardation: a review, in Clinical Approaches to the Mentally Disordered Offender. Edited by Howells K, Hollin CR. New York, Wiley, 1993, pp 111–144

Ellis A, Brancale R: The Psychology of Sex Offenders. Springfield, IL, Charles C Thomas, 1956

Emmanuel NP, Lydiard RB, Ballenger JC: Fluoxetine treatment of voyeurism (letter). Am J Psychiatry 148:950, 1991

Erickson TC: Erotomania (nymphomania) as an expression of cortical epileptiform discharge. Archives of Neurology and Psychiatry 53:226–231, 1945

Federoff JP, Peyser C, Franz ML, et al: Sexual disorders in Huntington's disease. J Neuropsychiatry Clin Neurosci 6:147–153, 1994

Freund K: Courtship disorder: is this hypothesis valid? Ann N Y Acad Sci 528:172–182, 1988

Freund K, Lanchard R: The concept of courtship disorder. J Sex Marital Ther 12:79–92, 1986

Gaffney GR, Berlin FS: Is there hypothalamic-pituitary-gonadal dysfunction in paedophilia? a pilot study. Br J Psychiatry 145:657–660, 1984

Gilby R, Wolf L, Goldberg B: Mentally retarded adolescent sex offenders. A survey and pilot study. Can J Psychiatry 34:542–548, 1989

Golden CJ: A standardized version of Luria's neuropsychological tests, in Handbook of Clinical Neuropsychology. Edited by Filskov SJ, Boll TJ. New York, Wiley, 1981

Goodman JD: Nymphomania and satyriasis, in Behavior in Excess. Edited by Mule SJ. New York, Free Press, 1981, pp 246–263

Gorman DG, Cummings JL: Hypersexuality following septal injury. Arch Neurol 49:308–310, 1992

Gottesman HG, Schubert DSP: Low-dose oral medroxyprogesterone acetate in the management of the paraphilias. J Clin Psychiatry 54:182–188, 1993

Graber B, Hartmann K, Coffman JA, et al: Brain damage among mentally disordered sex offenders, in International Research in Sexology. Edited by Lief HI, Hoch Z. New York, Praeger, 1984, pp 193–202

Harrison P, Stangeway P, McCann J, et al: Pedophilia and hyperprolactinemia. Br J Psychiatry 155:847–848, 1989

Harvey NS: Serial cognitive profiles in levodopa-induced hypersexuality. Br J Psychiatry 153:833–836, 1988

Henn FA, Herjanic M, Vanderpearl RH: Forensic psychiatry: profiles of two types of sexual offenders. Am J Psychiatry 133:694–696, 1976

Hoenig J, Kenna JC: EEG abnormalities and transsexualism. Br J Psychiatry 134:293–300, 1979

Hooshmand H, Brawley BW: Temporal lobe seizures with exhibitionism. Neurology 19:1119–1124, 1969

Hunter R, Logue V, McMenemy WH: Temporal lobe epilepsy supervening on long-standing transvestism and fetishism. Epilepsia 4:60–65, 1963

Huws R, Shubsachs APW, Taylor PJ: Hypersexuality, fetishism, and multiple sclerosis. Br J Psychiatry 158:280–281, 1991

Janus SS, Janus CL: The Janus Report on Sexual Behavior. New York, Wiley, 1993

Kafka MP, Prentsky R: Fluoxetine treatment of nonparaphilic sexual addictions and paraphilias in men. J Clin Psychiatry 53:351–358, 1992

Kafka MP, Prentsky R: Preliminary observations of DSM-III-R Axis I comorbidity in men with paraphilias and paraphilia-related disorders. J Clin Psychiatry 55:481–487, 1994

Kaplan HS: Disorders of Sexual Desire. New York, Simon & Schuster, 1979

Kolarsky A, Freund K, Machek J, et al: Male sexual deviation. Arch Gen Psychiatry 17:735–743, 1967

Kumar A, Koss E, Metzler D, et al: Behavioral symptomatology in dementia of the Alzheimer type. Alzheimer Dis Assoc Disord 2:363–365, 1988

Langevin R, Lang RA: The courtship disorders, in Variant Sexuality: Research and Theory. Edited by Wilson GD. Baltimore, MD, Johns Hopkins University Press, 1987, pp 202–228

Langevin R, Bain J, Wortzman G, et al: Sexual sadism: brain, blood, and behavior. Ann N Y Acad Sci 528:163–171, 1988

LeVay S: The Sexual Brain. Cambridge, MA, MIT Press, 1993

Lilly R, Cummings JL, Benson DF, et al: The human Klüver-Bucy syndrome. Neurology 33:1141–1145, 1983

Maden T, Swinton M, Gunn J: Psychiatric disorder in women serving a prison sentence. Br J Psychiatry 164:44–54, 1994

Masand PS: Successful treatment of sexual masochism and transvestic fetishism associated with depression with fluoxetine hydrochloride. Depression 1:50–52, 1993

Mellor CS, Farid NR, Craig DF: Female hypersexuality treated with cyproterone acetate (letter). Am J Psychiatry 145:1037, 1988

Miller BL, Cummings JL, McIntyre H, et al: Hypersexuality or altered sexual preference following brain injury. J Neurol Neurosurg Psychiatry 49:867–873, 1986

Mitchell W, Falconer MA, Hill D: Epilepsy with fetishism relieved by temporal lobectomy. Lancet 2:626–630, 1954

Money J: Lovemaps: Clinical Concepts of Sexual-Erotic Health and Pathology, Paraphilia and Gender Transposition in Childhood, Adolescence and Maturity. Amherst, MA, Prometheus Books, 1986

Monga TN, Monga M, Raina MS, et al: Hypersexuality in stroke. Arch Phys Med Rehabil 67:415–417, 1986

Moore SL: Satyriasis: a case study. J Clin Psychiatry 41:279–281, 1980

Ortego N, Miller BL, Itabashi H, et al: Altered sexual behavior with multiple sclerosis. Neuropsychiatry Neuropsychol Behav Neurol 6:260–264, 1993

Poeck K, Pilleri G: Release of hypersexual behavior due to lesion in the limbic system. Acta Neurol Scand 41:233–244, 1965

Prentky RA, Burgess AW, Rokous F, et al: The presumptive role of fantasy in serial sexual homicide. Am J Psychiatry 146:887–891, 1989

Rabins PV, Mace NL, Lucas MJ: The impact of dementia on the family. JAMA 248:333–335, 1982

Raine A: The Psychopathology of Crime. San Diego, CA, Academic Press, 1993

Regestein QR, Reich P: Pedophilia occurring after onset of cognitive impairment. J Nerv Ment Dis 166:794–798, 1978

Rich SS, Ovsiew F: Leuprolide acetate for exhibitionism in Huntington's disease. Mov Disord 9:353–357, 1994

Richfield EK, Twyman R, Berent S: Neurological syndrome following bilateral damage to the head of the caudate nuclei. Ann Neurol 22:768–771, 1987

Rooth G: Exhibitionism, sex violence, and pedophilia. Br J Psychiatry 122:705–710, 1973

Ryden MB: Aggressive behavior in persons with dementia who live in the community. Alzheimer Dis Assoc Disord 2:342–355, 1988

Schmidt G, Schorsch E: Psychosurgery of sexually deviant patients: review and analysis of new empirical findings. Arch Sex Behav 10:301–323, 1981

Tsuang MT: Hypersexuality in manic patients. Medical Aspects of Human Sexuality 9:83–89, 1975

Walinder J: Transvestism, definition and evidence in favor of occasional derivation from cerebral dysfunction. International Journal of Neuropsychiatry 1:567–573, 1965

Zohar J, Kaplan Z, Benjamin J: Compulsive exhibitionism successfully treated with fluvoxamine: a controlled case study. J Clin Psychiatry 55:86–88, 1994

Index

Page numbers printed in **boldface** type refer to tables or figures.

Aberrant Behavior Checklist (ABC),
175
Abnormal Involuntary Movement Scale
(AIMS), 340, 348, **354–356**
Abstinence, and substance abuse, 111,
120–121
Acetaldehyde, and alcohol abuse, 108
Acetylcholine, and aggression, 151
Acquired immunodeficiency syndrome
(AIDS). *See also* Human immuno-
deficiency virus central nervous
system diseases related to, **227**
homeless and, 321
prevalence of in prisons, 197
progression from dormancy to, 223
substance abuse and, 134
ACT. *See* Assertive Community
Treatment (ACT)
ADHD. *See* Attention-deficit/
hyperactivity disorder (ADHD)
Addison, Thomas, 24
Addison's disease, 24
Administration on Aging, 88
Adult day care, 90
Advocacy groups, and dementia, 89
Affective disorders, in homeless, 320
Age. *See also* Children; Elderly
dementia and, 69–70

tardive dyskinesia and, 338–339
Ageism, and treatment of older patients,
310
Aggression
dementia and, 80–81
neurochemistry and, 164–165
neuropsychiatric evaluation of,
165–174
pathophysiology of, 150–164
side effects of medications and, 56
state hospitals and, 51–53
traumatic brain injury and, 323
treatment of, 174–184
types of, 149
Aging, and differential diagnosis of
dementia, 73
AIDS. *See* Acquired immunodeficiency
syndrome (AIDS)
AIMS. *See* Abnormal Involuntary
Movement Scale (AIMS)
Akathisia, and neuroleptics, 58, 59, 177
Akinesia, and neuroleptics, 58
Alabama, and state hospitals, 49–50
Albumin, 307
Alcohol abuse and alcoholism. *See also*
Substance abuse
brain damage and, 116–117
dual diagnosis, 131

Alcohol abuse and alcoholism
(*continued*)
economic cost of, 105
elderly and, 295
history of mental health services and,
11
homeless and, 320–321
neuropsychiatric effects of, 107–115
prevalence of, 106
sexual deviations and, 368, 371
tardive dyskinesia and, 339
Alcoholic cerebellar degeneration, 113
Alcoholic dementia, 75
Alcoholic hallucinosis, 115
Alcoholic pellagra encephalopathy, 113
Alcohol-induced psychotic disorder
with delusions, 115
Alcohol-related brain damage (ARBD),
116–117
Algorithms
for detection of physical illness in
psychiatric patients, 32, **33–34**
for treatment of aggressive behavior,
178, 182
Alprazolam, 119
Alzheimer's Association, 89
Alzheimer's disease (AD)
cost of care for, 71
dementia and, 70–71, 73, 74
depression and, 81, 298
differential diagnosis of, 72
Down's syndrome and, 273
neuropsychological testing and, 306
self-care deficits, 82
side effects of medications in elderly,
85
tacrine for acetylcholine deficiency,
83
vitamin E and, 84
Amantadine, 58, 59, 182
Ambulatory care
for HIV, 238–241
for substance abuse, 133

American Academy of Neurology, **76,**
78, 229
American Association on Mental
Retardation, 259–260
American Medico-Psychological
Association, 15
American Psychiatric Association
recommendations on care of elderly
patients in state hospitals,
310–311
Task Force on Tardive Dyskinesia,
336, 352–353
Amitriptyline, 179
Amnesia, 73, 167
Amotivational syndrome, and cannabis
abuse, 126
Amphetamines, 107, 123
Amygdala, and aggression, 152–153
Anabolic steroids, 165
Analgesics, 123–125
Angelman syndrome, 276
Animal models, of aggression, 151, 153,
164, 165, 177, 208
Annual Nationwide Household Survey,
106
Antecedent behaviors, and aggression,
183
Anterior cingulum, and frontal
syndromes, **158–160**
Antianxiety agents
aggression and, 180
neuroleptics and, 59
schizophrenia and, 62
Antibodies, and HIV screening, 233
Anticholinergic medications, and tardive
dyskinesia, 341
Anticonvulsant agents
aggression and, 177, 180–181
behavioral and cognitive side effects
of, 155, 175
Antiepileptic drugs, 57, 155
Antinoradrenergic therapy, for
aggression, 181–182

Antipsychotic agents
  aggression and, 177
  dementia and, 85–87
  elderly and, 308–309
Antisocial personality disorder, 209,
  320, 368
Antistreptolysin O (ASO), 343
Anxiety. *See also* Anxiety disorders
  schizophrenia and, 62
  side effects of medications, 56
Anxiety disorders, and aggression, 180
Aphasia, 73
ARBD. *See* Alcohol-related brain
  damage (ARBD)
Arginine vasopressin systems, and
  aggression, 164
ASO. *See* Antistreptolysin O (ASO)
Asperger's syndrome, 262, 278–279
Assertive Community Treatment
  (ACT), 329
Assessment. *See also* Diagnosis;
  Neuropsychological assessment
  of aggression, 165–174
  of dementia, 87–88
  of HIV and central nervous system
    involvement, 226–235
  of late-onset depression and
    psychosis, 300–307
  in prison setting, 210–212
  of sexual deviations, 374–377
  of tardive dyskinesia, 348–349
Asylum, and history of mental health
  services
  organic psychiatry in, 8–12
  origins of, 3–5
  social role of psychiatry and, 12–17
Ataxia, and dementia, **77**
Atherosclerosis, 304
Atlantoaxial dislocation, and Down's
  syndrome, 273
Attention-deficit/hyperactivity disorder
  (ADHD), and aggression, 163–164,
  181

Autonomic arousal, and aggressive
  behavior, 52
Autopsy, and dementia, 79

Barbiturates, 57, 155, 175
Basal ganglia, lesions of, 345
Behavior. *See also* Aggression;
  Sexual behavior
  dementia and, 80–82, 88
  HIV and, **224, 225**
  temporal lobe epilepsy and interictal
    change, 155–157
Behavioral therapy
  for aggression, 183–184
  for developmental disabilities,
    267–268
Behavior Pharmacology Clinics of
  Colorado, 280
Benzodiazepines
  aggression and, 180
  dementia and, 86
  drug abuse and, 118–119
  schizophrenia and, 59–60, 62
β-Blockers
  aggression and, 165, 181
  dementia and, 86–87
  side effects of, 265
Bethlem Hospital (England), 8
Biofeedback, and HIV care, 239, 241
Biopsy, and dementia, 79
Bipolar disorder, 24
Bleuler, Eugen, 150
Blood banks, and HIV screening, 233
Blumer, G. Alder, 14
Boston, and study of homeless mentally
  ill, 326
Bradyphrenia, 298–299
Brain damage, alcohol-related,
  116–117
Brain function
  Jacksonian concept of hierarchical
    control of, 150
  prison populations and, 201–209

Brain shrinkage, and alcohol abuse, 111, 112
Brain tumors, 27, 369
Brainwashing, 268
Brief Psychiatric Rating Scale, 87
Bromocriptine, 58, 59, 87
Buckinghamshire Asylum (England), 8, 11
Bucknill, J. C., 6, 8, 16
Bucy, Paul, 152
Bureau of Health Care Delivery Assistance, 236
Buspirone, 86, 180
Butler Hospital (Rhode Island), 14

Calcium-channel blocking agents, 84
California
   history of mental health services in, 10
   sexual deviations in prison populations, 367
Canada, and prevalence of mental disorders in prisons, 199
Canadian Consensus Conference, **76**
Cannabis, and substance abuse, 107, 125–127
Carbamazepine
   aggression and, 175, 181
   dementia and, 87
   management of epilepsy, 57
   side effects of, 59, 155
Cardiovascular disease, and depression, 300
CARE. *See* Comprehensive AIDS Resources Emergency (CARE) Act
Caregivers
   dementia and, 71, 80, 82, 88–89, 90
   social supports for state hospital patients and, 61
Caring for People With Severe Mental Disorders (NIMH, 1991), 350
Case management systems, and dementia, 89

Case study, of cognitive impairment in homeless, 327–328
Castration, and sexual offenders, 378
CBF. *See* Cerebral blood flow (CBF)
CDC. *See* Centers for Disease Control and Prevention (CDC)
Center for Epidemiological Studies Depression Index, 88
Centers for Disease Control and Prevention (CDC), 222, 225, 233, 236
Central nervous system
   aggression and, **151**
   HIV and pathology of, 223–235
   side effects of medications, 55
Central pontine myelinolysis (CPM), 113–114
Cerebellar disease, 130, 342
Cerebellum degeneration, and alcohol abuse, 113
Cerebral atrophy, and cocaine abuse, 122
Cerebral blood flow (CBF)
   drug abuse and, 122, 127
   late-onset depression and psychosis, 305–306
   sexual deviation and, 372–373
Cerebral vasculitis, and amphetamine abuse, 123
Cerebrospinal fluid (CSF) examination
   dementia and, 78
   developmental syndromes and, 272
   HIV infection and, 234
   violent behavior and, 208
   Wernicke's encephalopathy and, 111
Cerebrovascular events, and AIDS, **227**
Child abuse, and developmental disabilities, 264
Children, and tardive dyskinesia, 337
Cholinergic abnormalities, and dementia, 83
Choreoacanthocytosis, 344

Choreoathetotic movements, and
dementia, **77**
Chromosomal abnormalities, and
aggression, 164
Chronic syndromes, and hallucinogens,
128
Cigarette smoking, 130–131
Clinical Dementia Rating Scale, 74
Clomipramine, 179, 378
Clorazepate, 119
Clozapine
aggression and, 177
medication-induced psychosis, 299
side effects of, 309
tardive dyskinesia and, 340–341, 349
Cluttering, and Fragile X syndrome, 274
Cocaine abuse, 107, 117, 119–123, 132,
321
Cognitive functions. *See also*
Neuropsychological deficits
alcohol abuse and, 116–117
dementia and, 74, 83–84
HIV and, **224, 225,** 226, **228–229**
homeless and, 324–326, 327–328
late-onset depression and psychosis,
297–300
state hospitals and impairment of,
53–54
traumatic brain injury and, 322
Colney Hatch Asylum (London), 8, 13
Columbia-Presbyterian Medical Center,
329
Coma, and alcohol abuse, 109
Committee on Aging of the Group for
the Advancement of Psychiatry,
84
Community mental health care
dementia and, 71
developmental disabilities and, 269,
279–281
prevalence of medical illness in
psychiatric patients, **29**
tardive dyskinesia and, 352

violent behavior and, 51
Comorbidity
dementia and, 80–82
developmental disabilities and,
263–265
homeless and, 320
late-onset depression in elderly and,
295
Competence, and legal status of
patients, 54–55
Compliance, with neuroleptic therapy,
57–60
Comprehensive AIDS Resources
Emergency (CARE) Act, 235–243
Computed tomography (CT). *See also*
Neuroimaging
aggression and, 173
alcohol abuse and, 111–112
dementia and, 78
screening programs for medical
illness in psychiatric patients
and, 31–32
Conduct disorder, 164
Conflict resolution strategies, and
aggression, 184
Consciousness, altered levels of, 37
Conversion disorder, 35, 343–344
Cook County Jail (Chicago), 199
Cornell Scale for Depression in
Dementia, 74
Cortical dementias, 73
Corticosteroids, 56
Cost
alcohol abuse and, 105
Alzheimer's disease and mental
hospitalization,
70–71
dementia and, 71–72, 84
screening programs for medical
illness in psychiatric patients
and, 32, 35
Countertransference, and treatment of
homeless mentally ill, 329

County of Lancaster Asylum (England), 8, 9, 11
Courtship, and sexual behavior, 365
CPA. *See* Cyproterone acetate (CPA)
CPM. *See* Central pontine myelinolysis (CPM)
Craniofacial abnormalities, and fetal alcohol syndrome, 115
Cranioscopy, 5
Creutzfeldt-Jakob disease, 78
Crichton Browne, James, 16
Crime. *See also* Homicide; Prisons
    brain function and, 201–209
    evaluation strategies for sexual offenders, 374–377
    neurological dysfunction in sexual offenders, 371–373
    rate of violent, 149
Critical Time Intervention Mental Health Program (CTI), 328–329
CSF. *See* Cerebrospinal fluid
CT. *See* Computed tomography
CTI. *See* Critical Time Intervention Mental Health Program (CTI)
Cushing's disease, 300
Cyproterone acetate (CPA), 378
Cytochrome P450 enzyme system, 308

Daily living, skills of, 307, 310
Dain, N., 6
Deafness, and differential diagnosis of dementia, 73
Defenses, and medical illness in psychiatric patients, 56
Degenerative dementias, 298
Deinstitutionalization, and elderly, 293
Delirium
    aggression and, 166
    cocaine-induced, 120
    dementia and, 73
    psychotic behavior in elderly and, 297
Delirium tremens, 109–110

Delusional depression, 308
Delusions, 81, 298, 374
Dementia
    alcohol abuse and, 106
    behavioral problems and comorbidity, 80–82
    depression and, 293
    differential diagnosis of, 72–80
    HIV-related, 241–242
    homeless and, 320
    late-onset depression and psychosis, 298
    neurobiology of, 82–83
    prevalence of, 69–70
    psychological management of, 87–92
    psychopharmacology for, 83–87
    service utilization and social costs of, 70–72
    sexual deviations and, 370, 374, 378
Dementia syndrome of depression, 72
Dementia with Lewy bodies, 74, 83
Denial, of medical illness in psychiatric patients, 56
Depression
    aggression and, 179
    dementia and, 72–73, 81–82, 88
    developmental disabilities and, 267
    late-onset in elderly, 291–311
    prisons and, 199
    traumatic brain injury and, 321, 322
Desire-phase sexual disorders, **366**
Developmental disabilities
    aggression and, 168, 174–175
    Asperger's syndrome, 278–279
    community psychiatrist and, 279–281
    comorbidity and, 263–265
    developmental syndromes, 270–272
    Down's syndrome, 272–274
    epidemiology and risk factors, 263
    Fragile X syndrome, 274–275
    myths concerning, 269–270
    phenylketonuria, 275–276

Prader-Willi syndrome, 276–277
treatment goals, 265–269
types of, 259–262
Williams syndrome, 277–278
Developmental history, 211, **376**. *See also* Patient history
Developmental syndromes, 270–272
Diabetes, 27, 323
Diagnosis. *See also* Assessment; Differential diagnosis; Neuropsychological assessment
asylums in nineteenth century and, 11–12, 13
developmental disabilities and psychiatric, 265–266
social role of psychiatry and, 13
state hospitals and, 50–51, 62–63
tardive dyskinesia and, 347
Diagnostic overshadowing, 50, 62, 270
Diazepam, 119
Diet, 275, 277. *See also* Malnutrition
Differential diagnosis. *See also* Diagnosis
aggression and, 170, 172–174
dementia and, 72–80
late-onset depression and psychosis, 297–300
tardive dyskinesia and, 341–347
Differential reinforcement of other behaviors (DRO), 184
DIS-CO. *See* Dyskinesia Identification System—Coldwater (DIS-CO)
Diuretics, 265
Divalproex, 181
Donepezil, 84
Dopamine agonists, and side effects of neuroleptics, 59
Dorsolateral convexity, and frontal syndromes, **158–160**
Dosages, of psychoactive medications
elderly and, 85, 307
tardive dyskinesia and, 340, 349, 357

Down's syndrome, 73, 270, 271, 272–274
DRO. *See* Differential reinforcement of other behaviors (DRO)
Drug abuse. *See also* Substance abuse
dual diagnosis, 131
neuropsychiatric effects of, 117–131
prevalence of, 106–107
Drug-disease interactions, 55–56
Drug-drug interactions, 55, 297
DSM-III, and antisocial personality disorder, 209
DSM-IV
Asperger's syndrome, 278–279
cannabis dependence, 125
depression, 294, 296
hallucinogens, 127
intermittent explosive disorder, 167–168
personality change due to traumatic brain injury, 322
tardive dyskinesia, 336
vascular dementia, 75
Dual diagnosis, and substance abuse, 131, 134
Dwarfism, 272
Dysarthria, and dementia, **77**
Dyskinesia Identification System—Coldwater (DIS-CO), 353
Dyskinesias, and cocaine abuse, 122
Dyslexia, 260–261
Dysmorphology, 260
Dysphoria, 231, 343
Dystonias, **77,** 342

ECA. *See* Epidemiologic Catchment Area (ECA)
ECGs. *See* Electrocardiograms (ECGs)
ECT. *See* Electroconvulsive therapy (ECT)
EEGs. *See* Electroencephalograms (EEGs)

Ecstasy. *See* 3,4-Methylenedioxy-
methamphetamine (MDMA;
ecstasy)
Education. *See* Psychoeducation
EE. *See* Expressed emotion (EE)
Elder abuse, and dementia, 80
Elderly. *See also* Elder abuse
benzodiazepines and, 118
depression and psychosis in, 292–297
dosages of medications for, 85, 307
history of mental health services and,
11
prevalence of medical illness in
psychiatric patients and, **29**
state hospitals and, 47–48, 310–311
tardive dyskinesia and, 339
Electrocardiograms (ECGs), 31
Electroconvulsive therapy (ECT), and
depression in elderly, 308
Electroencephalograms (EEGs)
dementia and, 78
prison populations and, 205–206,
212
sexual deviations and, 373
Eligible metropolitan areas (EMAs),
236, 237–243
ELISA. *See* Enzyme-linked
immunosorbent assay (ELISA)
Eltoprazine, 182
EMAs. *See* Eligible metropolitan areas
(EMAs)
Emergency room, 107, 132–133
Endocarditis, and cocaine abuse, 117
Endocrine disorders
depression and, 300
developmental disabilities and, 264
sexual deviations and, 373, 375
End-stage dementia, 91–92
Enzyme-linked immunosorbent assay
(ELISA), and HIV screening, 233
Epidemiologic Catchment Area (ECA)
study, 106, 199, 293
Epidemiology
of developmental disabilities, 263
of HIV infection, 222–223
of homelessness, 319–320
of late-onset depression and
psychosis, 292–294
of medical illnesses in psychiatric
patients, 24–41
of mental disorders in prisons,
198–201
of substance abuse, 106–107
of tardive dyskinesia, 338–341
Epilepsy. *See also* Temporal lobe
epilepsy
aggression and, 170, 206
developmental disabilities and, 264
history of mental health services and,
8–9, 11, 12
homeless and, 324
sexual deviations and, 370
state hospitals and, 56–57
EPS. *See* Extrapyramidal side effects
(EPS)
Episodic dyscontrol syndrome, 167,
206
Ergoloid mesylates, 83
Essential Medical Information Form,
39–40
Ethnicity
drug abuse and, 107
older population and, 292–293
tardive dyskinesia and, 339–340
Eugenics movement, 14
Evaluation. *See* Assessment; Diagnosis
Executive functions, 53–54, **232**
Executive Interview Test, 55
Excitement-phase sexual disorders, 365,
366
Exhibitionism, 365, 366–367, 368
Expressed emotion (EE), and dementia,
88
Extinction burst, 184
Extraocular movements, and dementia,
77

Extrapyramidal side effects (EPS), of
    neuroleptics, 340
Extrapyramidal signs, of dementia, **77**

Face sheet, of clinical record, 40
Family. *See also* Family history
    aggression and, 166
    dementia and, 71, 89–92
    social supports for state hospital
        patients and, 61
Family Burden Interview, 89
Family history. *See also* Family
    of alcohol abuse, 114
    of dementia, 73
    of mental retardation, 271
    neuropsychiatric evaluation in
        prisons and, 211
Felbamate, 175
Fenfluramine, 59
Ferrier, David, 16
Fetal alcohol syndrome, 115
Fetal effects. *See also* Obstetric
    complications; Perinatal factors;
    Pregnancy
    of benzodiazepine abuse, 122
    of cocaine abuse, 122–123
    treatment of substance abuse and,
        133
Fife and Kinross District Asylum
    (Scotland), 12
Financial resources, and patients of state
    hospitals, 61
Flashbacks, and hallucinogens, 127
Fluorescent treponema antibody test
    (FTA), 77
Fluoxetine, 208, 378
Folate deficiency, and depression, 300
Follicle-stimulating hormone, 373
Forced normalization, 156
Forensic issues, and sexual offenders,
    379
Foucault, Michel, 4
Fragile X syndrome, 164, 262, 274–275

France, and history of asylum, 4
Friends' Asylum (Pennsylvania), 6
Frontal lobe
    dysfunction of and legal status of
        patients, 54–55
    personality change and damage to,
        322
    subtypes of frontal syndromes, 157,
        158–160, 161–163
Frontal neocortex, and aggression,
    157–163
Fronto-temporal dementia (FTD), 75,
    298, 306
Frotteurism, 365, 368
FTA. *See* Fluorescent treponema
    antibody test (FTA)
FTD. *See* Fronto-temporal dementia
    (FTD)
Functional impairments, and tardive
    dyskinesia, 350–352

Gabapentin, 57
Gage, Phineas P., 161
Gait disorder, and dementia, **77**
Gall, Franz J., 5
Gastroesophageal reflux, and Down's
    syndrome, 273
Gender
    alcohol abuse and, 106
    tardive dyskinesia and, 339
General hospitals, and dementia, 70–71
General paresis of the insane (GPI),
    9–10
Genetics. *See also* Heredity
    criminal behavior and, 202–203
    developmental syndromes and, 271,
        274
George III, king of England, 3
Global Deterioration Scale, 232
Gowers, William, 9
GPI. *See* General paresis of the insane
    (GPI)
Granulomatous angiitis, 122

Gray, John, 11
Grob, Gerald, 12
Guardianship
  dementia and, 80
  state hospital patients and, 54, 55

Habilitation, 267
Habilitative Mental Healthcare Newsletter, The, 268
Hallucinations
  alcohol abuse and, 115
  Alzheimer's disease and, 298
  cocaine abuse and, 120
  dementia and, 81, 83
  hospitalization and, 51
Hallucinogens, 107, 127–130
Haloperidol, 85, 177
Halstead-Reitan Neuropsychological Test Battery, 230, 231
Hamilton Scales, 229
Hanwell Asylum (England), 8
Harlow, J. M., 161
Harris County Hospital District (Houston), 237
Head injury. *See also* Traumatic brain injury
  aggression and, 163
  alcohol abuse and, 108, 114
  criminal behavior and, 203–204
  dementia and, 73
  psychiatric symptoms and, 37
Health care professionals, and abuse of analgesics, 124
Health insurance, and HIV, 235–237
Health Resources and Services Administration (HRSA), 236
Hemorrhagic stroke, and cocaine abuse, 121
Heredity, and history of concepts of insanity, 7. *See also* Genetics
Heroin, 124–125
5-HIAA. *See* 5-Hydroxyindoleacetic acid (5-HIAA)

Histamine blockers, 265
History, of mental health services
  nature of insanity, 5–7
  organic psychiatry in asylums, 8–12
  origins of the asylum, 3–5
  perspective on, 1–3
  social role of psychiatry, 12–17
HIV. *See* Human immunodeficiency virus (HIV)
HIV-associated dementia complex, 226, 229, 241
HIV-associated minor cognitive-motor disorder, 226, 229, 230, 241
HIV encephalopathy, 223
Home-based hospice, 91–92
Homelessness
  AIDS and, 321
  epidemiology of, 319–320
  epilepsy and, 324
  neuropsychiatric problems among, 324–329
  schizophrenia and, 324
  substance abuse and, 320–321
  traumatic brain injury and, 321–323
Homemaker services, 90
Homicide. *See also* Crime
  mortality from in psychiatric patients, 24
  neuroimaging studies and, 205, 206, 207
  prefrontal dysfunction and, 163
  serotonin levels and, 208
  sexual deviations and, 366
Hospices, and dementia, 91–92
Houston, and neuropsychiatric AIDS care, 237–243
HRSA. *See* Health Resources and Services Administration (HRSA)
Human immunodeficiency virus (HIV). *See also* Acquired immunodeficiency syndrome
  central nervous system pathology, 223–226

cognitive-motor disorder, 226, 229, 230, 241
dementia and, 78, 226, 229, 241
encephalopathy, 223
epidemiology and risk factors, 222–223
neuroassessment of central nervous system involvement, 226–235
public health setting and, 235–243
substance abuse and tests for, 117, 134
Huntington's disease, 299, 344, 369
5-Hydroxyindoleacetic acid (5-HIAA), 164, 208
Hypersexuality, 364, 365, 369, 371
Hypertension, 56, 304, 323
Hyperthyroidism, 344
Hypochondriasis, 56
Hypometamorphosis, 153
Hypoparathyroidism, 344
Hypothalamic-pituitary-adrenal axis (HPA), and alcohol abuse, 108
Hypothalamus
aggression and, 150–152
Prader-Willi syndrome and, 276
Hypothyroidism, 35, 60, 264
Hysteria, 35

Ictal aggression, 154
Idiopathic orofacial dystonia, 342
Illinois, and prevalence of mental disorders in prisons, 200
Impulsivity, and serotonin levels, 208
Infants, and HIV screening, 233
Informed consent, 348
Inhalant abuse, 129–130
Inpatient care, for substance abuse, 133
Insanity, history of concepts of, 2, 5–7
Instrumental functions, and state hospitals, 53–54
Intelligence testing, 259
Interictal aggression, 154–155, 162–163

Intermittent explosive disorder, 163, 167–168
Intoxication states
alcohol abuse and, 108–109
amphetamine abuse and, 123
cannabis and, 125–126
cocaine abuse and, 120
hallucinogens and, 127, 128, 129
opioid abuse and, 124
Ischemic stroke, and cocaine abuse, 121

Jackson, Hughlings, 12, 16
Juvenile criminals, and neuro-psychological assessment, 207–208

Ketamine, 128–129
Kindling effect
alcohol withdrawal and, 108
epilepsy and behavior changes, 156–157
Klinefelter's syndrome, 164
Klüver, Heinrich, 152
Klüver-Bucy syndrome, 83, 153, 371
Korsakoff's syndrome, 106, 110–112
Kraepelin, Emil, 346

Laboratory tests
dementia and, 75–78
developmental disabilities and, 271
HIV and, 233–235
late-onset depression and psychosis, 301–302
screening for medical illness in psychiatric patient and, 30–31
sexual deviation and, **377**
tardive dyskinesia and, 348
Lamotrigine, 57, 181
Language impairment, 210, **232**
Late paraphrenia, 296
Learning disabilities, 260–262
Left hemisphere, psychopathy and dysfunction of, 210
Leuprolide, 165, 378

Levodopa, 345, 370
Lewy bodies, and dementia, 74
Limbic system, and aggression, 152–157
Lithium, 60, 180
Liver, and medications, 84, 307
Lorazepam, 119
Losses, elderly and depression, 295
LSD. *See* Lysergic acid diethylamide
    (LSD)
Lumbar puncture, 32, 78
Luria-Nebraska Neuropsychological
    Battery, 372
Luteinizing hormone, 373
Lysergic acid diethylamide (LSD), 107,
    127

MACS. *See* Multicenter AIDS Cohort
    Study (MACS)
Magnetic resonance imaging (MRI). *See
    also* Neuroimaging
    aggression and, 173
    alcohol abuse and, 111, 112
    dementia and, 78
    developmental syndromes and,
        271–272
    prison populations and, 212
Malingering, 343
Malnutrition, in homeless, 323. *See also*
    Diet
Mania
    Huntington's disease and, 299
    hypersexuality and, 371
    late onset of in elderly, 295, 300
    traumatic brain injury and, 322
Mapother, E., 14–15
Marchiafava-Bignami disease, 113
Marital violence, 163, 203–204
Masturbation, and history of causes of
    insanity, 7
Maternal rejection, and birth
    complications, 203
Maudsley, Henry, 6, 13
Maudsley Hospital (London), 14

McLean Hospital, 3, 7, 9–10
MDMA. *See* 3,4-Methylenedioxy-
    methamphetamine (MDMA;
    ecstasy)
Medical clearance, and state hospitals,
    50
Medical Evaluation Field Manual
    (Koran, 1991), 39, 40
Medical history. *See* Patient history
Medical illnesses, in psychiatric patients
    assessment of, 25–26
    depression in elderly and, 296
    developmental disabilities and, 264
    homelessness and, 320, 323, 325
    late-onset depression and psychosis,
        297–300
    prevalence of, 26–27, **28–29**
    psychiatric symptoms and, 24–25,
        35–38
    psychotic behavior in elderly and,
        297
    screening programs for, 29–35,
        39–41
    state hospitals and, 50–51, 55–57
Medicare and Medicaid, 63
Medroxyprogesterone acetate (MPA),
    165, 377–378
Meige's disease, 342
Memory
    alcohol abuse and, 108
    benzodiazepines and, 118–119
    HIV and, **232,** 239, 241
    schizophrenia and side effects of
        medications, 58
Memory and Behavior Problem
    Checklist, 87, 89
Meningeal carcinomatosis, 78
Mental health services
    aggression and, 150–184
    dementia and, 69–92
    developmental disabilities and,
        263–281
    history of, 1–17

homelessness and, 319–329
human immunodeficiency virus and, 222–243
late-onset depression and psychosis in elderly, 292–307
medical illnesses in psychiatric patients, 24–41
prisons and, 198–212
sexual deviations and, 366–380
state mental hospitals and, 47–63
substance abuse and, 106–135
tardive dyskinesia and, 336–358
Mental retardation
causes of, 260
criminal behavior and, 202
definition of, 259, 260
differential diagnosis of dementia, 73
history of mental health services and, 11
myths about, 269–270
prisons and, 201
sexual deviations and, 371, 374
Mental status examination. *See also* Mini-Mental State Exam
HIV and, 230
late-onset depression and, 301
sexual offenders and, 375
Mesoridazine, 266
Metabolic disorders, and alcohol abuse, 108
Methadone maintenance program, and benzodiazepines, 118
Methyldopa, 56
3,4-Methylenedioxymethamphetamine (MDMA; ecstasy), 107, 128
Methylphenidate, and aggression, 182
Metoclopramide, 343
Mini-Mental State Exam, 74, 84, 230, 240, 301, 305, 351
Minor brain injury, 323
Misidentification syndromes, and dementia, 81
Mitchell, S. Weir, 15

Mnemonic, for psychiatric symptoms of medical illness, 38
Mobile screening team, 39
Molindone, 59
Monoamine oxidase A, 202
Mood disorders. *See also* Depression
cocaine intoxication and symptoms of, 120
side effects of medications and, 56
Moral therapy, 4, 6–7
Morbidity
medical illness and rates of in psychiatric patients, 24–25
prisons and neurospychiatric, 200
Mortality
alcohol abuse and, 110
cocaine abuse and, 107
medical illness and rates of in psychiatric patients, 24–25
MPA. *See* Medroxyprogesterone acetate (MPA)
MRI. *See* Magnetic resonance imaging (MRI)
Multicenter AIDS Cohort Study (MACS), 230
Multi-infarct dementia, 75
Multiple sclerosis, 38, 369–370
Myoclonus, and dementia, **77**
Myxedema psychosis, 27

NADD Newsletter, The, 268
Nadolol, 181
National Hospice Organization, 91
National Hospital for the Paralysed and Epileptic (England), 9
National Institute of Mental Health, 350
National Institutes of Health, **76**
National Long-Term Care and Informal Caregivers Survey, 89
Negative EE, and dementia, 88
Neoplasia, and HIV, 225–226, **227**
Neurasthenia, 2

Neurobehavioral complications, of HIV
  infection, 223, **224, 225,** 230–232
Neurobiology, of dementia, 82–83
Neurochemistry, and aggression,
  164–165
Neurodevelopmental history, and
  aggression, 170, **172**
Neuroimaging. *See also* Computed
  tomography; Magnetic resonance
  imaging; Positron-emission
  tomography; Single photon
  emission computed tomography
  dementia and, 78–79
  HIV and, 234–235
  late-onset depression and psychosis,
    302–306
  prison populations and, 207, 212
  sexual deviations and, 372, 375
Neuroleptics
  aggression and, 177, 179
  dementia and, 85, 87
  extrapyramidal side effects of, 340
  nonadherence to treatment and side
    effects of, 57–60
  tardive dyskinesia and, 337–338,
    347–350, 357
Neuroleptic-withdrawal emergent
  dyskinesia, 338
Neurology
  cocaine abuse and complications of,
    121–122
  examination in prison setting,
    204–205
  late-onset depression and psychosis,
    300
  neuropsychiatry and development of,
    2–3
  sexual deviations and, 368–373,
    376–377
Neuropathy, and dementia, **77**
Neuropsychiatric Inventory, 74
Neuropsychiatry
  aggression and, 150–184

dementia and, 69–92
developmental disabilities and,
  263–281
history of mental health services and,
  1–17
homelessness and, 319–329
human immunodeficiency virus and,
  222–243
late-onset depression and psychosis
  in elderly, 292–307
medical illness in psychiatric patients
  and, 24–41
prisons and, 198–212
sexual deviations and, 366–380
state mental hospitals and, 47–63
substance abuse and, 106–135
tardive dyskinesia and, 336–358
Neuropsychological assessment. *See also*
  Assessment; Diagnosis
  benzodiazepine abuse and,
    118–119
  dementia and, 79
  late-onset depression and psychosis,
    306
  prisons and, 207–208
  sexual deviation and, **377**
Neuropsychological deficits. *See also*
  Cognitive functions
  alcohol abuse and, 112–113
  inhalant abuse and, 130
Neurosurgery, and sexual deviations,
  379
Neurosyphilis, 9–10, 73, 77
New York
  history of mental health services in,
    10
  HIV in prison population of, 197
  medical illness and homelessness in
    New York City, 320
Nicotine, 130–131
Nonverbal learning disabilities, 262
Norepinephrine, and aggression,
  165

Normal-pressure hydrocephalus (NPH), 75
North Riding Asylum (England), 7, 9
NPH. *See* Normal-pressure hydrocephalus (NPH)
Nursing homes
  dementia and, 70–72, 80, 81, 90–91
  HIV care and, 242–243
  sexual deviations and, 374
  syndromal depression and, 307
Nutritional therapies, and developmental disabilities, 269
Nymphomania, 364

OAS. *See* Overt Aggression Scale (OAS)
Obesity
  Prader-Willi syndrome and, 276, 277
  as side effect of neuroleptics, 58
Obsessive-compulsive disorder, 179
Obstetric complications, and criminal behavior, 202. *See also* Fetal effects; Perinatal factors; Pregnancy
Olanzapine, 299, 308, 341
Older Americans Act, 88
Omnibus Budget Reconciliation Act of 1987, 85–86
Opioids, and substance abuse, 107, 123–125
Opportunistic infections, and HIV, 225–226, **227**
Orbitofrontal cortex, and frontal syndromes, **158–160**
Organic brain syndrome
  alcohol abuse and, 110–114
  cannabis use and, 126–127
  cocaine abuse and, 122–123
  nicotine and, 131
  opioid abuse and, 124–125
Organic mental syndromes (OMS), and sexual deviations, 371
Orgasm, and sexual disorders, 365, **366**
Overdose, of benzodiazepines, 118

Overt Aggression Scale (OAS), 175, **176**
Oxazepam, 119
Oxytocin, and Prader-Willi syndrome, 276

Panic disorder, 180
Paranoia, late-onset, 303
Paranoid psychosis, 120
Paraphilias, 366–367
Paraphrenia, late-onset, 303
Parkinsonism, as side effect of neuroleptics, 58, 341–342
Parkinson's disease, 299, 370
Paroxetine, 308
Partial seizures, 153, **171**
Pathological aggression, 149
Pathological intoxication, 108–109
Pathophysiology, of aggression, 150–164
Patient. *See also* Compliance; Patient history
  homelessness and, 329–330
  labeling of as psychiatric or medical, 42
  legal status of in state hospitals, 54–55
  state hospitals and characteristics of, 48–50, 61–62
  support services for dementia, 89–92
Patient history
  aggression and, 166, **169**
  late-onset depression and, 301
  neuropsychiatric evaluation in prisons and, 211
  psychiatric symptoms and medical illness, 35–37
  screening for medical illness in psychiatric patient and, 29–35
  sexual deviations and, **376–377**
  tardive dyskinesia and, 348
PCP. *See* Phencyclidine (PCP)

PCS. *See* Postconcussive syndrome (PCS)
Pedophilia, 366, 367
Pemoline, 182
Pennsylvania Hospital for the Insane, 3
Pergolide, 59
Perinatal factors, and criminal behavior, 202–203. *See also* Fetal effects; Obstetric complications; Pregnancy
Peripheral neuropathy, and inhalation abuse, 130
Pervasive developmental disorder, 52
PET. *See* Positron-emission tomography (PET)
Pharmacodynamic interactions, 55
Phencyclidine (PCP), 128–129
Phenobarbital, and epilepsy, 60
Phenylalanine, 275
Phenylketonuria, 275–276
Phenytoin
    aggression and, 180–181
    clozapine-induced seizures and, 177
    side effects of, 57, 175, 264–265
Phrenology, 5
Physical complications, of tardive dyskinesia, 338
Physical examination
    developmental disabilities and, 264, 271
    late-onset depression and, 301
    prisons and, 211–212
    screening for medical illness in psychiatric patient and, 30, 37
    tardive dyskinesia and, 348
Physicians, primary care
    assessment of medical illness in psychiatric patients and, 25–26, 40
    homeless mentally ill patients and, 330
Pick's disease, 75
Pindolol, 181
Pinel, Philippe, 10

Police, and mental illness, 200
Polysomnography
    aggression and, 173
    dementia and, 79
    HIV and, 235
Porphyria, 38
Positron-emission tomography (PET), 111, 235. *See also* Neuroimaging
Postconcussive syndrome (PCS), 323
Posterior hypothalamotomy, 379
Postictal aggression, 154
Poststroke depression syndrome, 300
Posttraumatic stress disorder, 267
Prader-Willi syndrome, 271, 276–277
Pramipexole, 58–59
Pregnancy. *See also* Fetal effects; Obstetric complications; Perinatal factors
    alcohol abuse and, 115
    benzodiazepine abuse and, 119
Premature ejaculation, 365
Prenatal health care, and substance abuse, 133
Prevalence
    of AIDS in prison population, 197
    of alcohol abuse, 106
    of antisocial personality disorder in prisons, 209
    of brain diseases and brain dysfunction in state hospital patients, 47–48
    of depression in Alzheimer's disease, 298
    of drug abuse, 106–107
    of dyslexia, 260
    of homelessness, 319
    of late-onset depression and psychosis, 293–294
    of medical illness in psychiatric patients, 26–27, **28–29**
    of mental disorders in prisons, 199
    of mental retardation, 259

of psychiatric disorders in older
population, 293
of tardive dyskinesia, 336, 338
of white-matter abnormalities in
elderly patients, 303
Prisons. *See also* Crime
brain function and, 201–209
epidemiology of mental disorders in,
198–201
neuropsychiatric evaluations in,
210–212
prevalence of AIDS in, 197
psychopathy and, 209–210
sexual deviations and, 367, 375
Prochlorperazine, 343
Propranolol, 59, 181
Pseudodementia, 299, 300
Psychiatry
medical illness and psychiatric
symptoms, 24–25
neuropsychiatry and development of,
2–3
organic in asylums of nineteenth
century, 8–12
social role of and history of mental
health services, 117
substance abuse and, 133–135
Psychiatric disorders. *See also* specific
disorders
medical illness and symptoms of,
24–25, 35–38
prevalence of in homeless, 319
Psychoeducation
Asperger's syndrome and, 279
dementia and, 88–89
HIV and, 240
tardive dyskinesia and, 347
Psychopathy, and prisons,
209–210
Psychopharmacology. *See also*
Drug-drug interactions; Side
effects; Tardive dyskinesia
for aggression, 174–183

central nervous system side effects
of, 55
for dementia, 83–87
for developmental disabilities,
264–265, 266–267
homeless patients and, 328–329
for late-onset depression and
psychosis, 307–309
medical illness caused by, 24
nonadherence to treatment in state
hospitals, 57–60
for psychotic behavior in elderly, 297
for sexual deviation, 377–378
Psychosis
aggression and, 177
alcohol abuse and, 115
Alzheimer's disease and serotonin,
82–83
amphetamine abuse and, 123
cannabis-induced, 126
clozapine and tardive dyskinesia, 349
cocaine abuse and, 121
hallucinogens and, 127, 129
late-onset in elderly, 296–310
neuroleptics and dosage reduction
strategies, 357
traumatic brain injury and, 322–323
Psychosocial complications, of tardive
dyskinesia, 338, 350–351
Psychosocial therapies, for late-onset
depression and psychosis, 310
Psychostimulants, and side effects of
neuroleptics, 59
Psychotherapy, and developmental
disabilities, 268
Psychotic depression, 295
Psychotic disorder not otherwise
specified (NOS), 303
Public health
HIV and, 235–243
substance abuse and, 105
Punishment, and behavior therapy,
267–268

Pyramidal tract signs, of dementia, 77

Quality of life, and side effects of
    medication, 59

Rabbit syndrome, 342
Rape, and sexual deviations, 363–364,
    365, 367–368, 375
Rapid eye movement (REM) sleep
    behavioral disorder (RBD), 167,
    173
RBD. See Rapid eye movement (REM)
    sleep behavioral disorder (RBD)
Recidivism rates, for sexual offenders,
    379. See also Relapse
Referrals
    of psychiatric patients for medical
        care, 40
    state hospitals and specialist
        consultation, 62–63
Relapse, and substance abuse, 134. See
    also Recidivism rates
REM. See Rapid eye movement (REM)
Respite services, for caregivers, 90
Retarded ejaculation, 365
Rewards, and behavioral therapy for
    aggression, 184
Rey-Osterreith Complex Figure, 231
Rheumatic fever, 343
Right hemisphere
    aggression and, 168–169
    alcohol abuse and, 112
Right-hemisphere learning disability,
    262
Risk-benefit analysis, and neuroleptics,
    349
Risk factors
    for developmental disabilities,
        263
    for HIV infection, 222–223
    for late-onset depression, 295
    for tardive dyskinesia, 338–341
Risperidone

elderly patients and, 85, 299, 308,
    309
tardive dyskinesia and, 341, 349
Rockland Tardive Dyskinesia Rating
    Scale, 353

Sadism, 368
St. Hans Rating Scale, 353
St. Louis City Insane Asylum
    (Missouri), 12
Satiety cells, 276
Satyriasis, 364, 378
Schizophrenia
    anxiety and, 62
    brain injury and, 323, 326, 327
    cannabis abuse and, 126
    dementia and, 73
    diagnosis of in state hospitals, 50
    early-onset and late-onset compared,
        296–297
    elderly patients and, 303
    homelessness and, 319, 324, 326
    neuroleptics and self-injurious
        behavior, 52
    prisons and, 199
    sexual deviations and, 374
    side effects of medication and, 56,
        58, 59–60, 346
    substance abuse and, 134
Schonecker, M., 336
SCL-90. See Symptom Checklist–90
    (SCL-90)
Screening
    for medical illnesses in psychiatric
        patients, 29–35, 39–41
    for tardive dyskinesia, 352–357
SCUs. See Special care units (SCUs)
Seizures. See also Epilepsy
    aggression and, 170
    alcohol intoxication and, 109
    behavior and frequency of, 156
    cocaine intoxication and, 120
    opioid abuse and, 124

Selective serotonin reuptake inhibitors
(SSRIs)
aggression and, 179–180
dementia and, 86
sexual deviations and, 378
side effects of, 308
violent behavior and serotonin levels,
208
Selegiline, 84
Self-care deficits, and dementia, 82
Self-injurious behavior, 51–53
Sensory-limbic hyperconnection, 156
Serenic agents, 182
Serotonin and serotonin agonists
aggression and, 164–165
dementia and, 82
nutritional therapy for developmental disabilities, 269
prison populations and, 208
Sertraline, 179, 308
Sexual behavior. See also Sexual
deviations
aberrant in residents of noncriminal
institutions, 373–374
anatomy and physiology of, 364–365
disorders of, 366
Sexual deviations. See also Sexual
behavior
brain dysfunction and model of, 364
definition of, 363
neurological disorders and, 368–373
rape and, 367–368
treatment and management of,
377–379
types of, 366–367
Sham rage, 150–151
Side effects, of medications. See also
Psychopharmacology; Tardive
dyskinesia
central nervous system and, 55
developmental disabilities and, 264,
266
drug-drug interactions, 55, 297

elderly and, 85, 307–308
nonadherence to neuroleptic therapy,
58
psychotic behavior and, 299
Single photon emission computed
tomography (SPECT), 173–174,
279. See also Neuroimaging
Skills training, for families of impaired
elders, 89
Sleep apnea, 79, 277
Social-emotional learning disabilities,
261–262
Social Security Disability Insurance
(SSDI), 61
Social skills training, 184
Somatization disorders, 35
Special care units (SCUs), in nursing
homes, 90–91
Specialist substance abuse services,
133–135
Special Programs of National
Significance (SPNS), 236
SPECT. See Single photon emission
computed tomography (SPECT)
Spitzka, E. C., 15–16
SPNS. See Special Programs of National
Significance (SPNS)
Spontaneous dyskinesia, 345–346
SSDI. See Social Security Disability
Insurance (SSDI)
SSRIs. See Selective serotonin reuptake
inhibitors (SSRIs)
Staff, of mental health services
aggressive behavior and, 166, 183
dementia and, 81
developmental disabilities and,
280–281
screening programs for medical
illness in psychiatric patients
and, 40–41
State hospitals
aggressiveness and self-injurious
behavior, 51–53

State hospitals *(continued)*
   brain diseases and brain dysfunction
      in patients of, 47–48
   deinstitutionalization, 293
   dementia and, 70
   diagnosis and, 50–51
   elderly and, 310–311
   financial resources of patients, 61
   functional impairment and, 53–54
   legal status of patients, 54–55
   medical illness and, 55–57
   nature of patient population, 48–50
   neurodiagnostic technology and
      specialist consultation, 62–63
   patients' preferences for
      hospitalization, 61–62
   prevalence of medical illness in
      psychiatric patients, **28–29**
   setting of priorities for, 51
   social supports for patients of, 61
   statistics on, 47
Stereotactic hypothalamotomy, 379
Stimulants, abuse of, 119–123
Strokes, 121, 300
Structured interviews, and
   neuroassessment of HIV, 229
Subcortical dementia, 73, 298–299, 306
Subdural hematomas, 114
Substance abuse. *See also* Alcoholism
   and alcohol abuse; Drug abuse
   dual diagnosis, 131
   epidemiology of, 106–107
   history of mental health services and,
      11
   HIV and, 240
   homelessness and, 319, 320–321
   neuropsychiatric problems in,
      132–135
   prisons and, 199, 211
   as public health problem, 105
   sexual deviations and, 371, 375
Suicide and suicidal ideation
   depression in elderly and, 296

   Huntington's disease and, 299
   mortality from in psychiatric
      patients, 24
   serotonin levels and, 208
   tardive dyskinesia and, 338
Support services, for dementia, 89–92
Sweden, and criminal behavior in
   mentally handicapped, 201
Switzerland, and castration of sexual
   offenders, 378
Sydenham's chorea, 343
Symptom Checklist–90, 240
Syndromal depression, 307
Syphilis, and history of neuropsychiatry,
   9–10, 12
Systemic lupus erythematosus, 38

Tacrine, 83
Tardive akathisia, 267, 342–343
Tardive dyskinesia (TD)
   clinical features of, 336–338
   developmental disabilities and,
      266–267
   differential diagnosis of, 341–347
   elderly patients and, 309
   epidemiology and risk factors for,
      338–341
   functional impairment and, 350–352
   management strategies for, 347–350
   neuroleptics and, 177, 337–338,
      347–350, 357
   prevalence of, 336
   screening strategies for, 352–357
   treatment strategies for, 357–358
Tardive dystonia, 342
Target behaviors, and aggression, 183,
   184
TBI. *See* Traumatic brain injury (TBI)
TD. *See* Tardive dyskinesia (TD)
Temazepam, 119
Temperamental aggression, 149
Temporal lobe epilepsy (TLE). *See also*
   Epilepsy

aggression and, 153–157, 162–163, 170

EEG studies of prison populations and, 206

sexual deviations and, 370

Temporal sequence, of psychiatric symptoms, 37–38

Testosterone
aggression and, 165, 208–209
sexual deviations and, 373

Tetrahydrocannabinol (THC), 125

Theophylline, 56

Therapeutic alliance, and developmental disabilities, 268

Thiamine, and alcohol abuse, 110

Thioridazine, 266

Thomas Street Clinic (Houston), 238, 239

Thymoleptics, 59

Thyroid disease and thyroid hormones
dementia and, 77–78
psychosis and, 27
screening programs for medical illness in psychiatric
patients and, 31, 35
thyroid hormone augmentation and, 59, 60

Ticehurst House Asylum (England), 3, 7, 9, 11–12

TLE. See Temporal lobe epilepsy (TLE)

Toluene abuse, 130

Tourette syndrome
behavioral therapy and, 267, 268
differential diagnosis of tardive dyskinesia and, 343
frontosubcortical system dysfunction in, 279
sexual deviations and, 371

Transvestic fetishism, 368

Traumatic brain injury (TBI). See also Head injury
aggression and, 161–163, 169–170, 177, 182

depression and, 300

homeless and, 321–323, 326–327

prisons and, 200, 211

sexual deviations and, 370

Traveling team, and treatment of developmental disabilities, 269

Trazodone, 86, 179

Treatment, of neuropsychiatric disorders. See also Behavioral therapy; Psychoeducation; Psychopharmacology; Psychotherapy
aggression and, 174–184
Asperger's syndrome, 279
developmental disabilities and, 265–269
homeless mentally ill and, 328–330
late-onset depression and psychosis in public health setting, 307–310
medications as causes of medical disorders, 24
sexual deviations and, 377–379
state hospitals and patient compliance, 57–60
tardive dyskinesia and, 347–350, 357–358

Triazolam, 119

Tuberculosis, and homeless, 323

Tuke, D. H., 6, 8

Turner's syndrome, 262

Tyrosine, 275

United Kingdom
history of neuropsychiatry and of asylums, 3, 4, 5, 7, 9, 11, 12, 14
prevalence of mental disorders in prisons, 200
sexual deviations and prison population, 367

University of Massachusetts
Neuropsychiatry Referral Center,
161–162
Urinary incontinence, and Alzheimer's
disease, 82
Utica Asylum (New York), 7, 8, 9, 11,
14

Valproate
aggression and, 175, 181
clozapine-induced seizures and, 177
dementia and, 86
management of epilepsy, 57
side effects of, 155
Vascular dementia
cocaine abuse and, 122
depression and, 300
differential diagnosis of, 73
DSM-IV and, 75
neuropsychological testing and, 306
prevalence of, 70
Venereal Disease Research Laboratory
test (VDRL), 77
Ventromedial hypothalamus, 151–152
Vigabatrin, 155
Violence and violent behavior, 80. *See
also* Aggression; Crime
Visuospatial deficits, in HIV, **232**
Vitamin B deficiency, 73, 75–76, 113,
300
Vitamin E supplements, 84, 349
Von Economo's disease, 370
Voyeurism, 365, 366, 368

Wassermann reaction, 12
Wechsler Adult Intelligence Scale, 231
Wechsler Full Scale IQ, 325–326
Wechsler Memory Scale, 231
Wernicke-Korsakoff syndrome,
110–112, 132
Wernicke's encephalopathy, 110, 111
Western Blot, and HIV screening, 233
West Riding Lunatic Asylum (England),
16–17
White, Ryan, 235, 236
White-matter hyperintensities (WMH),
302–305
Williams syndrome, 277–278
Wilson's disease, 344, 348–349
Window period, and HIV screening,
233
Wisconsin Card Sorting Test, 53,
326
Withdrawal
alcohol abuse and, 108, 109–110
benzodiazepines and, 118
inhalant abuse and, 131
nicotine and, 124
Withdrawal-emergent dyskinesia,
347
WMH. *See* White-matler intensities
Wyman, Dr. Morrill, 7

Xanomeline, 84
X rays, chest, 31

York Retreat (England), 3, 7, 8